THE HUMAN BRAIN

An introduction to its functional anatomy

The brain, and the brain alone, is the source of our pleasures, joys, laughter, and amusement, as well as our sorrow, pain, grief, and tears. It is especially the organ we use to think and learn, see and hear, to distinguish the ugly from the beautiful, the bad from the good, and the pleasant from the unpleasant. The brain is also the seat of madness and delirium, of the fears and terrors which assail by night or by day, of sleeplessness, awkward mistakes and thoughts that will not come, of pointless anxieties, forgetfulness and eccentricities.

Hippocrates, ca. 400 B.C.

The human mind can be described as a slow-clockrate modified-digital machine with multiple distinguishable parallel processing, all working in salt water.

Philip Morrison: The mind of the machine, Technology Review **75**:17, 1973

One of the difficulties in understanding the brain is that it is like nothing so much as a lump of porridge.

THE HUMAN BRAIN

An introduction to its functional anatomy

JOHN NOLTE, Ph.D.

Associate Professor of Anatomy, School of Medicine,
University of Colorado Health Sciences Center,
Denver, Colorado

With **379** *illustrations*

The C. V. Mosby Company

ST. LOUIS • TORONTO • LONDON   1981

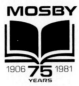

MOSBY

1906 **75** 1981
YEARS

A TRADITION OF PUBLISHING EXCELLENCE

Editor: John E. Lotz
Manuscript editor: Kendall Wills
Design: Diane Beasley
Production: Linda R. Stalnaker

Cover: Reproduction of a drawing by Rene Descartes in *De Homine*, 1662.
Descartes thought that the pineal gland was the seat of the
soul, monitoring the movement of "animal spirits" in sensory
nerves and controlling the movement of animal spirits
through motor nerves.

Printed in the United States of America

The C.V. Mosby Company
11830 Westline Industrial Drive, St. Louis, Missouri 63141

Library of Congress Cataloging in Publication Data

Nolte, John.
  The human brain.

  Includes bibliographies and index.
    1. Neuroanatomy. I. Title. [DNLM: 1. Nervous
system—Anatomy and histology. WL 101 N789n]
QM451.N64   611'.8   81-38337
ISBN 0-8016-3702-3   AACR2

GW/VH/VH   03/A/308

PREFACE

The human brain is a marvel in terms of what it allows us to do. Neurologists are fond of saying that the only really important function of the other parts of our bodies is to support the brain. Unfortunately, students often find the brain to be a marvel of complexity as well. I have tried to write a book that will lead beginning students through the basic aspects of the structure and function of their brains. It was designed primarily with students of the health sciences in mind, but I hope others will also find it useful.

In discussing the various parts of the nervous system and its environment, I have tried to restrict myself as much as possible to facts and details that can be correlated with function in some way. To bring home the correlation between structure and function, I have included numerous examples of clinical and experimental findings following damage to or manipulation of the nervous systems of humans and laboratory animals. Because of the difficulty of visualizing the structures and pathways of the brain in three dimensions, a wide variety of diagrams and photographs is also included.

A short and highly selective bibliography accompanies each chapter. The intent in choosing references was not only to document recent findings but also to provide access through those references to the vast neuroscientific literature. For these reasons, the emphasis is on recent reviews and research papers. Many classic and scientifically more important papers have been omitted, although some older or peripherally related articles that make interesting reading are listed.

This book was far from a solitary undertaking and could never have come about without the help and support of many people. I am especially grateful to my friends and colleagues Tom Finger, Claude Selitrennikoff, and Ted Tarby, who read parts (or all) of the manuscript for me and offered many helpful suggestions; to Gary Jenison, Stu Smith, and Jack Willson, who prepared some of the anatomic materials used for illustrations; to Shelley Frisch, Kris McInvaille, and Martha Potter, who watched my gesticulations and somehow came up with drawings; to Betty Aguilar and Sharon Ferdinandsen, who transformed my chicken scratchings into a manuscript; and to all the fellow students of the nervous system, cited in figure captions, who kindly provided illustrations. A very special thanks to Pam Eller, who prepared most of the anatomic materials, did most of the photography, read and commented on the manuscript, and patted me on the head a lot; without her help this would have been a lesser book or no book at all. Most of the photographs in the book depict materials developed for teaching purposes by my just-mentioned colleagues and me; I appreciate the cooperation of the University of Colorado Health Sciences Center in allowing them to be used in this book. Finally, I must acknowledge the students with whom it has been my pleasure to work at the University of Colorado Health Sciences Center; they have made teaching fun, and from the fun arose the notion of writing a book.

John Nolte

CONTENTS

THE HUMAN BRAIN
An introduction to its functional anatomy

CHAPTER 1

INTRODUCTION: THE CENTRAL NERVOUS SYSTEM

The object of this book is to present and explain some basic anatomical facts about how the brain is put together and to discuss a few aspects of how it works. This introductory chapter describes in a very general way the elements that make up the central nervous system (CNS) and some principles according to which these elements are connected to each other. In addition, there is a discussion of how the relatively simple embryonic nervous system is transformed into the much more complex CNS of the adult.

WHAT IS IN IT?

The principal cellular elements of the nervous system are *neurons* and *glial cells*, both present in enormous numbers. There are an estimated 100 billion neurons in the human brain and perhaps 10 times that many glial cells.

Neurons come in a great variety of sizes and shapes (Fig. 1-1); most of them have a long process called an *axon* that conducts information away from the neuronal cell body (or *soma*) and a series of smaller processes called *dendrites* that receive information from other neurons via *synaptic contacts* (or *synapses*). Certain aspects of somatic, dendritic, and axonal morphology give rise to a descriptive terminology for neurons. The vast majority of human neurons are *multipolar*, meaning that there are multiple dendritic projections from the cell body and almost always an axon as well (Fig. 1-1, *C* and *D*). Some are *unipolar* (Fig. 1-1, *A*) or *bipolar* (Fig. 1-1, *B*), having one or two processes, respectively. Neurons are also subdivided into *Golgi type I*, which have a long axon, and *Golgi type II*, which have a short axon or no axon at all.

Neurons may also be classified according to their con-

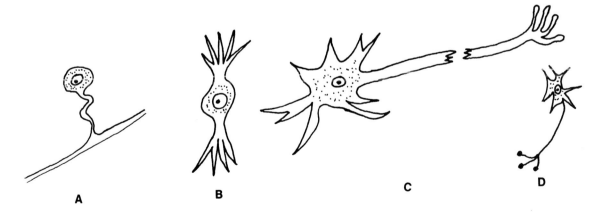

A   B   C   D

Fig. 1-1. Schematic illustrations of representative neurons. **A,** Unipolar neuron, like those found in the sensory ganglia of spinal and cranial nerves. **B,** Bipolar neuron, like those found in the retina. **C,** Multipolar cell with a long axon (Golgi type I), like the motor neurons found in the spinal gray matter. **D,** Multipolar cell with a short axon (Golgi type II), like the granule cells of the cerebral cortex.

nections. *Sensory neurons* are either directly sensitive to various stimuli (such as touch or temperature changes) or else receive direct connections from nonneuronal *receptor cells*. *Motor neurons* end directly on muscles or glands. *Interneurons* interconnect other neurons. In a strict sense, the CNS is composed almost entirely of interneurons: there are only about 5 million sensory fibers in all the spinal and cranial nerves combined, and only several hundred thousand motor neurons. Thus more than 99.99% of the neurons are interneurons. However, the words "sensory" and "motor" are often used in a much broader sense to refer to cells and axons that carry information related to sensory stimuli and to the generation of movements, respectively.

There are a variety of types of glial cells in the nervous system. Some of them (*oligodendroglia* in the CNS and *Schwann cells* in peripheral nerves) form *myelin sheaths*, which are spiral wrappings around axons that allow the axons to conduct information more rapidly. Other types of glia are thought to perform a variety of functions, such as regulating the composition of extracellular space, complementing neurons in certain metabolic activities, and devouring foreign materials that have gained access to the nervous system.

HOW IS IT ORGANIZED?

The CNS is composed of the *brain* and the *spinal cord* (Fig. 1-2). The brain, in turn, is composed of the *cerebrum*, the *cerebellum*, and the *brainstem*. There is general agreement on what the cerebellum is, but not all authors distinguish the cerebrum from the brainstem in the same way. In this book the cerebrum is treated as composed of the two massive *cerebral hemispheres* (separated by the *longitudinal fissure*) and the *diencephalon*; in an intact brain most of the diencephalon is hidden from view by the cerebral hemispheres. The brainstem is that part of the CNS, exclusive of the cerebellum, that lies between the cerebrum and the spinal cord. Many sources include the diencephalon with the brainstem, and some include small portions of the cerebral hemispheres as well.

For the most part, the CNS is easily divisible into *gray matter* and *white matter* (Figs. 2-15 to 2-21). Gray matter refers to areas where there is a preponderance of cell bodies and dendrites; it is actually a pinkish gray color because of its abundant blood supply. White matter refers to areas where there is a preponderance of myelinated axons; myelin is mostly lipid and so has a fatty white appearance.

Specific areas of gray matter are often called *nuclei*, particularly if the contained cell bodies are functionally related to one another. An area where gray matter forms a surface covering on some part of the CNS (and meets certain other technical criteria) is referred to as a

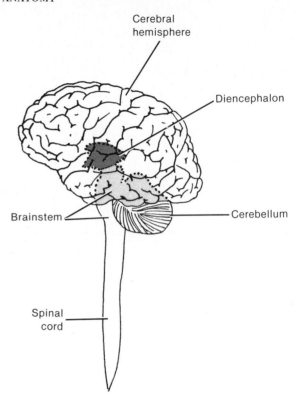

Fig. 1-2. Major divisions of the central nervous system. Stippled areas outlined by dotted lines are normally hidden from view by the massive cerebral hemispheres; they can be seen in a hemisected brain (Fig. 2-3).

cortex. The cerebral and cerebellar cortices are two prominent examples. Occasionally other names such as *body* or *center* are used for areas of gray matter, but these are relatively infrequent.

In contrast, subdivisions of white matter go by a bewildering variety of names, such as *fasciculus, funiculus, lemniscus, peduncle,* and, used most commonly, *tract.* Many tracts have two-part names that provide some free information about the nature of the tract: the first part of the name refers to the site of origin of the tract, and the second part refers to the site of its termination. Thus a spinocerebellar tract is one that starts in the spinal cord and ends in the cerebellum.

The spinal cord provides a reasonably clear example of the separation of neural tissue into gray matter and white matter (Fig. 1-3). Sensory axons, whose unipolar cell bodies are located in the dorsal root ganglia of spinal nerves, enter the spinal cord and divide into a large number of branches, most of which terminate in the spinal gray matter. Motor axons, whose multipolar cell bodies are located in the spinal gray matter, leave the spinal cord and enter spinal nerves. The white matter contains *long descending tracts* (from the brainstem and cerebrum), *long ascending tracts* (to the brainstem, cerebellum, and cerebrum), and local axons intercon-

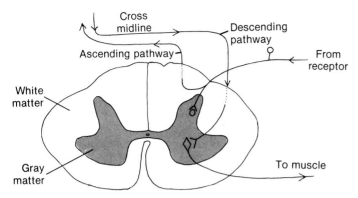

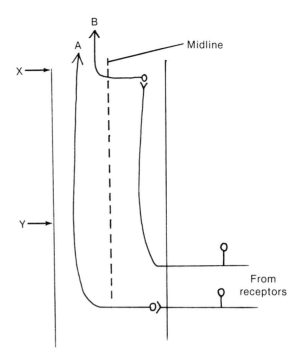

Fig. 1-3. Division of CNS into gray matter (stippled) and white matter, as illustrated by the spinal cord in cross section. Gray matter contains interneurons, motor neurons, and endings of sensory fibers. White matter contains ascending and descending pathways. Ascending pathways usually include interneurons, and descending pathways usually end on interneurons, but these links are omitted in this diagram. One axon in each ascending and descending pathway usually crosses the midline at some point.

Fig. 1-4. Different pathways may cross the midline at different points in the CNS. Damage to one side of the CNS at point *X* would cause both A- and B-type deficits on the side of the body contralateral to the lesion. Damage to one side of the CNS at point *Y* would cause an A-type deficit on the side of the body contralateral to the lesion and a B-type deficit on the side ipsilateral to the lesion. (The CNS is generally bilaterally symmetrical, but for simplicity pathways *A* and *B* are shown arising on one side only; damage at point *Y* should damage pathway B on the side of the lesion before it crossed.)

necting different spinal levels. The gray matter, on the other hand, contains motor neurons, the endings of incoming sensory axons and long descending tracts, local interneurons, and tract cells whose axons enter long ascending tracts. This division into white and gray matter is not absolute anywhere in the CNS; for example, axons in long descending tracts obviously must pass through some gray matter before reaching their targets.

Ascending (sensory) pathways usually cross to the opposite side of the CNS at some point before reaching the cerebrum (Fig. 1-3). That is, they become *contralateral* to the side on which they originate, so information from the right hand eventually reaches the left cerebral hemisphere.* This crossing of sensory pathways is a curious and unexplained fact of vertebrate evolution. It applies not only to those pathways representing spinal nerves but to those representing cranial nerves as well (except for olfaction; see Chapter 16). A number of hypotheses have been advanced to explain this phenomenon, including the notion that it is an early evolutionary mistake that is still awaiting correction.† Whatever its explanation, it would be even more peculiar if information from the *right* hand reached the left cerebral hemisphere, which in turn controlled the *left* hand. This is not the case, since decending pathways also cross the midline at some point between their origins and their terminations (Fig. 1-3).

It follows from this crossing pattern that damage to the appropriate regions of one cerebral hemisphere will cause sensory and/or motor deficits on the contralateral side. This is also frequently true of damage at lower levels such as the brainstem. However, different pathways cross at different levels within the CNS. Therefore it is possible for a single lesion to affect one pathway before it crosses and another pathway after it crosses (Fig. 1-4). The result would be the curious finding of one type of deficit on one side of the head or body and a second type of deficit on the other side.

As is generally the case, the generalization about crossing pathways has exceptions. Some sensory pathways (for example, auditory) ascend bilaterally, and some motor neurons (for example, trigeminal) are innervated by both cerebral hemispheres. The most outstanding exception is the cerebellum. Damage to one side of the cerebellum produces deficits on the same side of the body (that is, the side *ipsilateral* to the lesion). The anatomical bases of this ipsilaterality are discussed in Chapter 14.

---

*This does not mean that most ascending *axons* cross the midline. The pathway from a peripheral receptor to the cerebral cortex, as will be detailed in subsequent chapters, includes at least three serially arranged neurons; the axon of only one of these crosses the midline.
†Zill, Sasha N.: Personal communication, 1977.

HOW DO WE KNOW?

Inspection of Figs. 2-15 to 2-21 will reveal that gray matter and white matter have fairly uniform appearances, even though in any given section millions of axons interconnect a greater number of neurons. Yet the bulk of this book is concerned with a description of these connections in some detail. The question then arises of how we can know what is connected to what. A number of techniques are available that can help answer this question; some of these are newly devised and are contributing greatly to the current explosive growth of knowledge about the neurosciences.

Degeneration techniques have been used since the last century and are based on the reactions of neurons to injury. If an axon is severed, its formerly attached cell body undergoes a characteristic series of cytological changes *(chromatolysis)*. Therefore examining brain sections for chromatolytic cells can reveal the locations of the cell bodies of origin of the severed axons. While the cell body undergoes chromatolysis, the portion of the axon distal to the cut degenerates *(wallerian degeneration)*. The same changes occur if the damage is inflicted at the ultimate proximal location (that is, if the cell body is destroyed). Special staining methods can be used to selectively stain degenerating axons and/or their synaptic terminals. Therefore if a particular nucleus is destroyed, the path of axons originating there and the sites of their terminations can be determined.

Although a great deal of information has been gained over the years with the aid of degeneration techniques, their use is not without pitfalls. It is technically difficult, and sometimes impossible, to completely destroy a particular structure without damaging nearby structures as well. In addition, since the segregation of gray and white matter is not absolute, axons passing through a given nucleus can be destroyed along with the cell bodies forming the nucleus. For these and other reasons, various tracer techniques developed in recent years have been greeted with much enthusiasm. Most of these methods take advantage of the fact that under

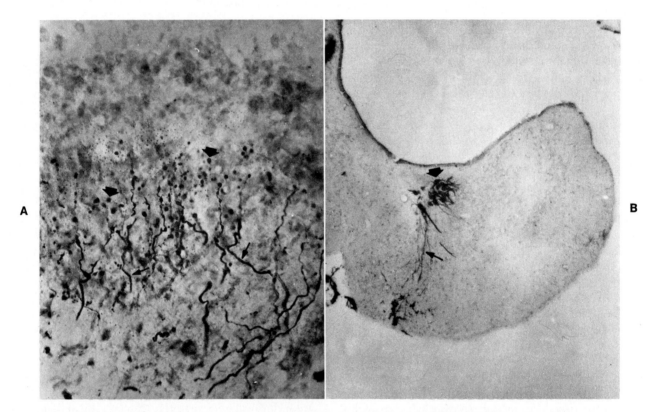

A

B

Fig. 1-5. Examples of the use of horseradish peroxidase (HRP) to label neuronal pathways. **A,** HRP applied to the proximal end of the lateral line nerve of a fish after cutting the nerve near its entrance into the brainstem; reaction product fills the entering fibers (thin arrows) and their synaptic endings (thick arrows) within the CNS. (Courtesy of Dr. Curtis Bell, Good Samaritan Hospital.) **B,** HRP applied to the proximal end of the hypoglossal nerve of a frog after cutting the nerve near its entrance into the brainstem; in this case the HRP was transported in a retrograde direction, and reaction product fills the hypoglossal motor neurons (thick arrow) and their axons (thin arrow). (Courtesy of Dr. Thomas Finger, Dr. Stephen Roper, and Barbara Taylor, University of Colorado Medical Center.)

normal circumstances substances are transported from a neuronal cell body down its axon toward its synapses *(anterograde transport)* and in the reverse direction as well *(retrograde transport)*. Appropriate radioactive substances (usually tritiated amino acids) introduced into a nucleus are taken up by the resident neurons, incorporated into macromolecules, and transported down the axons of these neurons. Eventually the synaptic terminals of these axons become radioactive.

In another method, a protein is introduced into areas of synaptic terminals. The terminals take up the protein, which is then transported back to the parent neurons. The protein of choice for such experiments is an enzyme called *horseradish peroxidase*, which can be detected with great sensitivity and resolution by appropriate histochemical procedures (Fig. 1-5).

Other anatomical methods utilize neural tissue that has not been experimentally manipulated prior to processing. The *Golgi technique* is a staining method that completely stains the cell bodies and processes of a small, random sample of neurons in the tissue (Fig. 11-2, *A*). This is useful for determining the sizes and

shapes of the cell types in a given area of the CNS. In addition, different classes of neurons have chemically different interiors, some of which can be distinguished by histochemical techniques. For example, neurons that use norepinephrine as the chemical transmitter at their synapses contain this substance throughout their axons and cell bodies. Appropriate fixation and processing causes these neurons to be fluorescent.

Finally, electrophysiological techniques have added a great deal of information about pathways and connections, much of which could not have been obtained by strictly anatomical studies. Such experiments range from those in which the electrical activity of various cortical areas is measured after stimulation of peripheral nerves and receptors to those in which the activity and connections of single neurons is measured.

HOW DID IT GET THAT WAY?

As complex as the human nervous system is, it has its embryonic origin as a simple, tubular, ectodermal structure. Its development provides some useful insights into its adult configuration and organization.

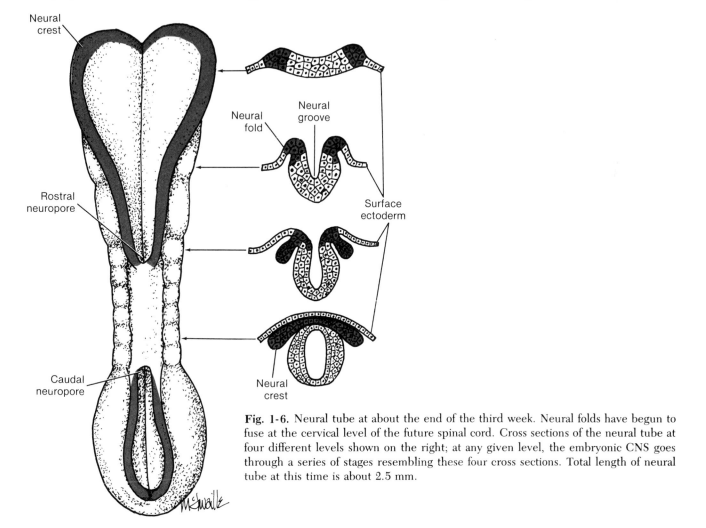

Fig. 1-6. Neural tube at about the end of the third week. Neural folds have begun to fuse at the cervical level of the future spinal cord. Cross sections of the neural tube at four different levels shown on the right; at any given level, the embryonic CNS goes through a series of stages resembling these four cross sections. Total length of neural tube at this time is about 2.5 mm.

Neural tube

During the third week of embryonic development a longitudinal band of ectoderm thickens to form the *neural plate*. Shortly thereafter the neural plate begins to fold inward, forming a longitudinal *neural groove* in the midline flanked by a parallel *neural fold* on each side (Fig. 1-6). The neural groove deepens, and the neural folds approach each other in the midline. At the end of the third week the two folds begin to fuse midway along the neural groove, forming the *neural tube*. As this fusion occurs, groups of cells from the crest of each neural fold are pinched off from the neural tube. These are appropriately called *neural crest cells*, which develop into a variety of cell types, including the sensory neurons of the ganglia of spinal and cranial nerves, the postganglionic neurons of the autonomic nervous system, and the Schwann cells and satellite cells of the peripheral nervous system. The neural tube, on the other hand, develops into the entire CNS; its cavity becomes the *ventricular system* of the brain.

The area of fusion of the two neural folds, which begins in the cervical region of the future spinal cord, rapidly expands rostrally (toward the future brain) and caudally (toward the sacral end of the future spinal cord). The *rostral neuropore*, the opening at the rostral end of the neural tube, closes completely in the middle of the fourth week; the *caudal neuropore* closes about 2 days later. As each successive bit of neural tube is formed by the progressive fusion of the neural folds, it becomes separated from the overlying ectoderm (Fig. 1-6).

Defective closure of the neural tube is a frequent cause of congenital malformations of the nervous system. Failure of the caudal neuropore to close can result in severe forms of *spina bifida*, in which the caudal walls of the neural tube are still continuous with the skin of the back, and the central cavity of the neural tube is open to the outside.

If the rostral neuropore fails to close, *anencephaly*, in which much of each cerebral hemisphere is absent, can result. As in spina bifida, the walls of the neural tube may be continuous with the skin of the head, and the central cavity of the neural tube may be open to the outside.

Sulcus limitans

During the fourth week a longitudinal groove appears in the lateral wall of the neural tube. This groove, called the *sulcus limitans*, extends throughout the future spinal cord and brainstem and subdivides the gray matter in the walls of the neural tube into a more dorsal *alar plate* and a more ventral *basal plate* (Fig. 1-7). This is a distinction of some functional importance, since alar plate derivatives are primarily concerned with sensory processes, while motor neurons are located in basal plate derivatives. In the adult spinal cord, even though the

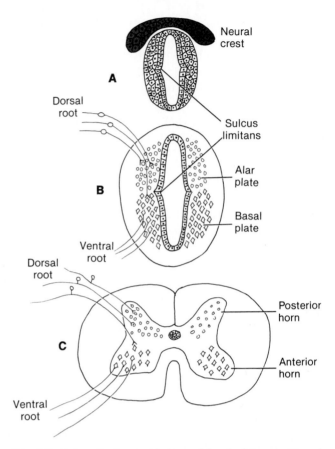

Fig. 1-7. Sulcus limitans and alar and basal plates. **A,** Neural tube during the fourth week. **B,** Embryonic spinal cord during the sixth week; dorsal root ganglion cells, derived from the neural crest, send their central processes into the spinal cord to terminate mainly on alar plate cells; basal plate cells become motor neurons, whose axons exit in the ventral roots. **C,** Adult spinal cord.

sulcus limitans can no longer be found, the central gray matter can be divided into a *posterior horn* and an *anterior horn* on each side (Fig. 1-7, *C*). The central processes of sensory neurons (derived from neural crest cells) end mainly in the posterior horn, which contains most of the cells that develop into ascending sensory pathways. In contrast, the anterior horn contains the cell bodies of motor neurons, whose axons leave the spinal cord and innervate skeletal muscles. The same distinction between sensory alar plate derivatives and motor basal plate derivatives holds true in the brainstem, as discussed briefly in this chapter and in more detail in Chapter 9. The sulcus limitans cannot be followed beyond the brainstem, and the entire cerebrum is considered to be an alar plate derivative.

Cerebral vesicles

Even before the rostral and caudal neuropores close, bulges begin to appear in the rostral end of the neural tube in the region of the future brain. During the fourth

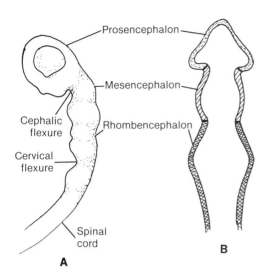

Fig. 1-8. Primary vesicles at the end of the fourth week.

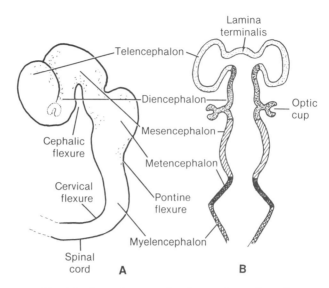

Fig. 1-9. Secondary vesicles during the sixth week.

TABLE 1

Derivatives of vesicles of the neural tube

Primary vesicle	Secondary vesicle	Neural derivatives	Cavity
Prosencephalon	Telencephalon	Cerebral hemispheres	Lateral ventricles
	Diencephalon	Thalamus, hypothalamus, etc.	Third ventricle
Mesencephalon	Mesencephalon	Midbrain	Cerebral aqueduct
Rhombencephalon	Metencephalon	Pons and cerebellum	Part of fourth ventricle
	Myelencephalon	Medulla	Part of fourth ventricle
			Part of central canal

week three bulges, or vesicles, are apparent and are referred to as the *primary vesicles* (Fig. 1-8, *B*). From rostral to caudal, these are the *prosencephalon* (forebrain), the *mesencephalon* (midbrain), and the *rhombencephalon* (hindbrain), which merges smoothly with the spinal portion of the neural tube. The prosencephalon develops into the cerebrum. The mesencephalon becomes the midbrain of the adult brainstem, and the rhombencephalon becomes the rest of the brainstem and the cerebellum (Table 1).

The three primary vesicles are not arranged in a straight line but rather are associated with two bends or flexures in the neural tube (Fig. 1-8, *A*). One of these, the *cervical flexure*, occurs between the rhombencephalon and spinal cord but does not persist in the adult CNS. The second, the *cephalic* (or *mesencephalic*) *flexure*, occurs between the mesencephalon and the prosencephalon; it persists in the adult as the bend between the axes of the brainstem and the forebrain (Fig. 2-1).

As the brain continues to develop, two of the primary vesicles become subdivided. During the fifth week five *secondary vesicles* can be distinguished (Fig. 1-9, *B*). The prosencephalon gives rise to the *telencephalon* and

the *diencephalon*; the mesencephalon remains undivided; the rhombencephalon gives rise to the *metencephalon* and the *myelencephalon*. The telencephalon becomes the cerebral hemispheres of the adult brain. The diencephalon gives rise to the *thalamus* (a large mass of gray matter interposed between the cerebral cortex and other structures), the *hypothalamus* (an autonomic control center), the neural part of the eye, and several other structures. The metencephalon becomes the *pons* (part of the brainstem) and the cerebellum. The myelencephalon becomes the *medulla* (the part of the brainstem that merges with the spinal cord).

In addition, a *pontine flexure* appears in the dorsal surface of the brainstem between the metencephalon and the myelencephalon (Fig. 1-8, *A*). This flexure does not persist as a bend in the axis of the brainstem, but it does have important consequences for the configuration of the caudal brainstem. As the flexure develops, the walls of the neural tube spread apart to form a diamond-shaped cavity (hence the name "rhombencephalon") so that only a thin membranous roof remains over what will become the *fourth ventricle* (Fig. 1-10). Thus the alar and basal plates, still separated by the sulcus limitans,

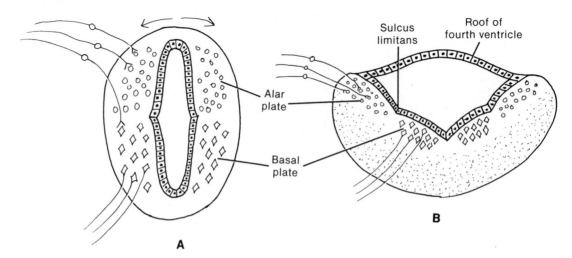

Fig. 1-10. Formation of the floor of the fourth ventricle. Walls of the neural tube are spread apart by the pontine flexure so that they and the sulcus limitans become the floor of the ventricle and the roof becomes a thin membrane.

come to lie in the floor of the fourth ventricle. The result is that in the corresponding part of the adult brainstem (rostral medulla and caudal pons), sensory nuclei are located lateral, rather than posterior, to motor nuclei. As discussed further in Chapter 9, this is of some utility in making sense of the arrangement of cranial nerve nuclei.

Lateral portions of the alar plate in the rostral metencephalon thicken considerably to form the *rhombic lips.* These continue to enlarge, finally fusing in the midline to form a transverse ridge that will eventually become the cerebellum.*

Further development

Subsequent events are dominated by the tremendous growth of the telencephalon. This portion of the neural tube begins as two swellings connected across the midline by a thin membrane, the *lamina terminalis* (Fig. 1-9). The basal part of the wall of the telencephalon, adjacent to the diencephalon, thickens to form the primordia of gray masses called the *basal ganglia* or *basal nuclei*. At the same time, the walls of the diencephalon thicken to form the thalamus and hypothalamus, separated by the *hypothalamic sulcus*. With continued growth, the telencephalon folds down alongside the diencephalon until eventually the two fuse (Fig. 1-11). The telencephalic surface overlying the area of fusion develops into a portion of the cerebral cortex called the *insula*. The remainder of the telencephalon grows rapidly in all available directions (Fig. 1-12), until the insula

---

*Although the cerebellum develops from the alar plate, it is involved in motor functions in the sense that cerebellar lesions cause impairments of posture and movement but not of sensation (see Chapter 14).

is completely hidden from view and each cerebral hemisphere has the shape of a great arc encircling the insular cortex (Fig. 1-11; compare Figs. 2-2 and 2-4). As discussed and demonstrated in the next chapter, knowledge of this growth of each cerebral hemisphere in a great **C** shape is of considerable importance for understanding the anatomical organization of the forebrain.

Ventricles and choroid plexus

The cavity of the neural tube persists as the ventricular system of the adult brain (Fig. 4-1). Except for the rudimentary central canal of the spinal cord and caudal medulla, the ventricles comprise a continuous, fluid-filled series of spaces extending through all the major divisions of the CNS. The cavity of the pons and rostral medulla is the fourth ventricle; that of the diencephalon is the *third ventricle;* a large **C**-shaped *lateral ventricle* occupies each cerebral hemisphere. Each lateral ventricle communicates with the third ventricle through an *interventricular foramen* (Fig. 1-11), and the third ventricle communicates with the fourth ventricle through the *cerebral aqueduct* of the midbrain.

Where the walls of the rhombencephalon spread apart to form the fourth ventricle, the roof of the ventricle becomes extremely thin (Fig. 1-10). An area covering the roof of the third ventricle and extending onto the surface of the telencephalon becomes similarly thin (Fig. 1-13). At each of these locations, tufts of small blood vessels invaginate the ventricular roof to form the *choroid plexus*, which is responsible for the production of most of the *cerebrospinal fluid* that fills the ventricles. As each cerebral hemisphere grows around in a **C** shape, so too does the choroid plexus, which protrudes into its lateral ventricle.

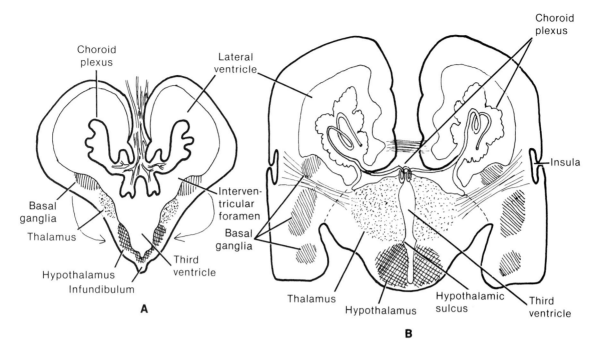

Fig. 1-11. Formation of choroid plexus and of the fusion between diencephalon and telencephalon. **A,** Condition at the end of the second month; vascular connective tissue has invaginated the third and lateral ventricles to form choroid plexus, and rapid growth of telencephalon begins to fold its basal ganglia down toward diencephalon, as indicated by arrows. **B,** Condition at the end of the third month; telencephalon and diencephalon have fused, as indicated by dashed line, and the insula, overlying the point of fusion, begins to be overgrown by other cerebral cortex. (Modified from Carpenter, M.: Human neuroanatomy, ed. 7, Baltimore, 1976, The Williams and Wilkins Co.)

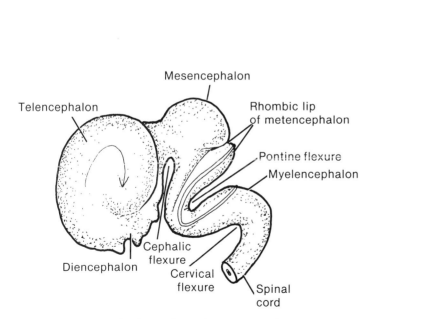

Fig. 1-12. Neural tube at the end of the second month. Development from this point is dominated by rapid growth of telencephalon in a C shape, as indicated by arrow.

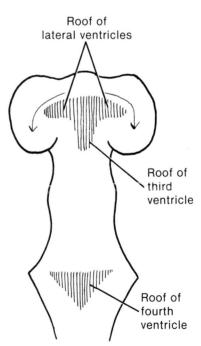

Fig. 1-13. Sites of formation of choroid plexus. As each cerebral hemisphere grows around in a C shape (indicated by arrows), so does its choroid plexus.

ADDITIONAL READING

Crelin, E.S.: Development of the nervous system, CIBA Clin. Symp. **26**(2), 1974.

Goochee, C., Rasband, W., and Sokoloff, L.: Computerized densitometry and color coding of [^{14}C] deoxyglucose autoradiographs, Ann. Neurol. **7**:150, 1980. *A new technique for studying the relative levels of activity of different areas of the brain based on the contrasting metabolic requirements of active and inactive neurons.*

Lemire, R.J., et al.: Normal and abnormal development of the human nervous system, New York, 1975, Harper and Row, Publishers, Inc.

Mesulam, M.-M.: Tracing neural connections of human brain with selective silver impregnation: observations on geniculocalcarine, spinothalamic, and entorhinal pathways, Arch. Neurol. **36**:814, 1979.

Moore, K.L.: The developing human, ed. 2, Philadelphia, 1977, W.B. Saunders Co.

Peters, A., Palay, S.L., and Webster, H.deF.: The fine structure of the nervous system: the neurons and supporting cells, Philadelphia, 1976, W.B. Saunders Co.

Robertson, R.T., editor: Neuroanatomical research techniques, New York, 1978, Academic Press, Inc.

Sokoloff, L.: Mapping of local cerebral functional activity by measurement of local cerebral glucose utilization with [^{14}C] deoxyglucose, Brain **102**:653, 1979.

Tuchmann-Duplessis, H., Auroux, M., and Haegel, P.: Illustrated human embryology, vol. III. Nervous system and endocrine glands. New York, 1974, Springer-Verlag, Inc.

CHAPTER 2

GROSS ANATOMY

The human central nervous system is composed of the brain and spinal cord. This chapter briefly discusses the major surface and internal structures of the brain. Together with the following four chapters, it lays the groundwork for the more detailed consideration of the functional anatomy of the CNS in ensuing chapters.

Planes and directions

Before considering the parts of the brain in more detail, it is necessary to discuss the terms used for planes and directions in the nervous system. The *sagittal* plane divides the brain into two symmetrical halves. *Parasagittal* planes are those parallel to the sagittal plane. *Frontal* planes (also called *coronal* planes) are parallel to the long axis of the body and perpendicular to the sagittal plane. These terms are fairly straightforward and have the same meaning with respect to any part of the nervous system. However, directional terms such as "*anterior*," "*dorsal*," and "*rostral*" change their relative meanings in different parts of the nervous system. The reason for this, as indicated in Fig. 2-1, is the bend of about 100° between the long axes of the brainstem and the cerebrum. This bend is a consequence of the cephalic flexure, which appears early in the embryological development of the nervous system and persists in the mature brain. The result is that in the brainstem (and spinal cord), "anterior" has the same meaning as "ventral," and "superior" has the same meaning as "rostral." In the cerebrum, on the other side of the cephalic flexure, "anterior" has the same meaning as "rostral," and "superior" has the same meaning as "dorsal." Rostral/caudal terminology may cause additional confusion because it has a functional connotation for many, so that the posterior end of the cerebral hemispheres could be considered rostral to all parts of the diencephalon. Use of anterior/posterior and superior/inferior (or dorsal/ventral) terminology in reference to the cerebrum avoids any ambiguity.

Medial surface

The cerebral hemispheres conceal most of the rest of an intact brain (Fig. 2-2). Hemisection reveals many parts of the diencephalon, brainstem, and cerebellum and additional features of the cerebral hemispheres as well (Fig. 2-3). The cephalic flexure is visible at the junction between the brainstem and the diencephalon. The brainstem itself is subdivided into (1) the *midbrain*, which is continuous with the diencephalon, (2) the *pons*, and (3) the *medulla*, which is continuous with the spinal cord. The two cerebral hemispheres are joined by a huge fiber bundle, the *corpus callosum*, which has an enlarged and rounded posterior *splenium*, a *body*, and an anterior, curved *genu*, which tapers gently into a ventrally directed *rostrum*.

Finally, the nervous system develops embryologically from a neuroectodermal tube; the cavity of the tube persists in the adult as a system of ventricles (Fig. 4-1), part of which is apparent in the sagittal plane (Fig. 4-2). Portions of the medial walls of the diencephalon define the narrow, slitlike *third ventricle*, which opens into the large *lateral ventricle* of each cerebral hemisphere through an *interventricular foramen* (or *foramen of Monro*). Posteriorly the third ventricle is continuous with a narrow channel through the midbrain, the *cerebral aqueduct* (or *aqueduct of Sylvius*). The aqueduct in turn is continuous with the *fourth ventricle* of the pons and medulla, and the fourth ventricle is continuous with the *central canal* of the caudal medulla and the spinal cord.

SURFACE FEATURES OF THE CEREBRAL HEMISPHERES

A striking aspect of human cerebral hemispheres is the degree to which their surface is folded and convoluted. Each ridge is called a *gyrus*, and each groove between the ridges is called a *sulcus;* particularly deep sulci are often called *fissures*. This folding into gyri and

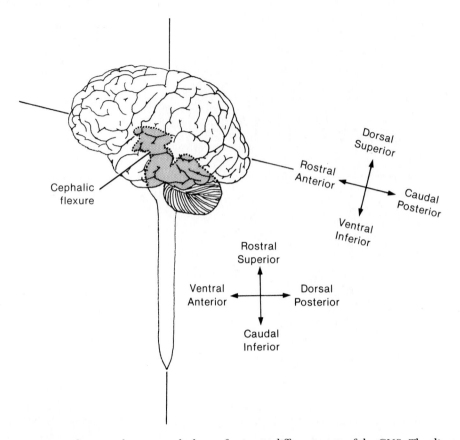

Fig. 2-1. Various directional terms used when referring to different parts of the CNS. The diencephalon and much of the brainstem, normally hidden from view in an intact brain, are drawn with dashed lines.

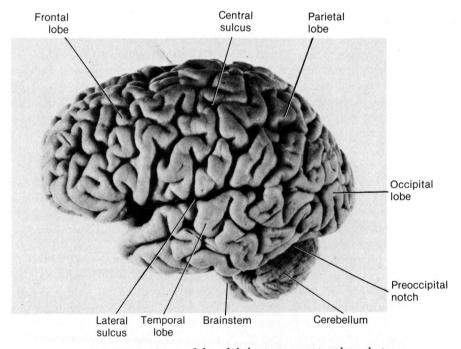

Fig. 2-2. Major regions of the adult brain as seen in a lateral view.

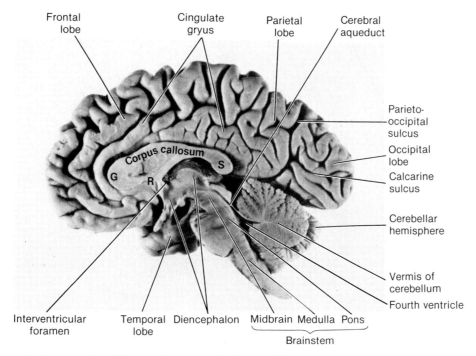

Frontal lobe — Cingulate gryus — Parietal lobe — Cerebral aqueduct

Corpus callosum — G — R — S

Parieto-occipital sulcus — Occipital lobe — Calcarine sulcus — Cerebellar hemisphere — Vermis of cerebellum — Fourth ventricle

Interventricular foramen — Temporal lobe — Diencephalon — Midbrain Medulla Pons — Brainstem

Fig. 2-3. Major regions of the cerebrum, cerebellum, and brainstem as seen in the sagittal plane. *R,* *G,* and *S* indicate the rostrum, genu, and splenium, respectively, of the corpus callosum.

sulci appears to be a mechanism for increasing the total cortical area: each person has about 2.5 sq ft of cortex, two thirds of which is hidden from view in the walls of sulci. The appearance of various gyri and sulci varies considerably from one brain to another, to the point where they may not even be continuous structures (for example, a particular gyrus may be transected by one or more sulci). Major features are, however, reasonably constant.

In the following account the principal surface features of the hemispheres are described, with some broad generalizations regarding the function of various cortical areas. These functional descriptions are highly oversimplified and are merely offered for purposes of initial orientation. Cortical function is discussed in more detail in Chapter 15.

Cerebral lobes

Four prominent sulci—the *central sulcus,* the *lateral sulcus,* the *parietooccipital sulcus,* and part of the *calcarine sulcus*—and the *preoccipital notch* are used to divide each cerebral hemisphere into four lobes (Figs. 2-2 and 2-3).

1. The *frontal lobe* extends from the anterior tip of the brain (the *frontal pole*) to the central sulcus (or *sulcus of Rolando*). Inferiorly it ends at the lateral sulcus (*fissure of Sylvius*). On the medial surface of the brain, it extends posteriorly to an imaginary line from the top of the central sulcus to the corpus callosum.

2. The *parietal lobe* extends from the central sulcus to an imaginary line from the top of the *parietooccipital fissure* to the preoccipital notch. Inferiorly it is bounded by the lateral fissure and the imaginary continuation of this fissure to the posterior boundary of the parietal lobe. On the medial surface of the brain, it is bounded inferiorly by the corpus callosum and calcarine sulcus, anteriorly by the frontal lobe, and posteriorly by the parietooccipital sulcus.

3. The *temporal lobe* extends superiorly to the lateral sulcus and the line forming the inferior boundary of the parietal lobe; posteriorly it extends to the line connecting the top of the parietooccipital sulcus and the preoccipital notch. On the medial surface its posterior boundary is an imaginary line from the preoccipital notch to the region of the splenium of the corpus callosum.

4. The *occipital lobe* is bounded anteriorly by the parietal and temporal lobes on both the lateral and medial surfaces of the hemisphere.

These separations do not correspond to precise functional subdivisions but merely provide a basis for discussion and reference.

An additional area of cerebral cortex not usually included in any of the four lobes discussed above lies buried in the depths of the lateral sulcus, concealed from view by portions of the frontal, parietal, and temporal lobes. This cortex, called the *insula,* overlies the site where the telencephalon and diencephalon fused during embryological development (Chapter 1). It can be re-

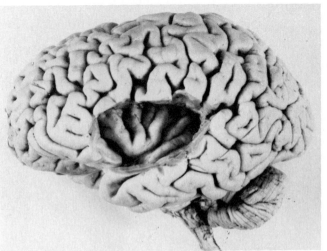

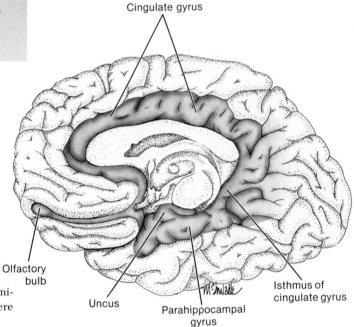

Fig. 2-4. Location of the insula. The frontal, temporal, and parietal opercula were removed from the brain shown in Fig. 2-2 in order to expose this cortical area.

Fig. 2-5. Limbic lobe as seen on the medial surface of a hemisected brain from which the brainstem and cerebellum were removed.

vealed by prying open the lateral sulcus or by removing the overlying portions of other lobes (Fig. 2-4). The portion of a given lobe overlying the insula is called an *operculum* (Latin = lid); there are frontal, parietal, and temporal opercula. A *circular sulcus* outlines the insula and marks its borders with an opercular cortex.

The *cingulate gyrus*, immediately superior to the corpus callosum, can be followed posteriorly to the splenium of the corpus callosum, where it turns inferiorly as the narrow *isthmus* of the cingulate gyrus and continues as the *parahippocampal gyrus* of the temporal lobe. These two gyri give the appearance of encircling the diencephalon and they, together with the *olfactory bulb, olfactory tract,* and certain other small cortical areas, are often separately referred to as the *limbic lobe* (Latin, limbus = border) (Fig. 2-5). The limbic lobe and many of the structures with which it is interconnected comprise the *limbic system,* which is important in emotional responses.

Frontal lobe. Four gyri make up the lateral surface of the frontal lobe (Fig. 2-6). The *precentral gyrus* is ante-

rior to the central sulcus and parallel to it, extending to the *precentral sulcus*. The *superior, middle,* and *inferior frontal gyri* are oriented parallel to one another and roughly perpendicular to the precentral gyrus. The superior frontal gyrus continues onto the medial surface of the hemisphere as far as the *cingulate sulcus*. The inferior frontal gyrus is visibly divided into three parts: (1) the *orbital part,* which is most anterior and is continuous with the inferior (*orbital*) surface of the frontal lobe; (2) the *opercular part,* which is most posterior and forms a portion of the frontal operculum; and (3) the wedge-shaped *triangular part,* which lies between the other two. The inferior or orbital surface of the frontal lobe is mostly occupied by a group of gyri of variable appearance that are collectively called *orbital gyri.* The only named gyrus on this surface is the *gyrus rectus,* which is most medial and extends onto the medial surface of the hemisphere. Between the gyrus rectus and the orbital gyri is the *olfactory sulcus,* containing the olfactory bulb and tract. The medial surface of the lobe contains part of the cingulate gyrus, extensions of the superior frontal

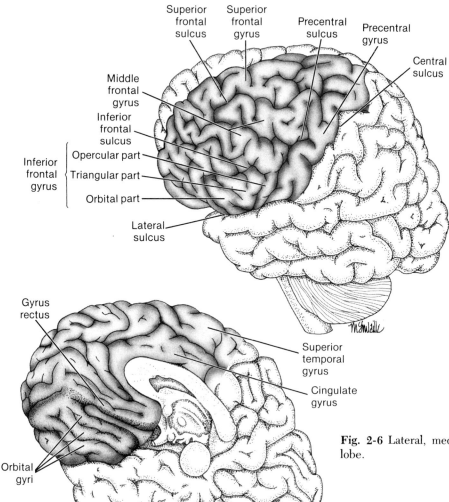

Superior
frontal
sulcus

Superior
frontal
gyrus

Precentral
sulcus

Precentral
gyrus

Central
sulcus

Middle
frontal
gyrus

Inferior
frontal
sulcus

Inferior
frontal
gyrus
{
Opercular part

Triangular part

Orbital part
}

Lateral
sulcus

Gyrus
rectus

Orbital
gyri

Superior
temporal
gyrus

Cingulate
gyrus

Fig. 2-6 Lateral, medial, and inferior surfaces of the frontal lobe.

gyrus and gyrus rectus, and certain small cortical areas near the rostrum of the corpus callosum that are related to the limbic system.

The frontal lobe is divided into four general functional areas:

1. The *primary motor cortex* is made up of much of the precentral gyrus and contains many of the cells of origin of descending motor pathways.
2. The *premotor area* is made up of the remainder of the precentral gyrus together with adjacent portions of the superior and middle frontal gyri and is also functionally related to motor systems.
3. *Broca's area*, the opercular and triangular parts of the inferior frontal gyrus of one hemisphere (usually the left), is important in the motor aspects of language production.
4. The *prefrontal cortex*, a very large and somewhat confusingly named area comprising the remainder

of the frontal lobe, is involved with what may very generally be described as personality, insight, and foresight.

Parietal lobe. The lateral surface of the parietal lobe is divided into three areas: the *postcentral gyrus* and the *superior* and *inferior parietal lobules* (Fig. 2-7). The postcentral gyrus is posterior to the central sulcus and parallel to it, extending to the *postcentral sulcus*. The *intraparietal sulcus* runs posteriorly from the postcentral sulcus toward the occipital lobe, separating the superior and inferior parietal lobules. The inferior parietal lobule in turn is composed of the *supramarginal gyrus*, which caps the upturned end of the lateral sulcus, and the *angular gyrus*, which similarly caps the *superior temporal sulcus*. The angular gyrus is typically broken up by small sulci and may overlap the supramarginal gyrus. The medial surface of the parietal lobe contains a portion of the cingulate gyrus and the medial extension of the postcentral gyrus. It is completed by an area called the *pre-*

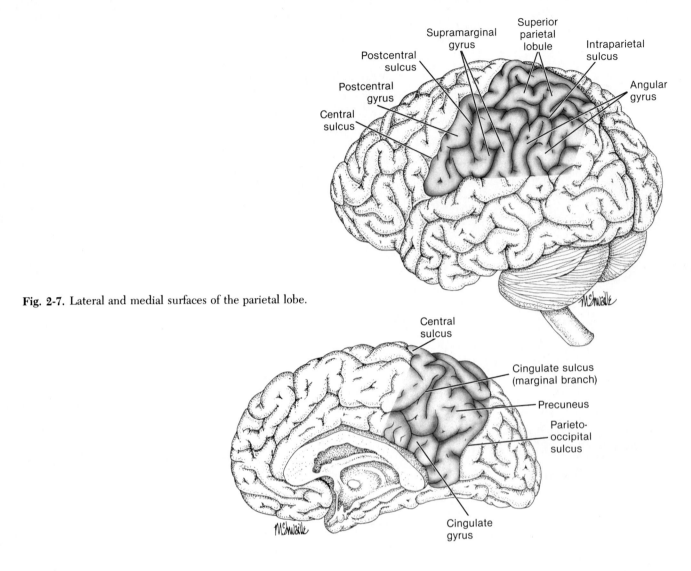

Fig. 2-7. Lateral and medial surfaces of the parietal lobe.

cuneus, which is bounded by the cingulate gyrus, the parietooccipital sulcus, and the *marginal branch* of the cingulate sulcus. The extensions of the precentral and postcentral gyri onto the medial surface of the hemisphere are sometimes referred to together as the *paracentral lobule,* which is partly in the frontal lobe and partly in the parietal lobe.

The parietal lobe is associated, in a very general sense, with three functions:

1. The postcentral gyrus more or less coincides with *primary somatosensory cortex;* that is, it is concerned with the initial cortical processing of tactile and proprioceptive (sense of position) information.
2. Much of the inferior parietal lobule of one hemisphere (usually the left), together with portions of the temporal lobe, are involved in language functions.
3. The remainder of the parietal cortex subserves complex aspects of orientation of the individual in space and time.

Temporal lobe. The lateral surface of the temporal lobe is composed of the *superior, middle,* and *inferior temporal gyri* (Fig. 2-8). The superior temporal gyrus continues into the lateral sulcus where it forms one of its walls. Thus part of the superior temporal gyrus comprises the temporal operculum. The inferior temporal gyrus continues onto the inferior surface of the lobe. The rest of the inferior surface is made up of the broad and often discontinuous *occipitotemporal (fusiform) gyrus* and the parahippocampal gyrus, separated from one another by the *collateral sulcus.* The occipitotemporal gyrus, as its name implies, is partly in the occipital lobe and partly in the temporal lobe. The parahippocampal gyrus is continuous with the cingulate gyrus around the splenium of the corpus callosum by way of the isthmus of the cingulate gyrus. The anterior end of the parahippocampal gyrus turns backward and forms a medially directed bump called the *uncus.* The superior border of the parahippocampal gyrus is the *hippocampal sulcus* (Figs. 2-5 and 2-8). Folded into the temporal lobe at the

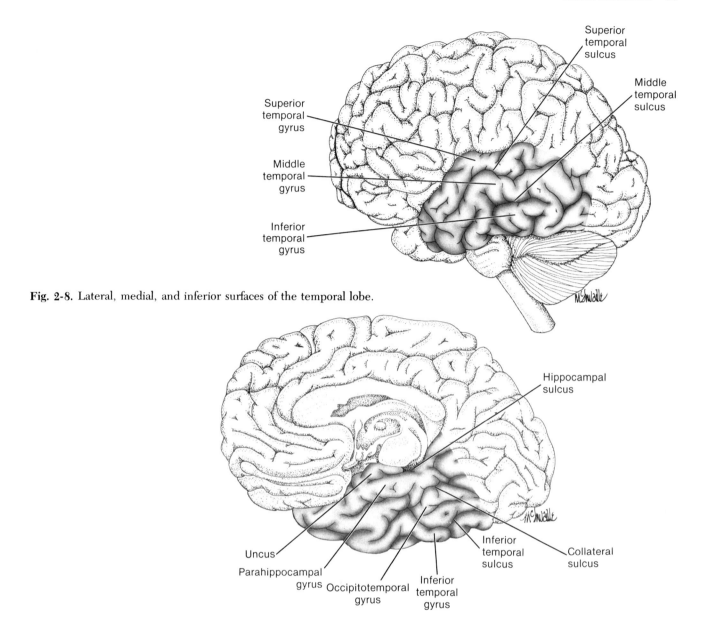

Fig. 2-8. Lateral, medial, and inferior surfaces of the temporal lobe.

hippocampal sulcus is an area of cortex called the *hippocampus*, which is part of the limbic system. The hippocampus cannot be seen without sectioning or dissecting the brain (Figs. 2-9 and 2-18).

The temporal lobe is associated in a general way with three functions:

1. A small area of that portion of the superior temporal gyrus that lies in the lateral sulcus is *primary auditory cortex.*
2. The parahippocampal gyrus and hippocampus, as parts of the limbic system, are involved in emotional and visceral responses.
3. The temporal lobe is involved in complex aspects of learning and memory recall.

The second and third functions may overlap to some degree. For example, portions of the limbic system, particularly the hippocampus, are thought by many to be important for memory processes.

Occipital lobe. The lateral surface of the occipital lobe is of variable configuration, and its gyri are usually referred to simply as *lateral occipital gyri.* On the medial surface, the wedge-shaped area between the parieto-occipital and calcarine sulci is called the *cuneus* (Latin = wedge) (Fig. 2-10). The gyrus inferior to the calcarine sulcus is the *lingual gyrus.* The lingual gyrus is adjacent to the posterior portion of the occipitotemporal gyrus, separated from it by the collateral sulcus, and usually continuous anteriorly with the parahippocampal gyrus. The transition from lingual to parahippocampal gyrus occurs at the isthmus of the cingulate gyrus (Fig. 2-5).

The occipital lobe is more or less exclusively concerned with visual functions. *Primary visual cortex* is

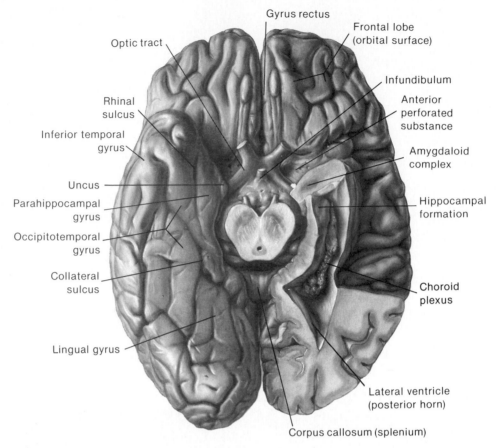

Fig. 2-9. Dissection of the temporal lobe to demonstrate the hippocampus. The hippocampus is a cortical area that has folded into the inferior horn of the lateral ventricle in the temporal lobe. The anterior perforated substance is an area of the base of the brain where many small blood vessels enter the cerebrum. The rhinal sulcus is an anterior continuation of the collateral sulcus. (From Mettler, F.A.: Neuroanatomy, ed. 2, St. Louis, 1948, The C.V. Mosby Co.)

contained in the walls of the calcarine sulcus and a bit of the surrounding cortex. The remainder of the lobe is referred to as *visual association cortex* and is involved in higher order processing of visual information.

DIENCEPHALON

The diencephalon has four divisions: *thalamus, hypothalamus, epithalamus,* and *subthalamus.* Portions of three of these divisions can be seen on a hemisected brain (Fig. 2-11); the subthalamus is an internal structure that can only be seen in sections through the brain.

The thalamus is an oval nuclear mass, part of which borders on the third ventricle. The line of attachment of the roof of this ventricle is marked by a horizontally oriented ridge, the *stria medullaris thalami.* Posteriorly the thalamus protrudes over the most rostral portion of the brainstem. Anteriorly it abuts the interventricular foramen. The thalamus is a nuclear mass of major importance in both sensory and motor systems. No sensory information, with the exception of olfactory information, reaches the cerebral cortex without prior processing in

thalamic nuclei. In addition, the complex anatomical loops characteristic of motor systems, which involve pathways between the cerebellum and cerebral cortex and between basal ganglia and cerebral cortex, typically involve thalamic nuclei as well.

The hypothalamus is inferior to the thalamus, separated from it by the hypothalamic sulcus in the wall of the third ventricle. It also forms the floor of the ventricle, and its inferior surface is one of the few parts of the diencephalon visible on an intact brain. This inferior surface (Fig. 2-13) includes the *infundibular stalk* and two rounded protuberances, the *mammillary bodies.* The hypothalamus is the major visceral control center of the brain and is involved in limbic system functions as well.

The epithalamus comprises the midline *pineal gland* and several small neural structures visible in sections.

BRAINSTEM

The brainstem is divided into the midbrain, the pons, and the medulla (Fig. 2-3). The *tectum* of the midbrain,

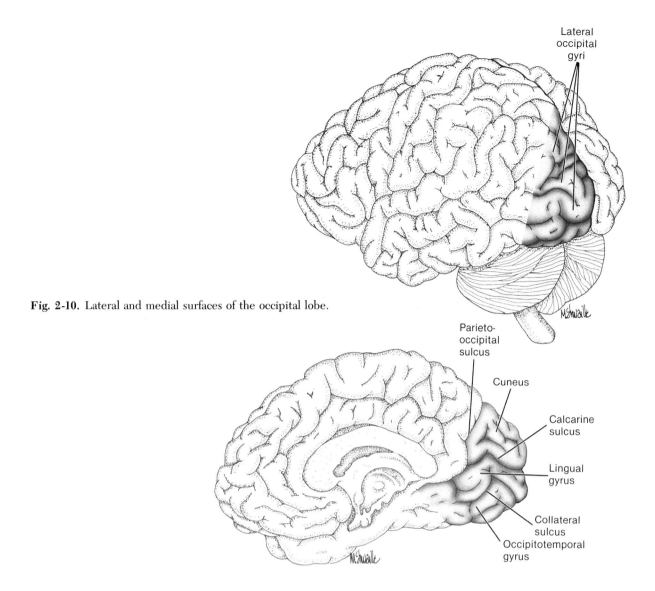

Fig. 2-10. Lateral and medial surfaces of the occipital lobe.

Lateral occipital gyri

Parieto-occipital sulcus

Cuneus

Calcarine sulcus

Lingual gyrus

Collateral sulcus

Occipitotemporal gyrus

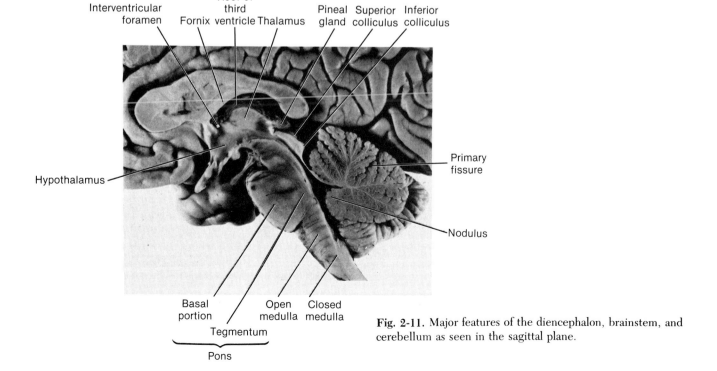

Interventricular foramen

Fornix

Roof of third ventricle

Thalamus

Pineal gland

Superior colliculus

Inferior colliculus

Primary fissure

Hypothalamus

Nodulus

Basal portion

Tegmentum

Open medulla

Closed medulla

Pons

Fig. 2-11. Major features of the diencephalon, brainstem, and cerebellum as seen in the sagittal plane.

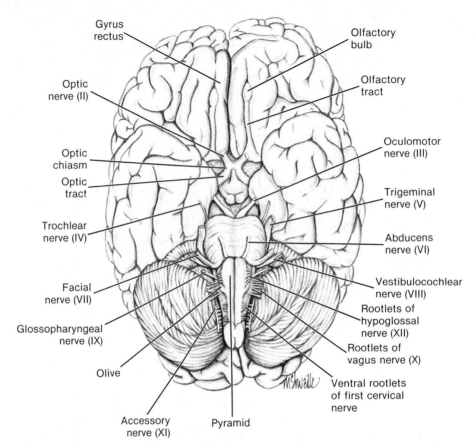

Fig. 2-12. Inferior surface of the brain, indicating the locations of the cranial nerves.

that portion dorsal to the cerebral aqueduct, consists of the *superior* and *inferior colliculi*. The paired *cerebral peduncles* constitute the remainder of the midbrain. The pons consists of a protruding *basal portion*, oval-shaped in sagittal section, and the overlying *pontine tegmentum*, which forms part of the floor of the fourth ventricle. The medulla consists of a rostral *open* portion, containing part of the fourth ventricle, and a caudal *closed* portion, continuous with the spinal cord (Fig. 2-11).

The points of attachment of most cranial nerves, as well as additional brainstem structures, can be seen in an inferior view of the brain (Figs. 2-12 and 2-13). The olfactory tract is located in the olfactory sulcus, medial to the gyrus rectus, and is attached directly to the cerebral hemisphere. *Cranial nerve I (olfactory)* is actually a collection of very fine axons called *fila olfactoria* that terminate in the olfactory bulb at the anterior end of the tract. Slightly posterior to the attachment points of the olfactory tracts, the *optic nerves (cranial nerve II)* join to form the *optic chiasm*, in which half the fibers of each nerve cross to the opposite side. The *optic tract* proceeds from the optic chiasm to a thalamic nucleus. Embryologically the optic nerves are outgrowths of the diencephalon (Chapter 1) and properly are tracts of the

CNS, but they are treated as cranial nerves because of their course outside the rest of the brain. Considered in this way, cranial nerve II is the only one that projects directly to the diencephalon.

Located farther posteriorly are the cerebral peduncles of the midbrain, each of which contains a massive fiber bundle that carries a great deal of the descending projection from the cerebral cortex to the brainstem and spinal cord. *Cranial nerve II (oculomotor)* emerges into the *interpeduncular fossa* between the cerebral peduncles. *Cranial nerve IV (trochlear)* emerges from the dorsal surface of the brainstem just caudal to the inferior colliculi, then proceeds anteriorly through the space between brainstem and cerebral hemisphere.

Caudally the cerebral peduncles disappear into the transversely oriented basal portion of the pons. Dorsolaterally this part of the pons narrows into a large fiber bundle that enters the cerebellum. This is the *middle cerebellar peduncle (brachium pontis)*, which carries the major input from the cerebral hemispheres to the cerebellum by way of relays in nuclei of the pons. *Cranial nerve V (trigeminal)* emerges from the lateral aspect of the basal portion of the pons. *Cranial nerve VI (abducens)* emerges near the midline at the caudal edge of

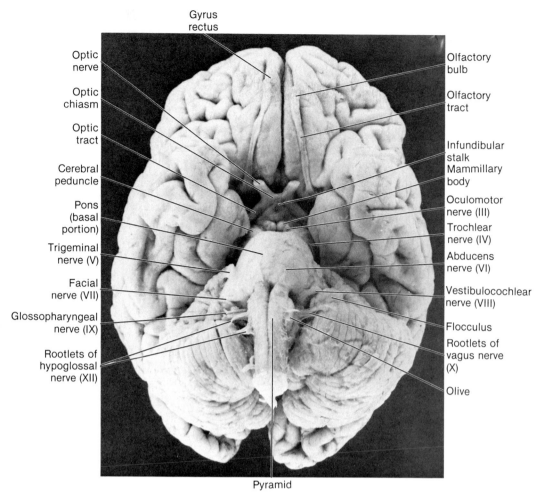

Gyrus
rectus

Optic
nerve

Optic
chiasm

Optic
tract

Cerebral
peduncle

Pons
(basal
portion)

Trigeminal
nerve (V)

Facial
nerve (VII)

Glossopharyngeal
nerve (IX)

Rootlets of
hypoglossal
nerve (XII)

Olfactory
bulb

Olfactory
tract

Infundibular
stalk
Mammillary
body

Oculomotor
nerve (III)

Trochlear
nerve (IV)

Abducens
nerve (VI)

Vestibulocochlear
nerve (VIII)

Flocculus

Rootlets of
vagus nerve
(X)

Olive

Pyramid

Fig. 2-13. Inferior surface of the brain, illustrating the attachment points of the cranial nerves as well as other surface features of the diencephalon, brainstem, and cerebellum. (Dissection by Pam Eller, University of Colorado Medical Center.)

the pons. *Cranial nerves VII (facial)* and *VIII (vestibulocochlear)* emerge more laterally near the cerebellum and also at the caudal edge of the pons. The area of attachment of cranial nerves VII and VIII is called the *cerebellopontine angle* and is a common site of development of tumors, such as tumors of the sheaths of these cranial nerves.

Caudal to the pons are two thick fiber bundles somewhat resembling the cerebral peduncles but considerably smaller. These are the *pyramids* of the medulla, which carry those fibers of the cerebral peduncles that are directed to the spinal cord. The two pyramids decussate* in the area of transition from brainstem to spinal cord. Dorsolateral to each pyramid is an oval protuberance called the *olive. Cranial nerve XII (hypoglossal)* emerges from the sulcus between the pyramid and the

olive. The more or less continuous series of filaments that will form *cranial nerves IX (glossopharyngeal), X (vagus)*, and part of *XI (accessory)* emerge from the sulcus dorsal to the olive.

CEREBELLUM

The cerebellum can be subdivided in several different ways, two of which will be briefly considered here. In one sense, the cerebellum comprises a midline *vermis*, which is hemisected in a hemisected brain (Fig. 2-3), and a much larger *lateral hemisphere* on each side (Fig. 2-2). Using any other method of subdividing the cerebellum, a given division has both a vermal and a hemispheral component.

Lobes of the cerebellum, which roughly correspond to separate functional areas, are also recognized. The *anterior lobe* is that portion anterior to the primary fissure (Fig. 2-11). This lobe receives afferent inputs from the spinal cord and seems to be predominantly concerned with postural adjustments. The *flocculonodular*

---

*A *decussation* is a site where nerve fibers joining unlike areas of the CNS cross, such as here where fibers cross on their way from one side of the cerebrum to the opposite side of the spinal cord. In contrast, a *commissure* is a crossing site for fibers connecting like areas.

lobe consists of three small components: the *nodulus*, which is the vermal portion of the lobe (Fig. 2-11), and a small *flocculus* on each side near the vestibulocochlear nerve (Fig. 2-13). The nodulus is actually continuous with the flocculus of each side, but this continuity is difficult to see without dissecting the cerebellum. The flocculonodular lobe receives afferent inputs from the vestibular system and is involved in postural adjustments to gravity. All of the cerebellum posterior to the primary fissure, exclusive of the flocculonodular lobe, constitutes the *posterior lobe*, which is the largest of the three. The posterior lobe receives the majority of the afferent input from the cerebral cortex by way of relays in *pontine nuclei* and transmission through the middle cerebellar peduncle. This lobe is involved in the coordination of voluntary movements. In reality, cerebellar function is not quite so neatly parcelled out among the anatomical subdivisions; the details of cerebellar function will be considered in Chapter 14.

INTERNAL STRUCTURES

Prior to consideration of the internal structures of the brain, it is useful to discuss certain consequences of the shape of the cerebral hemispheres. As a result of the embryological development of the hemispheres (Chapter 1), the cortical lobes are arranged in a C shape from the frontal lobe, through the parietal and occipital lobes, and into the temporal lobe (Fig. 2-14). A number of other structures, such as the lateral ventricles (Figs. 4-1 and 4-2), are similarly C shaped, with the result that sections through the brain may cut these structures in two different places. The hippocampus, together with its efferent fiber bundle (the *fornix*) (Fig. 16-9), is another example. The hippocampus is folded into the temporal lobe, forming part of the wall of the lateral ventricle there (Fig. 2-18). It becomes smaller as the temporal lobe curves into the parietal lobe, and it ends near the splenium of the corpus callosum. The fornix continues this curved course (Fig. 2-11), arching anteriorly under the corpus callosum, then turning inferiorly and posteriorly toward the hypothalamus, where many of its fibers end in the mammillary bodies.

Basal ganglia

The basal ganglia are a group of nuclei that form part of each cerebral hemisphere. They are internal structures of the hemisphere, visible only in sections. Use of the term varies, but the major basal ganglia are the *amygdala*, the *caudate nucleus*, and the *lentiform nucleus*. The amygdala lies beneath the uncus of the temporal lobe (Fig. 2-17). The caudate nucleus, another example of a C-shaped structure, has an enlarged *head* deep in the frontal lobe, and its increasingly attenuated *body* and *tail* follow the lateral ventricle around into the temporal lobe, where it finally fuses with the amygdala (Fig. 13-4). The lentiform nucleus, which is subdivided into the *putamen* and the *globus pallidus*, lies lateral, and partially anterior, to the thalamus. It is separated from the thalamus and from much of the head of the caudate nucleus by a thick sheet of fibers called the *internal capsule*. The internal capsule contains most of the fibers interconnecting the cerebral cortex and deep structures such as the thalamus and basal ganglia.

Figs. 2-15 to 2-21 are intended to introduce the beginning student to the configuration of internal structures of the brain. Each section is in a coronal plane and has been stained with Mulligan's stain, which differentiates gray matter from white matter. In each case the anterior surface of the section is shown, and the plane of this anterior surface is indicated on the right side of each photograph. Only major structures are labeled.

Text continued on p. 26.

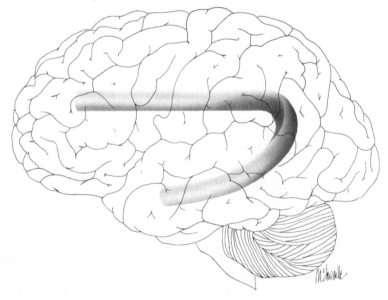

Fig. 2-14. General configuration of C-shaped structures such as the lateral ventricle, the caudate nucleus, and the hippocampus-fornix system.

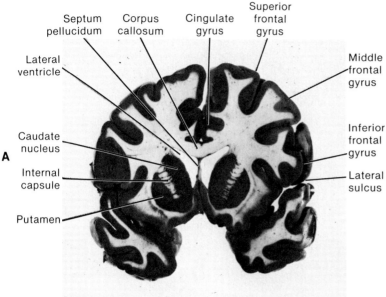

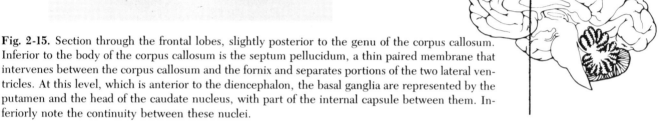

Septum
pellucidum

Corpus
callosum

Cingulate
gyrus

Superior
frontal
gyrus

Lateral
ventricle

Middle
frontal
gyrus

Caudate
nucleus

Inferior
frontal
gyrus

Internal
capsule

Lateral
sulcus

Putamen

A

B

C

Fig. 2-15. Section through the frontal lobes, slightly posterior to the genu of the corpus callosum. Inferior to the body of the corpus callosum is the septum pellucidum, a thin paired membrane that intervenes between the corpus callosum and the fornix and separates portions of the two lateral ventricles. At this level, which is anterior to the diencephalon, the basal ganglia are represented by the putamen and the head of the caudate nucleus, with part of the internal capsule between them. Inferiorly note the continuity between these nuclei.

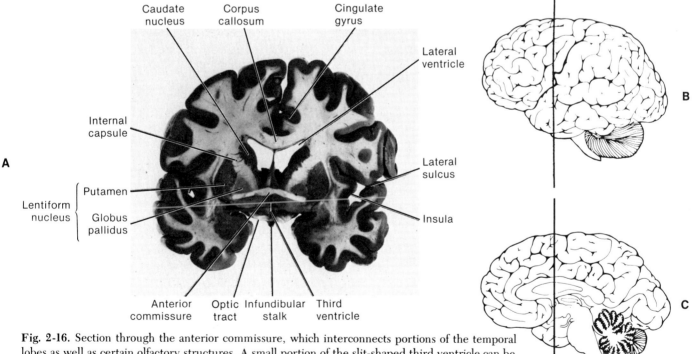

Caudate
nucleus

Corpus
callosum

Cingulate
gyrus

Lateral
ventricle

Internal
capsule

Lentiform
nucleus

Putamen

Globus
pallidus

Lateral
sulcus

Insula

A

B

Anterior
commissure

Optic
tract

Infundibular
stalk

Third
ventricle

C

Fig. 2-16. Section through the anterior commissure, which interconnects portions of the temporal lobes as well as certain olfactory structures. A small portion of the slit-shaped third ventricle can be seen between the anterior commissure and the optic chiasm. At this level both parts of the lentiform nucleus (the putamen and the globus pallidus) are present. The section is slightly anterior to both the interventricular foramen and the thalamus.

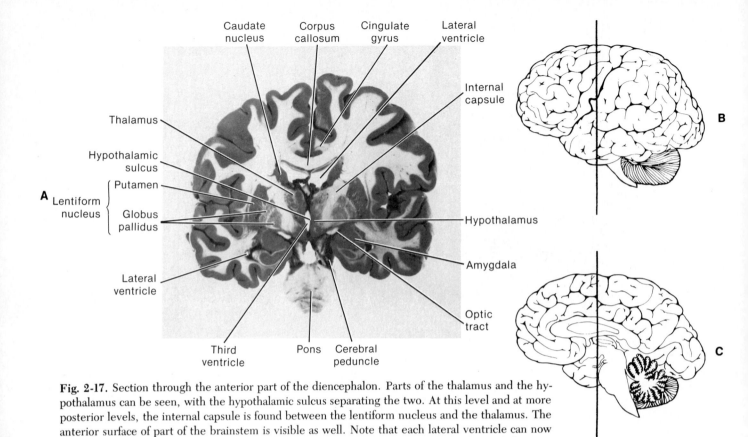

Fig. 2-17. Section through the anterior part of the diencephalon. Parts of the thalamus and the hypothalamus can be seen, with the hypothalamic sulcus separating the two. At this level and at more posterior levels, the internal capsule is found between the lentiform nucleus and the thalamus. The anterior surface of part of the brainstem is visible as well. Note that each lateral ventricle can now be seen in two places; because of their C shape, they were transected twice in this and the next three sections.

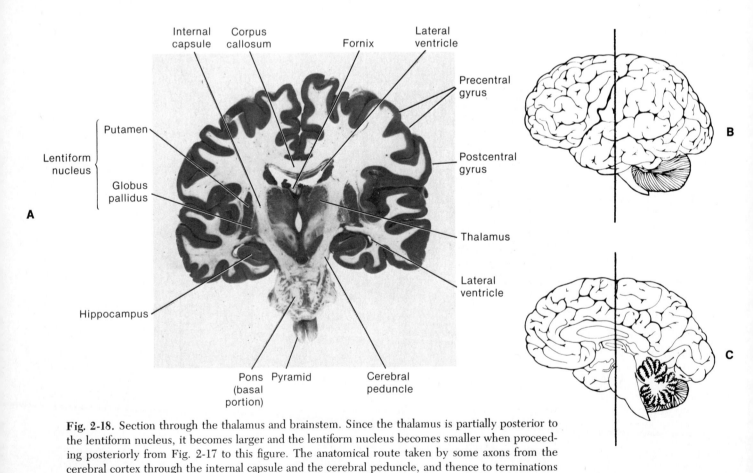

Fig. 2-18. Section through the thalamus and brainstem. Since the thalamus is partially posterior to the lentiform nucleus, it becomes larger and the lentiform nucleus becomes smaller when proceeding posteriorly from Fig. 2-17 to this figure. The anatomical route taken by some axons from the cerebral cortex through the internal capsule and the cerebral peduncle, and thence to terminations in the brainstem or spinal cord, is apparent.

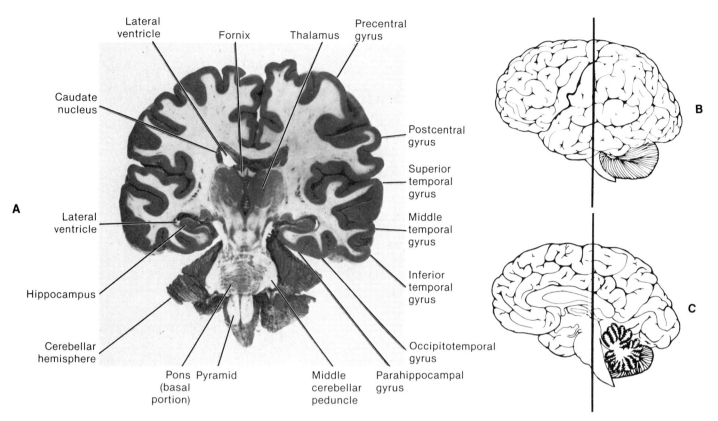

Fig. 2-19. Section through the brainstem and posterior thalamus. This level is posterior to the lentiform nucleus; the few scattered clumps of gray matter in its former location are bridges of gray matter that extend from the putamen to the caudate nucleus.

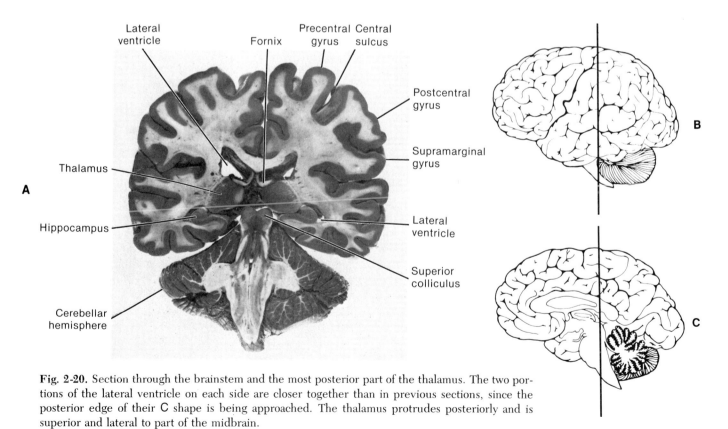

Fig. 2-20. Section through the brainstem and the most posterior part of the thalamus. The two portions of the lateral ventricle on each side are closer together than in previous sections, since the posterior edge of their C shape is being approached. The thalamus protrudes posteriorly and is superior and lateral to part of the midbrain.

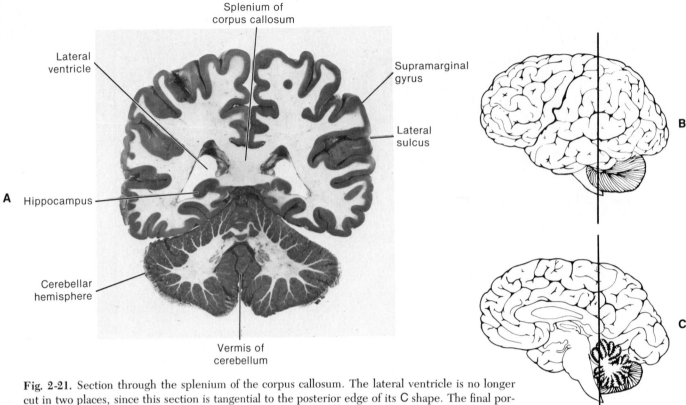

Fig. 2-21. Section through the splenium of the corpus callosum. The lateral ventricle is no longer cut in two places, since this section is tangential to the posterior edge of its C shape. The final portion of the hippocampus can be seen as it ends near the splenium.

ADDITIONAL READING

DeArmond, S.J., Fusco, M.M., and Dewey, M.M., Structure of the human brain: a photographic atlas, ed. 2. New York, 1976, Oxford University Press.

Gluhbegovic, N., and Williams, T.H.: The human brain: a photographic guide, New York, 1980, Harper and Row, Publishers, Inc.

Igarashi, S., and Kamiya, T.: Atlas of the vertebrate brain: morphological evolution from cyclostomes to mammals, Baltimore, 1972, University Park Press. *Ever wonder what an anteater's brain looks like?*

Ludwig, E., and Klingler, J.: Atlas cerebri humani, Boston, 1956, Little, Brown and Co. *A series of technically spectacular dissections of human brains.*

Nieuwenhuys, R., Voogd, J., and van Huijzen, C.: The human central nervous system: a synopsis and atlas, New York, 1978, Springer-Verlag, Inc. *Includes many beautiful drawings of the brain and various subsystems of the CNS, as well as a brief but up-to-date text portion.*

Roberts, M., and Hanaway, J.: Atlas of the human brain in section, Philadelphia, 1970, Lea & Febiger.

CHAPTER 3

MENINGEAL COVERINGS OF THE BRAIN AND SPINAL CORD

Living brain is on the soft and mushy side. Without support of some kind it would be unable to maintain its shape, particularly in the presence of head movements and outside pressures. The brain and spinal cord are protected from outside forces by their encasement in the skull and vertebral column, respectively. In addition, the CNS is suspended within a series of three membranous coverings, the *meninges* (Greek, meninx = membrane), that stabilize the shape and position of nerve tissue in two different ways during head and body movements. First, the brain is mechanically suspended within the meninges, which in turn are anchored to the skull so that the brain is constrained to move in parallel with the head. Second, there is a layer of *cerebrospinal fluid* within the meninges; the buoyant effect of this fluid environment greatly decreases the tendency of various forces (such as gravity) to distort the brain. Thus a brain weighing 1500 grams in air effectively weighs less than 50 grams in its normal cerebrospinal fluid environment, where it is easily able to maintain its shape. In contrast, an isolated fresh brain, unsupported by its usual surroundings, becomes seriously distorted and may even tear under the influence of gravity.

The three meninges, from the outermost layer inward, are the *dura mater*, the *arachnoid*, and the *pia mater* (Fig. 3-1). In common usage the dura mater and pia mater are often referred to simply as the dura and pia. The dura mater is by far the most substantial of the three meninges and for this reason is also called the *pachymeninx* (Greek, pachy = thick, as in pachyderms). The arachnoid and pia mater, in contrast, are thin and delicate. They are similar to and continuous with each other and so are sometimes referred to together as the pia-arachnoid or the *leptomeninges* (Greek, lepto = thin, fine). The dura mater is attached to the inner surface of the skull, and the arachnoid adheres to the inner surface of the dura mater. The pia mater is attached to

the brain, following all its contours, and the space between the arachnoid and pia mater is filled with cerebrospinal fluid.

Because of the differences between cranial and spinal meninges, those of the spinal cord are described separately at the end of this chapter.

DURA MATER

The cranial dura is a thick, tough, collagenous membrane that adheres firmly to the inner surface of the skull (Latin, dura = hard, as in durable). It is often described as consisting of two layers: an outer layer that serves as the periosteum of the inner surface of the skull and an inner layer, the true dura. Since these two layers are tightly fused with no sharp histological boundary between them, the entire complex is ordinarily referred to as dura mater.

No space exists on either side of the dura under normal circumstances, since one side is attached to the skull and the other side is adjacent to the arachnoid. However, two *potential* spaces, the *epidural* and *subdural* spaces, are associated with the dura (Fig. 3-12). Epidural space refers to the potential space between the cranium and the periosteal layer. Subdural space is commonly described as the potential space between dura and arachnoid and is said to contain a thin film of fluid. However, recent electron microscopic evidence indicates that when the dura and arachnoid appear to separate, the splitting actually occurs within the innermost cellular layers of the dura. Parts of these potential spaces can become actual fluid-filled cavities in certain pathological conditions, most often as a result of hemorrhage.

Dural reflections

There are several places where the inner dural layer is reflected as sheetlike protrusions, called *dural reflections* or *dural septa*, into the cranial cavity. The principal

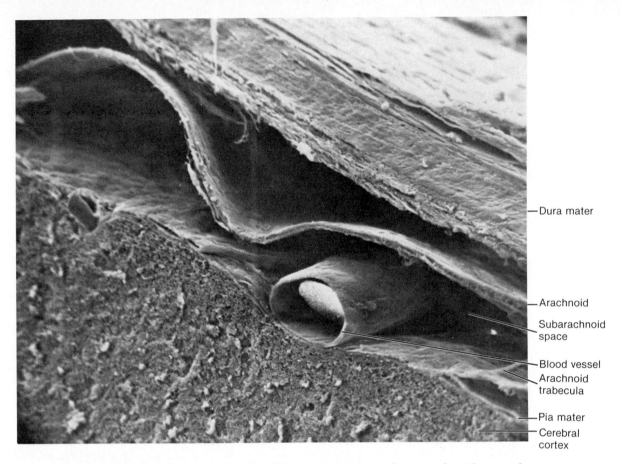

—Dura mater

—Arachnoid

—Subarachnoid space

—Blood vessel

—Arachnoid trabecula

—Pia mater

—Cerebral cortex

Fig. 3-1. Scanning electron micrograph of the cranial meninges of a young dog. The space between the dura mater and the arachnoid is an artifact of processing and would not normally be present. (Courtesy of Dr. Delmas J. Allen, Medical College of Ohio.)

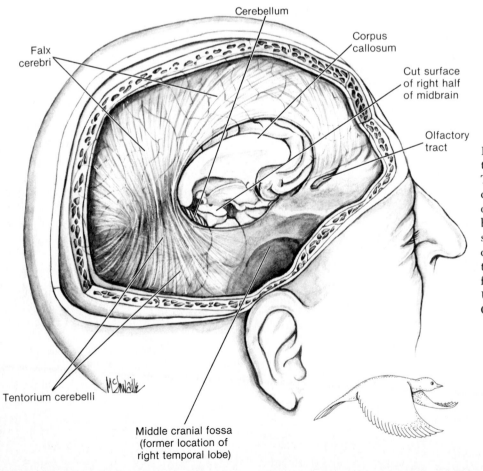

Cerebellum

Corpus callosum

Cut surface of right half of midbrain

Falx cerebri

Olfactory tract

Tentorium cerebelli

Middle cranial fossa (former location of right temporal lobe)

Fig. 3-2. Shape and spatial relationships of the dural reflections. The cerebellum and part of the left cerebral hemisphere are drawn in on the other side of the falx cerebri and tentorium cerebelli. The small bird in the corner reminds certain individuals of the shape of the tentorium cerebelli. (Drawn from a dissection by Gary Jenison, Univeristy of Colorado Medical Center.)

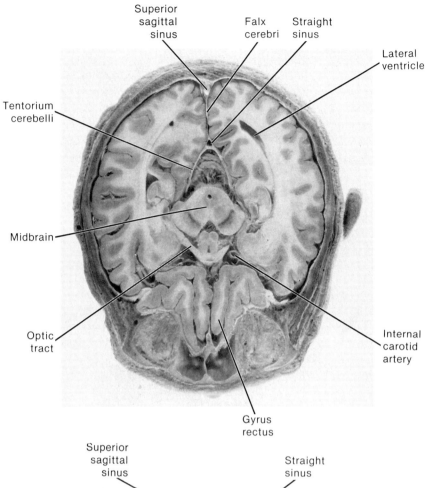

Fig. 3-3. Horizontal section near the top of the tentorium cerebelli. The superior sagittal sinus can be seen in one attached edge of the falx cerebri and the straight sinus in the other attached edge. Notice the manner in which the tentorium partially surrounds the midbrain, forming the tentorial notch. (Courtesy of Dr. John T. Willson, University of Colorado Medical Center.)

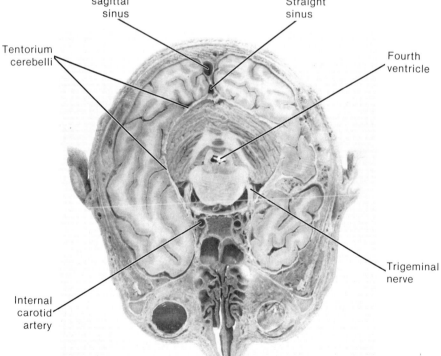

Fig. 3-4. Horizontal section at a level just above the confluence of the sinuses. The straight sinus is about to join the superior sagittal sinus. Note again how close the brainstem is to the tentorium as it passes through the tentorial notch. (Courtesy of Dr. John T. Willson, University of Colorado Medical Center.)

dural reflections are the *falx cerebri,* which intervenes between the two cerebral hemispheres, and the *tentorium cerebelli,* which intervenes between the cerebral hemispheres and the cerebellum (Fig. 3-2). The *falx cerebelli* is a small reflection that partially separates the two cerebellar hemispheres. The *diaphragma sellae,* another small reflection, covers the pituitary fossa, admitting the infundibulum through a small perforation.

The falx cerebri (Latin, falx = sickle) is a long, arched,

vertical dural sheet (Figs. 3-2 and 3-3) that occupies the longitudinal fissure and separates the two cerebral hemispheres. Anteriorly it is attached to the crista galli of the ethmoid bone. The falx curves posteriorly and fuses with the middle of the tentorium cerebelli at the internal occipital protuberance. The inferior, free edge of the falx generally parallels the corpus callosum, but the falx is somewhat broader posteriorly than it is anteriorly, so this free edge comes closer to the splenium of the corpus

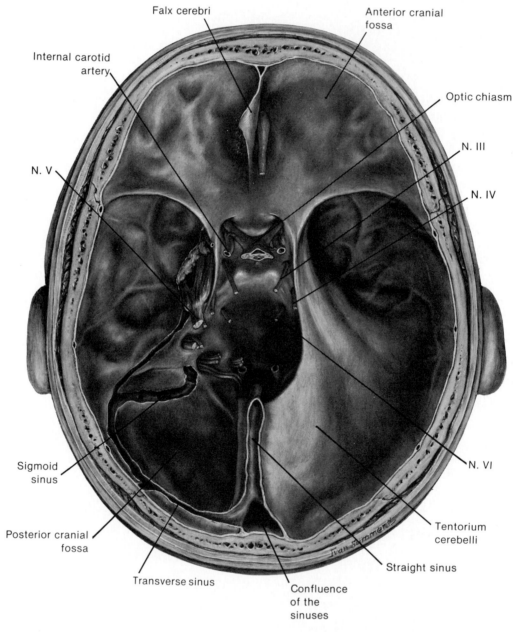

Fig. 3-5. Dural lining of the base of the skull. The falx has been removed except for a small anterior portion. The left half of the tentorium has also been removed, exposing the posterior fossa (where the cerebellum was). Compare to Figs. 3-3 and 3-4. (From Mettler, F.A.: Neuroanatomy, ed. 2, St. Louis, 1948, The C.V. Mosby Co.)

callosum than to the genu (Fig. 3-2). The anterior portion of the falx is frequently incomplete, containing a number of perforations.

The tentorium cerebelli separates the superior surface of the cerebellum from the occipital lobes, defining *supratentorial* and *infratentorial* compartments. Because the interval between the cerebrum and cerebellum is not horizontal or flat, neither is the tentorium. Rather, it is roughly the shape of a bird with its wings extended in front of it; the bird's body would correspond to the midline region where the falx joins the tentorium, and its wings would correspond to the rest of the tentorium, which is prolonged anteriorly (Figs. 3-2 to 3-4). Posteriorly the tentorium is attached mainly to the occipital bone. This line of attachment continues anteriorly and inferiorly along the petrous temporal bone. The free edge of the tentorium also curves anteriorly on each side, almost encircling the midbrain (Figs. 3-4 and 3-5). This space in the tentorium through which the brainstem passes is called the *tentorial notch*, (or *tentorial incisure*) and is of great clinical significance, as discussed later in this chapter.

Dural sinuses

As noted previously, the two layers of the cranial dura are tightly fused, and there are no pathological conditions in which an intradural space (that is, a space between the two layers) develops. However, at some edges of dural reflections (most often attached edges), the two layers are normally separated to form channels, called *dural venous sinuses*, into which the cerebral veins empty. These sinuses are roughly triangular in cross section and are lined with endothelium (Figs. 3-6 and 3-7). The locations of the major sinuses can be inferred by considering the lines of attachment of the falx and the tentorium. The *superior sagittal sinus* is found along the attached edge of the falx, the *left* and *right transverse sinuses* are found along the posterior line of attachment of the tentorium, and the *straight sinus* is found along the line of attachment of the falx and tentorium to each other (Figs. 3-3, 3-4, and 5-8). All four of these sinuses meet in the *confluence of the sinuses* (also called the *torcular*, or *torcular Herophili*) near the internal occipital protuberance. Venous blood flows posteriorly in the superior sagittal and straight sinuses into the con-

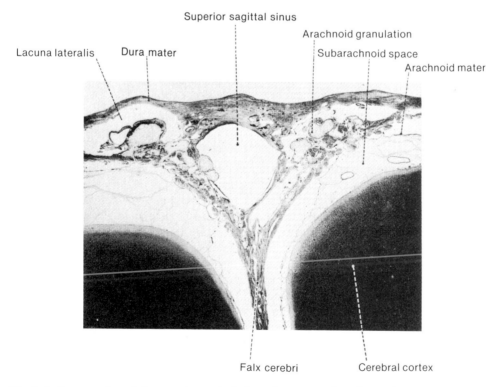

Fig. 3-6. Cross section of the superior sagittal sinus showing arachnoid granulations. Note the fine arachnoid trabeculae spanning the subarachnoid space. Lacunae laterales are lateral extensions of venous sinuses, particularly the superior sagittal sinus, into which many of the arachnoid granulations protrude. (From Hamilton, W.J.: Textbook of human anatomy, ed. 2, St. Louis, 1976, The C.V. Mosby Co., p. 595. By permission of Macmillan Press, London and Basingstoke.)

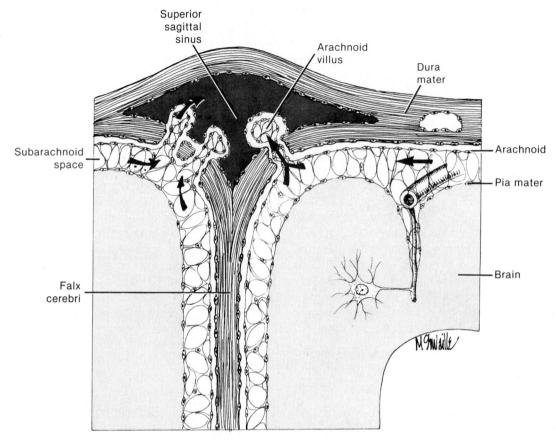

Fig. 3-7. Section through the superior sagittal sinus showing the movement of cerebrospinal fluid from subarachnoid space, through the arachnoid villi, and into the sinus. The apparent subdural space shown in this drawing would not normally be present; it merely illustrates the distinction between dura and arachnoid. (Modified from Hamilton, W.J.: Textbook of Human Anatomy, ed. 2, St. Louis, 1976, The C.V. Mosby Co. By permission of Macmillan Press, London and Basingstoke.)

fluence, and from there through the transverse sinuses. Each transverse sinus continues, from the point where it leaves the tentorium, as the *sigmoid sinus*, which proceeds anteriorly and inferiorly through an S-shaped course and empties into the internal jugular vein (Figs. 3-5, 3-8, and 5-8).

The confluence of the sinuses is generally not a symmetrical structure. Usually blood from the superior sagittal sinus flows into the right transverse sinus, while blood from the straight sinus flows into the left transverse sinus (Figs. 3-8 and 5-14). In an extreme case, the two transverse sinuses may not be interconnected at all.

In addition to receiving cerebral veins, the major dural sinuses mentioned above are interconnected with several smaller sinuses (Fig. 5-8). The *inferior sagittal sinus*, in the free edge of the falx cerebri, empties into the straight sinus. The small *occipital sinus*, in the attached edge of the falx cerebelli, empties into the confluence of the sinuses. The *superior petrosal sinus*, in the

edge of the tentorium attached to the petrous temporal bone, carries blood from the cavernous sinus to the transverse sinus at the point where the latter leaves the tentorium to become the sigmoid sinus. The *inferior petrosal sinus* follows a groove between the temporal and occipital bones, carrying blood from the cavernous sinus to the internal jugular vein.

Dural vasculature and innervation

The arterial supply of the dura comes from a large number of meningeal arteries. These are somewhat misnamed because they travel in the periosteal layer of the dura and function mainly in supplying the bones of the skull; however, many small arterial branches penetrate the dura itself. The largest of the meningeal arteries is the *middle meningeal artery*, a branch of the maxillary artery, which ramifies over most of the lateral surface of the cerebral dura. Anteriorly the dura is supplied by branches of the ophthalmic artery, and posteriorly it is

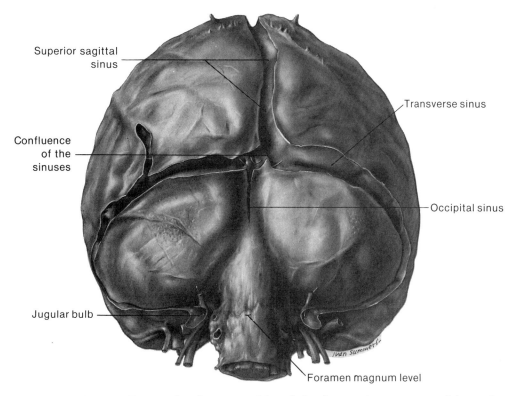

Superior sagittal
sinus

Transverse sinus

Confluence
of the
sinuses

Occipital sinus

Jugular bulb

Foramen magnum level

Fig. 3-8. The brain, still encased in dura, viewed from behind. Note the asymmetry of the conflu-ence of the sinuses (compare to Fig. 5-14). Note also the jagged line at the foramen magnum level corresponding to the cut edge of the periosteal layer of the cranial dura. Below this line, a single-layered dural sheath continues around the spinal cord. (From Mettler, F.A.: Neuroanatomy, ed. 2, St. Louis, 1948, The C.V. Mosby Co.)

supplied by branches of the occipital and vertebral ar-teries. Meningeal veins, also located in the periosteal layer, generally parallel the arteries.

Most of the cranial dura, except for that of the pos-terior fossa, receives sensory innervation from the tri-geminal nerve. Dural nerves follow the meningeal arter-ies and end either near the arteries or near the dural sinuses. Areas of dura between branches of meningeal arteries are innervated poorly, if at all. Deformation of these endings causes pain and is presumably the cause of certain types of headache. Interestingly, the way the pain is perceived depends on whether endings near meningeal arteries or endings near dural sinuses are stimulated. In the former case, the pain is accurately localized to the site of stimulation; in the latter case, the pain is referred to portions of the peripheral distribution of the trigeminal nerve such as the temple or forehead.

The dura of the posterior fossa is supplied by fibers of the second and third cervical nerves.* These fibers travel within the posterior fossa in the sheaths of the vagus and glossopharyngeal nerves, which probably

accounts for older reports that these cranial nerves con-tribute to the innervation of the dura.

ARACHNOID

The arachnoid is a thin avascular membrane composed of a few layers of cells interspersed with bundles of col-lagen. It is semitransparent and resembles a substantial cobweb, for which it is named (Greek, arachne = spi-der's web). Mesothelial cells cover both the inner and outer surfaces of the arachnoid. Small strands of meso-thelium-covered arachnoid tissue, called *arachnoid trabeculae*, leave the inner surface and extend to the pia, with which they merge (Figs. 3-6 and 3-7). Arachnoid trabeculae presumably serve to help keep the brain sus-pended within the meninges, much the way the Lillipu-tians stabilized Gulliver's position.*

Subarachnoid cisterns

Because the arachnoid is attached to the inner surface of the dura mater, it, like the dura, conforms to the general shape of the brain but does not dip into sulci or

---

*The first cervical nerve rarely has a sensory component.

*I thank Dr. Theodore J. Tarby for the analogy.

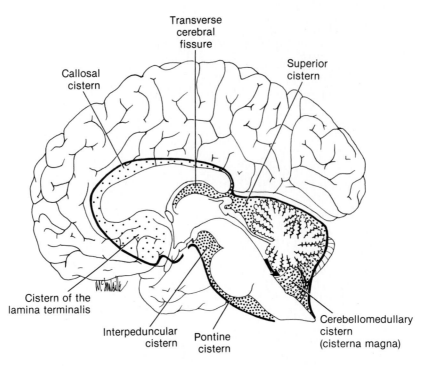

Fig. 3-9. Hemisected brain in which the falx was split, with the locations of the major subarachnoid cisterns indicated. The density of the dotted pattern is roughly proportional to the amount of fluid in a particular cistern. The heavy line represents the edge of the arachnoid, which would have been cut through during the hemisection. An arrow is shown passing from the fourth ventricle, through its median aperture, and into cisterna magna. This is one of the three routes (discussed in the next chapter) by which cerebrospinal fluid escapes from the ventricles into subarachnoid space.

follow the more intricate contours of the surface of the brain. There is, therefore, a *subarachnoid space*, filled with cerebrospinal fluid, between the arachnoid and the pia mater, since the pia closely covers all the external surfaces of the central nervous system. This is the only substantial fluid-filled space normally found around the brain. The subarachnoid space is nonexistent over the surfaces of gyri, relatively small where the arachnoid bridges over small sulci, and much larger in certain locations where it bridges over large surface irregularities. An example of such a location is the space between the inferior surface of the cerebellum and the dorsal surface of the medulla. Regions such as this, which contain a considerable volume of cerebrospinal fluid, are called *subarachnoid cisterns*. This particular example is called the *cerebellomedullary cistern* on anatomical grounds and, since it is the largest cranial cistern, it is also referred to as *cisterna magna*. Other prominent cisterns are indicated in Fig. 3-9 and include (1) the *pontine cistern*, around the anterior surface of the pons and medulla, which is continuous posteriorly with the cerebellomedullary cistern; (2) the *interpeduncular cistern*, between the cerebral peduncles, which contains the arterial circle of Willis (Fig. 5-1); and (3) the *superior cistern*,

a radiological landmark above the midbrain (Fig. 4-12, *B*). The superior cistern is also referred to as the *cistern of the great cerebral vein*, the *quadrigeminal plate cistern*, and *cisterna ambiens*.

Arachnoid villi

The cerebrospinal fluid contained in the subarachnoid space is generally separated from the venous blood in dural sinuses by a layer of arachnoid, a thick layer of dura, and the endothelial lining of the sinus. However, at many locations along dural sinuses, particularly along the superior sagittal sinus, small evaginations of the arachnoid, called *arachnoid villi*, protrude into the sinus. At these sites the connective tissue of the dura is lacking, and only a loose layer of arachnoid cells and a layer of endothelium intervene between subarachnoid space and venous blood (Figs. 3-7, 3-10). Large arachnoid villi are called *arachnoid granulations*, and those that become calcified with age are referred to as *pacchionian bodies*. The villi are especially numerous in laterally directed dilations of the superior sagittal sinus, called *venous lacunae* or *lateral lacunae* (Fig. 3-6), but some are found along all the sinuses and even along some cerebral veins.

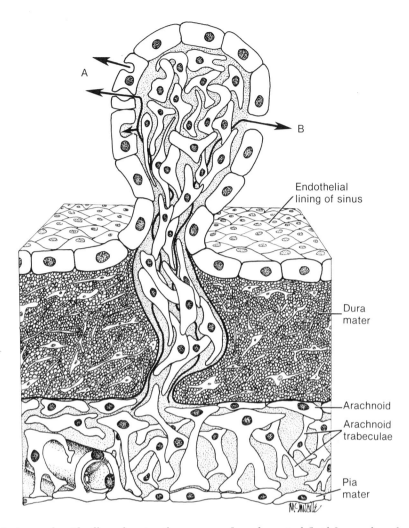

Fig. 3-10. An arachnoid villus, showing the passage of cerebrospinal fluid from subarachnoid space into a dural venous sinus. **A,** Cerebrospinal fluid movement through large vacuoles in endothelial cells, as described by some workers. **B,** Movement through channels between cells, as described by other workers. (Modified from Shabo, A.L., and Maxwell, D.S.: The morphology of the arachnoid villi: a light and electron microscopic study in the monkey, J. Neurosurg. **29:**451, 1968.)

The arachnoid villi are the major sites of reabsorption of cerebrospinal fluid into the venous system. Functionally, they behave like one-way valves, allowing flow from subarachnoid space into venous blood but not in the reverse direction. Since cerebrospinal fluid pressure is ordinarily greater than venous pressure, the villi normally allow continuous movement of cerebrospinal fluid, more or less as though by bulk flow, into the sinuses; however, even if the pressure gradient reverses, the flow does not. The exact mechanism of this flow has been the subject of debate for many years. Some authors have described continuous open channels, micrometers in diameter, through the walls of the arachnoid villi, but most deny their existence. It has recently been suggested that giant vacuoles originating on the subarachnoid side of the endothelial cells, traveling across to the

venous side, and sometimes being transiently open to both sides simultaneously, are responsible for the flow.

Arachnoid barrier layer

The central nervous system is insulated in some respects from the rest of the body and lives in a tightly controlled environment (discussed in more detail in Chapters 4 and 5). This control is achieved partly by a system of barriers between the extracellular space in and around the nervous system and extracellular space elsewhere. One such barrier is that between the cerebrospinal fluid in the subarachnoid space and the extracellular fluids of the dura. Marker substances injected into the middle meningeal artery spread throughout the dura but do not enter the subarachnoid space. The barrier apparently resides in those cellular layers of the arachnoid closest to the dura, where the cells are connected to each other by a series of tight junctions that occlude extracellular space (Fig. 3-12).

PIA MATER

The pia mater is a second delicate membrane (Latin, pia = tender) that, unlike the arachnoid, closely invests all surfaces, following all the contours of the brainstem and all the folds of the cerebral and cerebellar cortices.

Arachnoid trabeculae span the subarachnoid space and merge with the pia mater so subtly that it is difficult to decide where the arachnoid ends and the pia begins. The area of the pia immediately adjacent to nervous tissue is a very thin layer of collagen and scattered cells and is considered separately as the *intima pia* by some authors. The intima pia merges with a more superficial region, which consists of loose connective tissue closely resembling the arachnoid. Those who recognize the intima pia as a separate entity designate this more superficial region the *epipial* layer. Others, however, consider

the intima pia to represent the true pia mater and the epipia to be part of the arachnoid. Still others speak of the entire leptomeningeal complex as one entity, the pia-arachnoid.

The pia mater is often referred to as a vascular membrane, but in fact the cranial epipial layer is rather sparse, and the cerebral arteries and veins travel in subarachnoid space before penetrating the brain. The vessels essentially rest on the intima pia, held there by small strands of connective tissue. A cuff of pia surrounds each small vessel as it enters the brain, enclosing a shell of subarachnoid space around the vessel. This is the *perivascular space* (or *space of Virchow-Robin*), which ends abruptly at the point at which the vessel becomes a capillary.

SPINAL MENINGES

The meningeal coverings of the spinal cord are fundamentally similar to those of the brain, but there are several important differences.

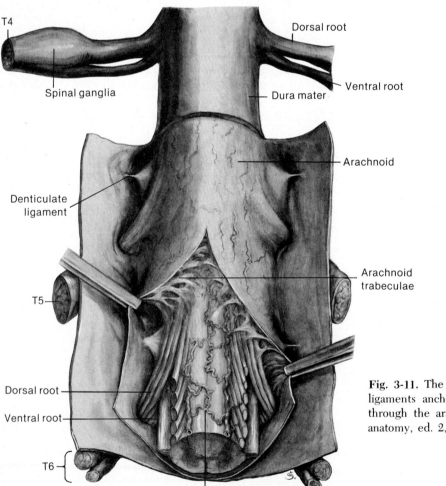

Fig. 3-11. The spinal meninges, showing how dentate ligaments anchor the spinal cord to its dural sheath through the arachnoid. (From Mettler, F.A.: Neuroanatomy, ed. 2, St. Louis, 1948, The C.V. Mosby Co.)

The spinal dura mater is a single-layered membrane, lacking the periosteal component of the cranial dura. The inner layer of the cranial dura is continuous at the foramen magnum with the spinal dural sheath, which is separated from the vertebral periosteum by an epidural space (Fig. 3-8). Thus there are two basic differences between cranial and spinal epidural spaces:

1. Cranial epidural space is a potential space, while spinal epidural space is an actual space.
2. Cranial epidural space, when present, is located between periosteum and cranium, while spinal epidural space is located between periosteum and dura. This spinal epidural space is filled with fatty tissue and a vertebral venous plexus.

The spinal arachnoid, like its cranial counterpart, is closely applied to the inner surface of the dura, leaving a cerebrospinal fluid–filled subarachnoid space between itself and the spinal cord (Fig. 3-11). The spinal dural sheath (and its arachnoid lining) ends at about the second sacral vertebra, whereas the spinal cord itself ends at about the level of the disk between the first and second lumbar vertebrae (Fig. 7-3). There is therefore a large subarachnoid cistern, the *lumbar cistern*, between these two points. This is the favored site for sampling cerebrospinal fluid, since a needle can be inserted here with relatively little risk of damaging the central nervous system.

The epipial layer around the spinal cord is relatively thick and gives rise to a toothed longitudinal projection on each side called the *dentate (denticulate) ligament*. The dentate ligament anchors the spinal cord to the arachnoid and through it to the dura. In addition, another pial projection, the *filum terminale*, anchors the caudal end of the spinal cord (the *conus medullaris*) to the caudal end of the spinal dural sheath (Fig. 7-2). The caudal end of the dural sheath, in turn, is anchored to the caudal end of the vertebral canal.

SOME FUNCTIONAL ASPECTS OF THE MENINGES

As discussed previously, the three meningeal coverings of the brain have various real or potential spaces associated with them (Fig. 3-12). There is no space between pia and brain, but there is a subarachnoid space between pia and arachnoid, along with potential subdural and epidural spaces. Both of these potential spaces can become actual fluid-filled spaces under certain conditions.

The meningeal arteries run in the periosteal layer of the dura. If one of these arteries is torn (typically as a result of traumatic skull injury), bleeding occurs between the periosteum and the skull, opening up the potential epidural space and causing an *epidural hematoma*. As the hematoma expands, it compresses and dis-

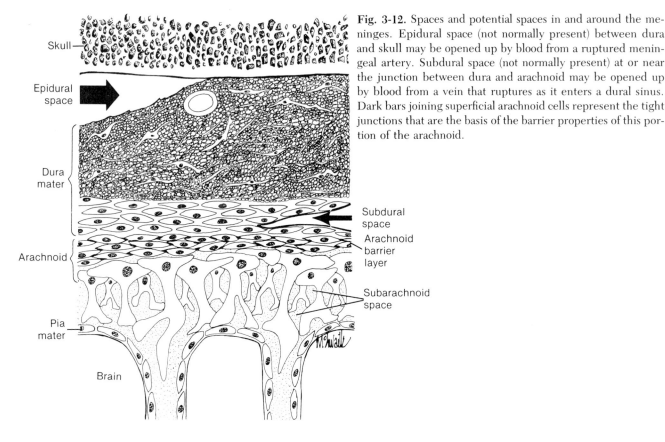

Skull

Epidural space

Dura mater

Arachnoid

Pia mater

Brain

Subdural space

Arachnoid barrier layer

Subarachnoid space

Fig. 3-12. Spaces and potential spaces in and around the meninges. Epidural space (not normally present) between dura and skull may be opened up by blood from a ruptured meningeal artery. Subdural space (not normally present) at or near the junction between dura and arachnoid may be opened up by blood from a vein that ruptures as it enters a dural sinus. Dark bars joining superficial arachnoid cells represent the tight junctions that are the basis of the barrier properties of this portion of the arachnoid.

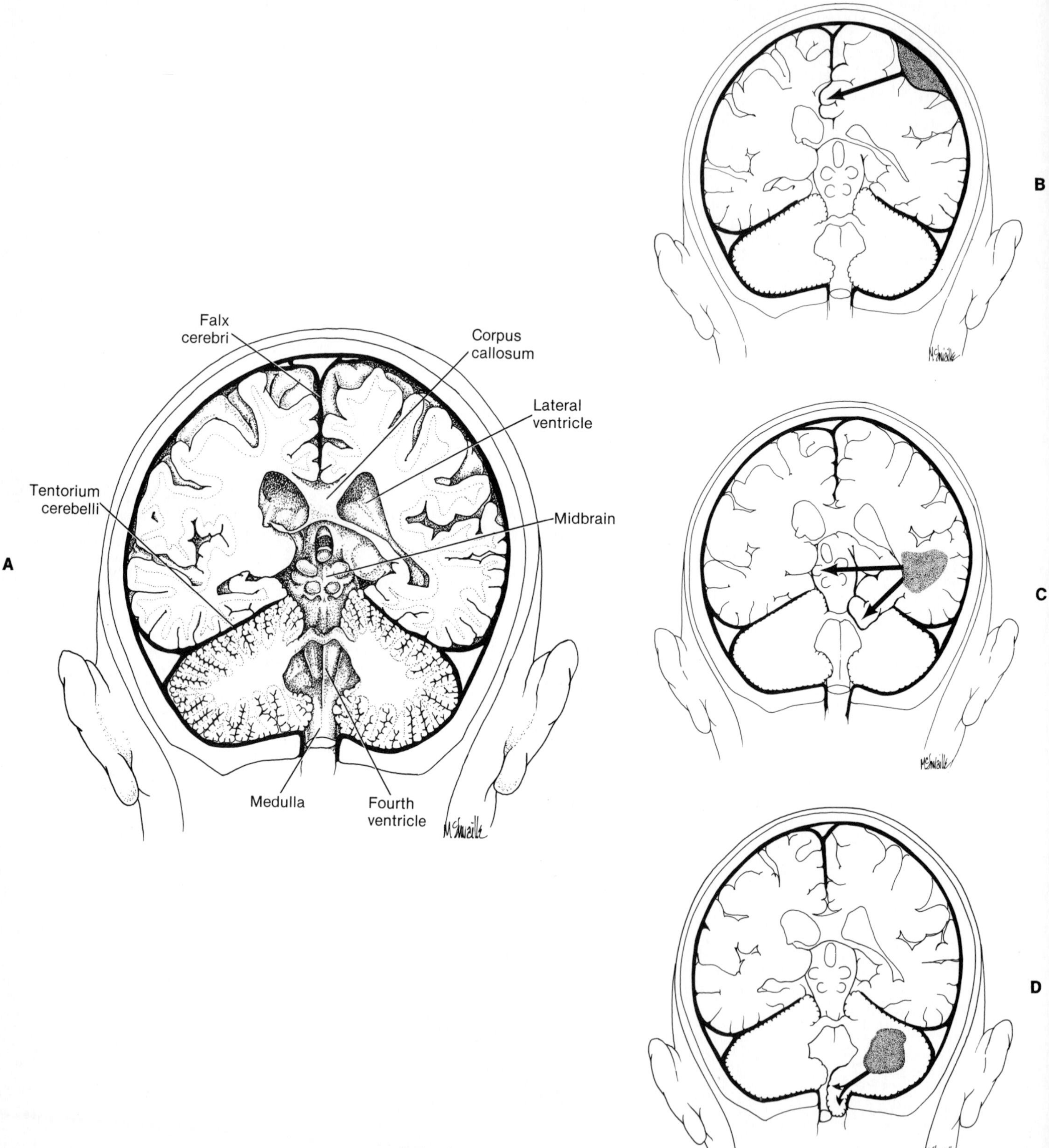

Fig. 3-13. For legend see opposite page.

Fig. 3-13. The three most common ways in which portions of the brain herniate from one compartment into another. **A,** The normal configuration in a plane approximately parallel to the long axis of the brainstem. **B,** As a result of pressure from a subdural hematoma, one cingulate gyrus has slipped under the falx cerebri and is pressing on the opposite cingulate gyrus; this can happen with no serious neurological consequences. **C,** As a result of pressure from an expanding tumor in one temporal lobe, part of the medial temporal lobe has herniated through the tentorial notch and is pressing the midbrain against the free edge of the tentorium. The midbrain contains structures essential for consciousness, and this type of herniation typically produces coma, often followed by death. **D,** As a result of pressure from a cerebellar tumor, one tonsil of the cerebellum has herniated through the foramen magnum, compressing the medulla against the margin of the foramen. The medulla contains respiratory and cardiovascular centers, and pressure on it is usually rapidly fatal.

---

torts the underlying brain and is almost always fatal unless promptly treated surgically.

Bleeding can also occur into the potential subdural space, resulting in a *subdural hematoma.* The most common cause is the tearing of a cerebral vein as it enters a dural sinus. Some subdural hematomas are acute and produce symptoms much like those of an epidural hematoma, while others may progress very slowly and become surprisingly large before producing symptoms.

Dural reflections such as the falx cerebri and the tentorium cerebelli are firmly attached to the cranium. These reflections are stretched rather taut, which allows them to perform their mechanical support function, but this very tautness can result in additional problems in cases of increasing intracranial pressure (for example, subdural hematoma or an expanding tumor). The midbrain may be pushed against the edge of the tentorium as it passes through the tentorial notch, causing damage to a cerebral peduncle and one or more cranial nerves. Also, depending on where the expanding mass causing the increased pressure is located, certain portions of the brain may herniate from one side of a dural reflection to another (Fig. 3-13). For example, increased pressure on the lateral surface of one cerebral hemisphere can cause the hemisphere to be displaced inferiorly and medially, causing the uncus and adjacent portions of the temporal lobe to herniate through the tentorial notch and compress the midbrain. Such pressure could also cause one cingulate gyrus to herniate under the falx. Similarly, downward pressure can cause portions of the cerebellum to herniate into the foramen magnum and compress the medulla. Herniations that compress the brainstem are likely to have very grave consequences.

ADDITIONAL READING

Alksne, J.F., and Lovings, E.T.: Functional ultrastructure of the arachnoid villus, Arch. Neurol. **27**:371, 1972.

Davson, H., Hollingsworth, G., and Segal, M.B.: The mechanism of drainage of the cerebrospinal fluid, Brain **93**:665, 1970. *Recent physiological experiments supporting the concept of bulk flow of cerebrospinal fluid through arachnoid villi.*

Kimmel, D.L.: Innervation of spinal dura mater and dura mater of the posterior cranial fossa, Neurol. **11**:800, 1961.

Livingston, R.B.: Mechanics of cerebrospinal fluid. In Ruch, T.C., and Patton, H.D., editors: Physiology and biophysics ed. 19, Philadelphia, 1965, The W.B. Saunders Co. *Explains why a brain suspended in cerebrospinal fluid has an effective weight of only 50 grams.*

May, P.R.A., et al.: Woodpecker drilling behavior: an endorsement of the rotational theory of impact brain injury, Arch. Neurol. **36**:370, 1979. *Not closely related to the meninges but an interesting discussion of suspension of the brain within the cranium and protection of the brain from injury. Imagine what would happen to you if you banged your beak on a tree as often and as hard as a woodpecker does.*

Meyer, A.: Herniation of the brain, Arch. Neurol. Psychiatr. **4**:387, 1940.

Millen, J.W., and Woollam, D.H.M.: On the nature of the pia mater, Brain **84**:514, 1961. *A lucid discussion of the appearance of the pia at the light microscopic level and of the differences between epipia and intima pia.*

Nabeshima, S., et al.: Junctions in the meninges and marginal glia, J. Comp. Neurol. **164**:127, 1975. *Ultrastructural appearance of the meninges, the arachnoid barrier layer, and subdural space.*

Pease, D.C., and Schultz, R.L.: Electron microscopy of rat cranial meninges, Am. J. Anat. **102**:301, 1958.

Penfield, W., and McNaughton, F.: Dural headache and innervation of the dura mater, Arch. Neurol. Psychiatr. **44**:43, 1940. *A long but interesting account of the gross anatomy of dural innervation, headaches resulting from dural distortion, and the surgical relief of such headaches.*

Shabo, A.L., and Maxwell, D.S.: The morphology of the arachnoid villi: a light and electron microscopic study in the monkey, J. Neurosurg. **29**:451, 1968.

Tripathi, B.J., and Tripathi, R.C.: Vacuolar transcellular channels as a drainage pathway for cerebrospinal fluid, J. Physiol. **239**:195, 1974.

Waggener, J.D., and Beggs, J.: The membranous coverings of neural tissues: an electron microscopy study, J. Neuropath. Exp. Neurol. **26**:417, 1967.

CHAPTER 4

VENTRICLES AND CEREBROSPINAL FLUID

The hollow core of the embryonic neural tube develops into a continuous fluid-filled system of ventricles, lined with *ependymal cells,* in the adult; each division of the CNS contains a portion of this ventricular system. Within each cerebral hemisphere is a relatively large *lateral ventricle.* The paired lateral ventricles communicate with the *third ventricle* of the diencephalon through the *interventricular foramina* (or *foramina of Monro*). The third ventricle in turn communicates with the *fourth ventricle* of the pons and medulla through the narrow *cerebral aqueduct* (or *aqueduct of Sylvius*) of the midbrain. The fourth ventricle continues caudally as the tiny *central canal* of the spinal cord and caudal medulla; this canal is usually not patent over much of its extent.

Cerebrospinal fluid is formed within the ventricles, fills them, and emerges from apertures in the fourth ventricle to fill the subarachnoid space.

VENTRICLES
Lateral ventricle

The lateral ventricle follows a long C-shaped course through all the lobes of the cerebral hemisphere. It is customarily divided into five parts (Figs. 4-1 and 4-2): (1) an *anterior* (or *frontal*) *horn,* in the frontal lobe anterior to the interventricular foramen; (2) a *body,* in the frontal and parietal lobes, extending posteriorly to the region of the splenium of the corpus callosum; (3) a *posterior* (or *occipital*) *horn,* projecting backward into the occipital lobe; (4) an *inferior* (or *temporal*) *horn,* curving down and forward into the temporal lobe; and (5) a *collateral trigone* (or *atrium*), the region near the splenium where the body and the posterior and inferior horns meet.

Various structures form the borders of the lateral ventricle in its course through the cerebral hemisphere;

Fig. 4-1. Drawing of a cast of the ventricular system.

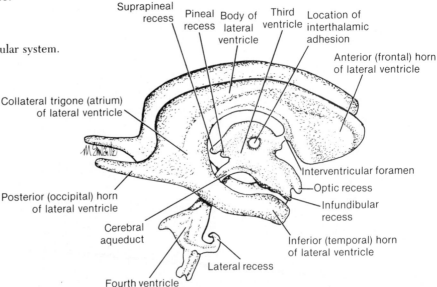

Suprapineal recess — Pineal recess — Body of lateral ventricle — Third ventricle — Location of interthalamic adhesion — Anterior (frontal) horn of lateral ventricle — Collateral trigone (atrium) of lateral ventricle — Interventricular foramen — Optic recess — Infundibular recess — Posterior (occipital) horn of lateral ventricle — Cerebral aqueduct — Inferior (temporal) horn of lateral ventricle — Lateral recess — Fourth ventricle

40

many of them can be easily seen in coronal sections (Figs. 2-15 to 2-21) or in brains dissected from above (Fig. 4-3). The *caudate nucleus* is a constant feature in sections through the ventricle. Its enlarged head is the lateral wall of the anterior horn (Fig. 2-15), its somewhat smaller body is most of the lateral wall of the body of the ventricle (Fig. 2-17), and its attenuated tail lies in the roof of the inferior horn (Fig. 4-6, *D*). Proceeding posteriorly, as the caudate nucleus becomes smaller, the thalamus becomes larger and forms the floor of the body of the ventricle (compare Figs. 2-15 and 2-19). The *corpus callosum* and *septum pellucidum* give a good indica-

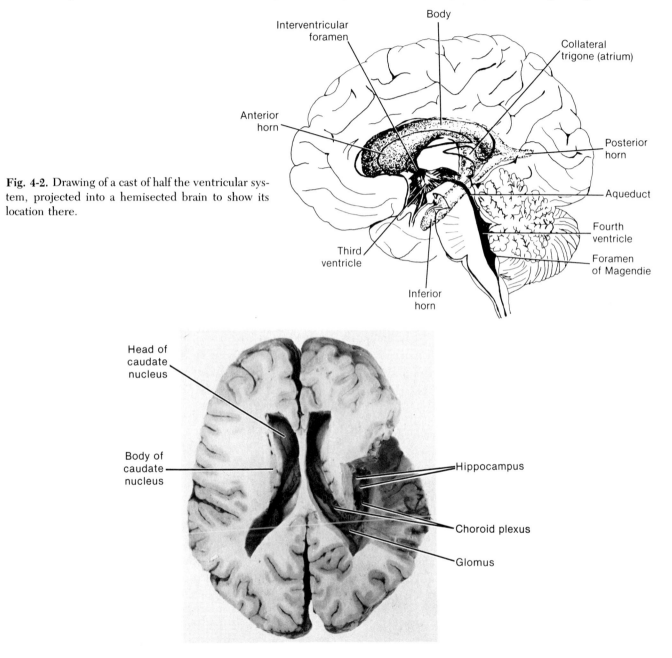

Fig. 4-2. Drawing of a cast of half the ventricular system, projected into a hemisected brain to show its location there.

Fig. 4-3. Dissection demonstrating the lateral ventricles. A horizontal cut was made to expose the ventricles, and most of the corpus callosum was removed. Some white matter was removed on both sides to expose the posterior horns. On the right side, the insula and superior portions of the temporal lobe were also removed so that the inferior horn could be seen. Continuous choroid plexus follows a C-shaped course from the inferior horn through the collateral trigone, through the body of the ventricle, and into the interventricular foramen (not visible from this angle). There is no choroid plexus in the anterior or posterior horn.

tion of the size and location of the anterior horn and body of the ventricle. The body of the corpus callosum forms the roof of these parts of the ventricle, and the genu of the corpus callosum curves downward to form the anterior wall of the anterior horn. The septum pellucidum forms the medial wall of the body and anterior horn, and its termination near the splenium marks the site where the bodies of the ventricles diverge from the midline and begin to curve around into the inferior horns (Compare Figs. 2-18 and 2-21).

The posterior horn is phylogenetically the most recently developed part of the lateral ventricle and is also the most variable in size, sometimes being rudimentary. A number of asymmetries between the cerebral hemispheres of the human brain have been discovered (or rediscovered) in recent years, and it appears that the left posterior horn tends to be longer than the right, particularly in right-handed individuals. The two lateral ventricles are otherwise quite symmetrical.

The *hippocampus* forms most of the floor and medial wall of the inferior horn (Fig. 4-6), which ends anteriorly at about the level of the uncus.

Third ventricle

The narrow, slit-shaped third ventricle occupies most of the midline region of the diencephalon, and so its entire outline can be seen in a hemisected brain (Figs. 2-11 and 4-2). It often looks like a misshapen doughnut in casts of the ventricular system (Fig. 4-1). The hole in the doughnut corresponds to the *interthalamic adhesion,* which crosses the ventricle in most human brains.

Anteriorly the third ventricle ends at the lamina terminalis, the adult remnant of the rostral end of the neural tube. Much of the medial surface of the thalamus and hypothalamus forms the wall of the third ventricle, and part of the hypothalamus forms its floor. It has a thin membranous roof containing choroid plexus (discussed in the next section). At the posterior end of the mammillary bodies, the third ventricle narrows fairly abruptly to become the *cerebral aqueduct,* which traverses the midbrain. The interventricular foramen, in the anterior part of the wall of the third ventricle, is an important radiological landmark, since its location can be visualized by several different methods, and it bears a known anatomical relationship to a number of deep structures.

An outline of the third ventricle reveals four protrusions, called *recesses* (Fig. 4-1), corresponding to structures that have evaginated from the diencephalon. Inferiorly the *optic recess* lies in front of the optic chiasm, at the base of the lamina terminalis; the *infundibular recess* lies just behind the chiasm. Superiorly the *pineal recess* invades the stalk of the pineal gland, and the *suprapineal recess* lies just anterior to this stalk.

Fourth ventricle

The fourth ventricle is sandwiched between the cerebellum posteriorly and the pons and rostral medulla anteriorly (Figs. 2-11 and 4-2). It is shaped like a tent

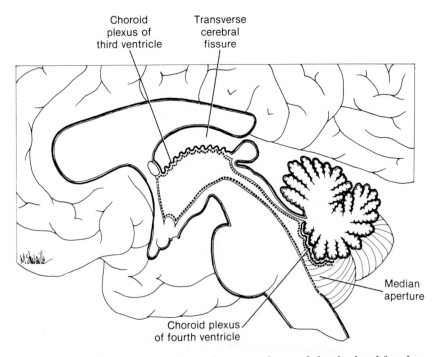

Fig. 4-4. Disposition of the pia mater and ependyma in and around the third and fourth ventricles. The solid line represents the edge of the pia mater that would have been cut during hemisection. The dashed line represents the cut edge of the ependymal lining.

with a peaked roof, the peak protruding into the cerebellum. The floor is relatively flat, and since it narrows rostrally into the aqueduct and caudally into the central canal, it is somewhat diamond shaped (Fig. 8-3, *A*). For this reason, the floor is sometimes referred to as the *rhomboid fossa*. At the location where the lateral point of the diamond would be expected, the entire ventricle becomes a narrow tube that proceeds anteriorly and curves around the brainstem, ending adjacent to the flocculus of the cerebellum. This tubular prolongation is the *lateral recess* of the fourth ventricle (Figs. 4-1 and 8-8). The portion of the roof of the ventricle rostral to the peak is the *superior medullary velum*, and the portion caudal to the peak is the *inferior medullary velum*. The superior medullary velum is a thin layer of white matter related to the cerebellum, while the inferior medullary velum is a membrane containing choroid plexus and is similar to the roof of the third ventricle.

The lateral and third ventricles are closed cavities, communicating only with other parts of the ventricular system. In contrast, there are three apertures in the fourth ventricle through which the ventricular system communicates freely with subarachnoid space. These are the unpaired *median aperture* (or *foramen of Magendie*) and the two *lateral apertures* (or *foramina of Luschka*) of the fourth ventricle. The median aperture is simply a hole in the inferior medullary velum (Fig. 4-4); it is as though the caudal end of the membrane, where it should have closed off the ventricle at its junction with the central canal, had instead been lifted up and attached to the inferior surface of the cerebellar vermis. The result is a funnel-shaped opening from the subarachnoid space (the *cerebellomedullary cistern*) into the ventricle. The inferior medullary velum also covers the lateral recess, and at the end of each recess is another opening in the velum, the lateral aperture.

Ventricular size

The ventricles are both smaller and more variable in size than one might expect. Although there is an average total of approximately 130 ml of cerebrospinal fluid within and around the brain and spinal cord, only about 20 ml of this fluid is contained within the ventricles. The rest occupies subarachnoid space. The third and fourth ventricles together have a volume of only about 2 ml, so the lateral ventricles contain nearly all the ventricular cerebrospinal fluid. The total volume of 20 ml is only an average figure, and the ventricles of some apparently normal brains have been found to have total volumes of less than 10 ml or more than 50 ml (however, volumes greater than 30 ml are usually considered suspicious).

CHOROID PLEXUS

All four ventricles contain strands of highly convoluted and vascular membranous material called *choroid plexus*

that secretes most of the cerebrospinal fluid. The composition of choroid plexus can be appreciated by first considering, for example, the anatomy of the roof of the third ventricle (Figs. 1-11 and 4-5). This roof is simply a layer of ependymal cells overlain by a layer of pia. As in all other locations, the pial layer also faces subarachnoid space, where the blood supply of the brain is located. At certain locations this pia-ependyma complex invaginates into the ventricle along with a collection of arterioles, venules, and capillaries (Fig. 4-5). At these locations, the ependymal layer assumes the appearance of cuboidal epithelium (*choroid epithelium*), and the whole ependyma-pia-capillary complex is called the choroid plexus. There is a long continuous band of choroid plexus in each lateral ventricle, extending from near the tip of the inferior horn, around in a C-shaped course through the body of the ventricle to the interventricular foramen (Figs. 1-13 and 4-3). There is no choroid plexus in the anterior or the posterior horn. The plexus is enlarged in the region of the collateral trigone, and here it is called the *glomus* (Latin, glomus = ball of thread). Choroid plexus tends to become calcified with advancing age, and the glomus can often be seen in x-ray studies (Fig. 4-12, *C*). The choroid plexus of each lateral ventricle grows through the interventricular foramen, forming its posterior wall, and becomes one of the two narrow strands of choroid plexus in the roof of the third ventricle (Fig. 4-6). It does not continue through the aqueduct, which is completely surrounded by neural tissue.

The choroid plexus of the fourth ventricle is formed from a similar invagination of the inferior medullary velum into the caudal half of the ventricle. It is T shaped, with the vertical part of the T consisting of two adjacent longitudinal strands of plexus. These frequently extend as far as the median aperture, where they would be directly exposed to subarachnoid space (Fig. 4-4). The transverse portion of the T consists of one strand of plexus, which extends into each lateral recess. Each end reaches the lateral aperture, where a small tuft of choroid plexus generally protrudes through the aperture and is exposed directly to subarachnoid space (Fig. 8-8).

Since one side of pia mater always faces subarachnoid space, choroid plexus must always be adjacent to subarachnoid space on its pial side and to intraventricular space on its choroid epithelial side. Although this may seem contrary to the plexus's apparent location deep within each cerebral hemisphere (Fig. 4-3), it can be easily demonstrated in coronal sections (Fig. 4-6). The location of the invagination of choroid plexus into the lateral ventricle is called the *choroid fissure*. The choroid fissure is a C-shaped slit of subarachnoid space that accompanies the fornix system of fibers from the inferior horn to the interventricular foramen. By the same reasoning, the space above the roof of the third ventricle, which continues laterally into the choroid

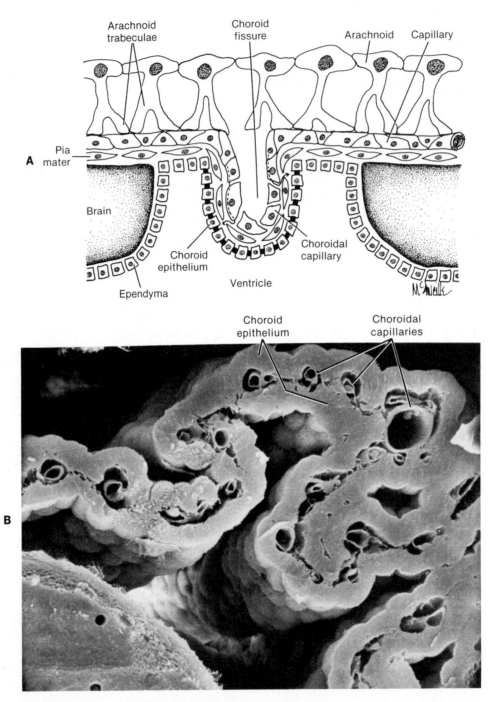

Fig. 4-5. A, Composition of choroid plexus. Spaces are shown between endothelial cells of the choroidal capillary as opposed to those of ordinary cerebral capillaries, indicating that substances can escape from blood into the choroid plexus. However, they are stopped by arrays of tight junctions (represented here as dark bars) between choroid epithelial cells. **B,** Scanning electron micrograph of freeze-fractured preparation of choroid plexus. Note that choroid epithelium almost completely surrounds the choroidal capillaries, being separated from the capillaries only by attenuated pial elements. (From Tissues and organs: a text-atlas of scanning electron microscopy by Richard G. Kessel and Randy H. Kardon. W.H. Freeman and Company. Copyright © 1979.)

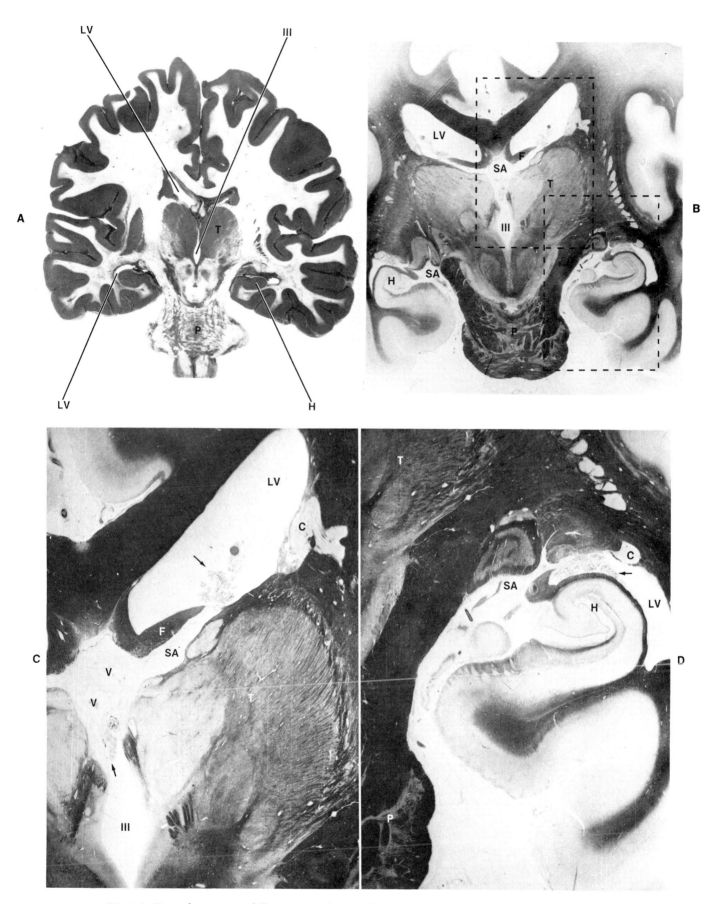

Fig. 4-6. Coronal sections at different magnifications demonstrating the relationship of choroid plexus to subarachnoid space on one side and ventricular space on the other. *C*, Caudate nucleus; *F*, fornix; *H*, hippocampus; *LV*, lateral ventricle; *P*, pons; *SA*, subarachnoid space; *T*, thalamus; *V*, vein in subarachnoid space; *III*, third ventricle; small arrows point to choroid plexus. The central part of the brain slice in **A** is enlarged in **B** (although the planes of section are not quite identical). The areas enclosed in the dotted rectangles in **B** are further enlarged in **C** and **D**.

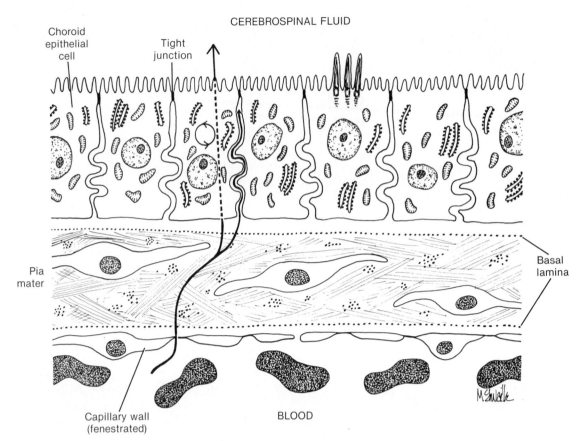

Fig. 4-7. Microscopic structure of choroid plexus showing the three layers of tissue between blood and cerebrospinal fluid. Substances pass through the fenestrated capillary and through the extracellular space of the pia mater but cannot pass through the bands of tight junctions between choroid epithelial cells. They must pass through these cells by an active transport system.

fissure, is also subarachnoid space (Figs. 4-4 and 4-6). This is the *transverse cerebral fissure,* a long finger of subarachnoid space trapped in the middle of the cerebrum by the growth of the cerebral hemispheres posteriorly over the diencephalon and brainstem. The transverse cerebral fissure continues posteriorly into the superior cistern.

Microscopic structure

Choroid plexus is functionally a three-layered membrane between blood and cerebrospinal fluid (Fig. 4-7). The first layer is the endothelial wall of the choroidal capillary. This wall is fenestrated, allowing easy movement of substances out of the capillary (in contrast to capillary walls elsewhere in the brain, which, as discussed in Chapter 5, are tightly sealed). The second layer, consisting of scattered pial cells and some collagen, is very incomplete. The third layer, continuous with the ependymal lining of the ventricles, is the choroid epithelium. The choroid epithelial cells look as though they are specialized for secretion because they

have many basal infoldings, numerous microvilli on the side facing the cerebrospinal fluid, and abundant mitochondria. In addition, adjacent cells are connected to one another by arrays of tight junctions that occlude the extracellular space around them. As in the case of the arachnoid barrier layer (Chapter 3), this is thought to prevent free access of substances to the brain by preventing their diffusion into the cerebrospinal fluid.

The surface area of the choroid plexus is increased not only by the folding of individual cell membranes into microvilli, but also by the macroscopic folding of the choroid plexus itself into numerous fronds and villi (Fig. 4-6). This folding is so extensive that the total surface area of the human choroid plexus, neglecting the contribution of the microvilli, is more than 200 sq cm, or about two thirds of the total ventricular surface area.

CEREBROSPINAL FLUID
Formation

Cerebrospinal fluid is a colorless liquid, low in cells and proteins, but generally similar to plasma in its ionic composition. For this reason it was considered for some time to be an ultrafiltrate of blood. However, careful analysis of the composition of cerebrospinal fluid reveals that its content of various ions differs from that of plasma in a way that is not consistent with its being an ultrafiltrate. For example, compared to plasma, cerebrospinal fluid contains an excess of sodium and magnesium ions and a deficiency of potassium and calcium ions. Furthermore, these concentrations are maintained at very stable levels in the face of changes in plasma concentrations—a constancy that would not be expected if cerebrospinal fluid were an ultrafiltrate. Finally, the formation of new cerebrospinal fluid is depressed by certain metabolic inhibitors, as would be expected if it were formed by an active, energy-requiring process. Therefore cerebrospinal fluid is now considered to be an actively secreted product whose composition is dictated by specific transport mechanisms.

Most of the cerebrospinal fluid is produced within the ventricular system, primarily by the choroid plexus. Production of fluid by the choroid plexus was demonstrated rather directly by the neurosurgeon Cushing early in the twentieth century. He noted, during procedures in which it was necessary to open and drain a lateral ventricle, that fluid could be seen accumulating on the surface of the choroid plexus; if he put a small silver clip on the artery supplying the choroid plexus, the fluid stopped appearing. A basically similar procedure has been used more recently to study the composition of newly formed cerebrospinal fluid: a micropipette in contact with oil-covered choroid plexus can collect the fluid as it is formed. Chemical analysis has shown that it is identical in composition to bulk cerebrospinal fluid in normal ventricles.

Cerebrospinal fluid apparently is formed by filtration of blood through the fenestrations of the choroidal capillaries, followed by the active transport of substances (particularly sodium ions) across the choroid epithelium into the ventricle. Water then flows passively across the epithelium to maintain osmotic balance. The barrier properties of the choroid epithelium prevent substances from diffusing across it in an uncontrolled manner. The total process is actually more complicated than this; it is known, for example, that some substances are transported in the reverse direction (that is, from cerebrospinal fluid to blood).

Although cerebrospinal fluid seems to be secreted primarily by choroid plexus, there is also evidence that this is not its only source. This has been shown most directly in monkeys from whose lateral ventricles all the choroid plexus had been removed; these ventricles still produce substantial quantities of cerebrospinal fluid, although less than normal. The source of this extrachoroidal cerebrospinal fluid is generally considered to be

the parenchyma of the brain, with fluid moving across the ependymal lining into the ventricle. The proportion of cerebrospinal fluid normally arising from this source is not known accurately, but most researchers estimate that at least 80% is made by the choroid plexus.

The rate of formation of new cerebrospinal fluid (an average of about 350 μl/minute in man) is relatively constant and little affected by blood pressure or intraventricular pressure. This means that the total volume of cerebrospinal fluid is renewed more than three times per day. Little is known about mechanisms available to modify the secretion rate, but some very recent experiments indicate that stimulation of the sympathetic supply to the choroid plexus can decrease this rate markedly.

Circulation

If the cerebrospinal fluid is turned over several times per day, it must circulate from its site of formation to a site of removal. We have already discussed all the elements of the system involved (Figs. 4-8 and 4-9): cerebrospinal fluid formed in the lateral ventricles passes through the interventricular foramina into the third ventricle, from there through the cerebral aqueduct into the fourth ventricle, and thence through the median and lateral apertures into cisterna magna and the pontine cistern. From the pontine cistern, the fluid slowly moves up over the cerebral hemispheres, through the arachnoid villi, and into the superior sagittal sinus. The flow should not be thought of as slow and steady, since arterial pulsations cause a constant ebb and flow, with a small net movement toward the superior sagittal sinus with each heartbeat. As would be expected from the rate of cerebrospinal fluid formation, it takes several hours for new cerebrospinal fluid to complete the journey.

In addition to this basic pattern of circulation, some cerebrospinal fluid moves from the cisterns around the fourth ventricle into the subarachnoid space around the spinal cord. It slowly makes its way caudally to the lumbar cistern, and then some of it slowly makes its way back rostrally. Along the way, most of this fluid is returned to the venous system through small arachnoid villi that are found in the dural sleeves accompanying spinal nerve roots.

Function

The cerebrospinal fluid in the subarachnoid space plays a supportive role because of the buoyant effect discussed previously. However, it seems apparent that an actively secreted, constantly renewed fluid with a closely regulated composition must have other functions as well. Most of the functions that have been suggested involve the regulation of the extracellular environment of neurons. This could happen in either or both of two ways.

Fig. 4-8. Path followed by cerebrospinal fluid through the ventricles. (Redrawn from Hamilton, W.J., editor: Textbook of human anatomy, ed. 2. St. Louis, 1976, The C.V. Mosby Co. By permission of Macmillan Press, London and Basingstoke.)

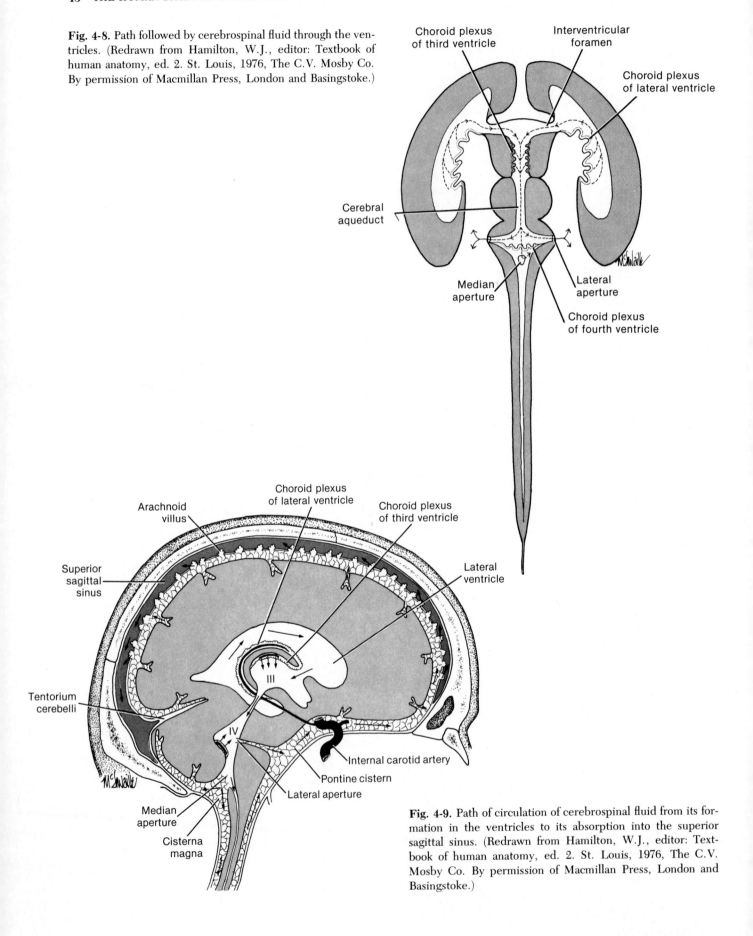

Fig. 4-9. Path of circulation of cerebrospinal fluid from its formation in the ventricles to its absorption into the superior sagittal sinus. (Redrawn from Hamilton, W.J., editor: Textbook of human anatomy, ed. 2. St. Louis, 1976, The C.V. Mosby Co. By permission of Macmillan Press, London and Basingstoke.)

First, the cerebrospinal fluid is known to be in free communication with the extracellular fluid of the brain, so secretion of controlled cerebrospinal fluid by the choroid plexus will secondarily control, to some extent, the composition of this extracellular fluid. Second, the cerebrospinal fluid system probably exerts a reverse sort of control by acting as a sink for substances produced by the brain, which would then be selectively absorbed from cerebrospinal fluid by the choroid plexus or nonselectively removed by flow through arachnoid villi. There have also been suggestions that the cerebrospinal fluid is a route for the spread of neuroactive hormones through the nervous system.

SOME FUNCTIONAL ASPECTS OF THE VENTRICULAR SYSTEM

Since the rate of production of cerebrospinal fluid is relatively independent of blood pressure and intraventricular pressure, the fluid will continue to be produced even if the path of its circulation is blocked or is otherwise abnormal. When this happens, cerebrospinal fluid pressure rises and ultimately the ventricles expand at the expense of surrounding brain, creating a condition known as *hydrocephalus*. In principle, hydrocephalus can result from excess production of cerebrospinal fluid, from blockage of cerebrospinal fluid circulation, or from a deficiency in cerebrospinal fluid reabsorption. All

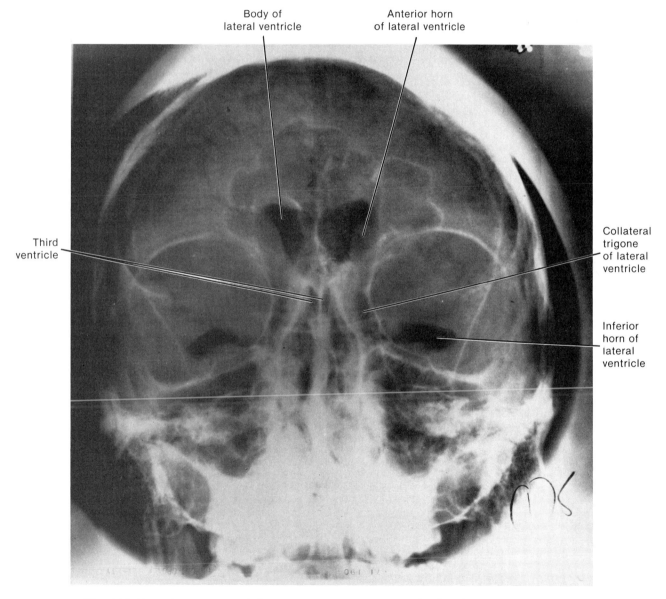

Fig. 4-10. Normal pneumoencephalogram, anterior-posterior view (as though you were looking into the patient's face). The body and inferior horn of each lateral ventricle are particularly dark because they are viewed approximately end-on, so that the x rays traverse a relatively long path through air. (Courtesy of Dr. John Stears, University of Colorado Medical Center.)

Body of
lateral ventricle

Third
ventricle

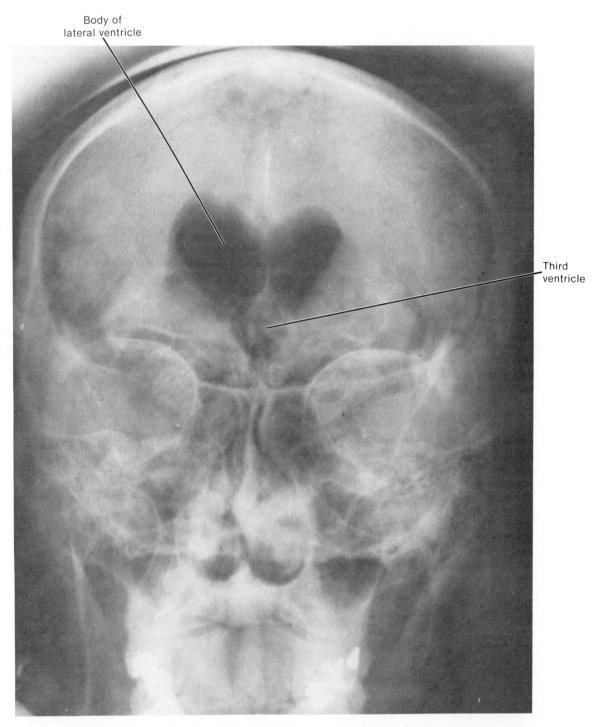

Fig. 4-11. Pneumoencephalogram of a patient with hydrocephalus, anterior-posterior view. Enlargement of the lateral and third ventricles is apparent. This patient had a shunt inserted into one lateral ventricle and improved markedly. (Courtesy of Dr. Michael Earnest, Denver General Hospital and University of Colorado Medical Center.)

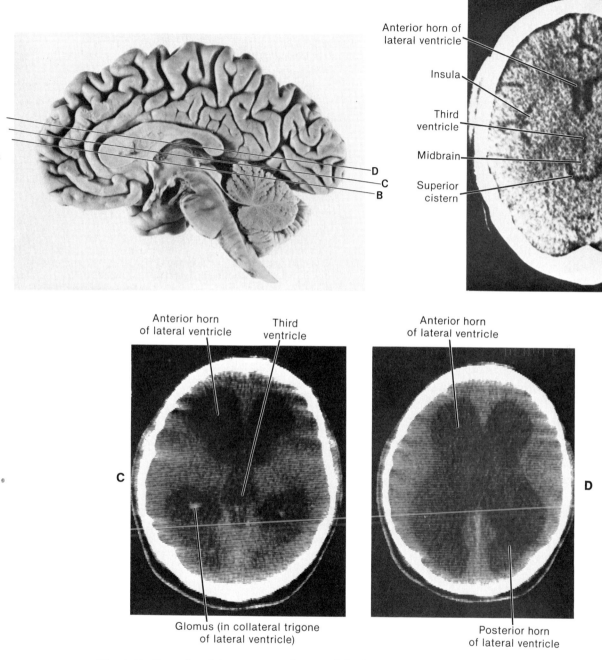

Fig. 4-12. Examples of CT scans. Cerebrospinal fluid is dark in these scans and fills the ventricular system, subarachnoid cisterns, and cerebral sulci around the edge of the brain. **A,** Planes of section produced by the computer. **B,** Normal CT scan. **C** and **D,** Scans of two different planes from a patient with hydrocephalus; the great enlargement of the lateral and third ventricles is obvious. (**B** courtesy of Dr. John Stears, University of Colorado Medical Center; **C** and **D** courtesy of Dr. Michael Earnest, Denver General Hospital and University of Colorado Medical Center.)

three types occur, but that caused by a blockage of circulation is by far the most common.

Tumors of the choroid plexus, called *papillomas*, are sometimes associated with hydrocephalus. In some of these cases, a much greater than normal production of cerebrospinal fluid has been directly shown and is believed to be the cause of the hydrocephalus.

Circulation of cerebrospinal fluid can be obstructed at any point in the pathway. A tumor can occlude one interventricular foramen (or both of them), in which case the lateral ventricle involved becomes hydrocephalic, while the remainder of the ventricular system remains normal. Tumors of the pineal gland sometimes push down on the midbrain, squeeze the aqueduct shut, and cause hydrocephalus of the third ventricle and both lateral ventricles (Fig. 4-11). In some congenital abnormalities, all three apertures of the fourth ventricle may either fail to develop or be occluded, resulting in hydrocephalus of the entire ventricular system. (Occlusion of only one or two of these apertures apparently has no effect.) Finally, circulation may be obstructed outside the ventricular system in subarachnoid space. For example, meningitis is sometimes followed by meningeal adhesions around the base of the brain that block the flow of cerebrospinal fluid through the tentorial notch. This too causes hydrocephalus of the entire ventricular system.

Defects in the reabsorption of cerebrospinal fluid are not common, but rare cases have been reported of apparent congenital absence of arachnoid villi associated with hydrocephalus. Also, obstruction of the superior sagittal sinus can cause hydrocephalus, presumably because venous pressure becomes high enough to prevent cerebrospinal fluid movement through the arachnoid villi.

Clinically hydrocephalus is divided into *communicating* and *noncommunicating* types, depending on whether or not both lateral ventricles are in communication with subarachnoid space. Thus occlusion of the superior sagittal sinus or blockage of flow through the tentorial notch would cause communicating hydrocephalus; stenosis of the aqueduct or occlusion of the apertures of the fourth ventricle would cause noncommunicating hydrocephalus.

Pneumoencephalography is a clinical test sometimes used to diagnose hydrocephalus. This test involves injecting air or oxygen into the lumbar cistern and then maneuvering it into the ventricles. Air is much less dense to x rays than is cerebrospinal fluid, so the shape of the ventricles can be recorded by x-ray photography (Figs. 4-10 and 4-11). The shape of the ventricles can yield information not only about the presence and location of hydrocephalus, but also about masses pushing against the brain and distorting the ventricles.

Pneumoencephalography is (for the patient) a very unpleasant procedure and has been largely supplanted by computerized tomography, or CT scanning. This new technique involves directing an x-ray beam through the patient's head from a number of different angles and comparing and processing the resulting collection of density profiles with a computer. Small density differences can be detected in this way, and newer machines can even differentiate between gray and white matter. Since the test is completely noninvasive and the radiation dosage small, it is ideal for many applications. Examples are shown in Fig. 4-12.

Once diagnosed, many cases of hydrocephalus can be treated surgically by implanting a shunt that extends from the locus of increased pressure to the peritoneal cavity or the internal jugular vein. The implanted catheter must contain a valve to prevent reverse flow. There were many early attempts to treat hydrocephalus by removing the choroid plexus, but they were generally unsuccessful, probably because of the continued extrachoroidal production of cerebrospinal fluid.

ADDITIONAL READING

Bito, L.Z., Davson, H., and Fenstermacher, J.D., editors: The ocular and cerebrospinal fluids, Exp. Eye Res. **25**(Suppl.), 1977.

Brightman, M.W., and Reese, T.S.: Junctions between intimately apposed cell membranes in the vertebrate brain, J. Cell. Biol. **40:** 648, 1969. *An interesting paper that discusses, among other things, the barrier properties of the choroid epithelium.*

Bull, J.W.D.: The volume of the cerebral ventricles, Neurol. **11:**1, 1961.

Cserr, H.F.: Physiology of the choroid plexus, Physiol. Rev. **51:**273, 1971.

Cushing, H.: Studies in intracranial physiology and surgery, London, 1926, Oxford University Press. *Contains the classic account of the direct observation of cerebrospinal fluid forming on the surface of human choroid plexus.*

Cutler, R.W.P., et al.: Formation and absorption of cerebrospinal fluid in man, Brain **91:**707, 1968. *Direct measurement of the rate of formation of cerebrospinal fluid in humans.*

Dandy, W.E.: Experimental hydrocephalus, Ann. Surg. **70:**129, 1919. *The classic description of the production of hydrocephalus by obstruction of an interventricular foramen, the cerebral aqueduct, or subarachnoid space around the base of the brain. It appears in the light of subsequent work that some of the experiments were technically flawed, but the conclusions are basically sound.*

Davson, H.: Physiology of the cerebrospinal fluid, Boston, 1967, Little, Brown and Co.

De Rougemont, J., et al.: Fluid formed by choroid plexus, J. Neurophysiol. **23:**485, 1960. *Experiments in which droplets of cerebrospinal fluid were collected, under oil, from the surface of the choroid plexus, and their composition analyzed.*

DiChiro, G.: Observations on the circulation of the cerebrospinal fluid, Acta. Radiol. (Diagn.) **5:**988, 1966. *Description of the time, course, and pattern of movement of tracer substances through subarachnoid space on their way toward the venous system.*

Dohrmann, G.J.: The choroid plexus: a historical review, Brain Res. **18:**197, 1970.

Dohrmann, G.J., and Bucy, P.C.: Human choroid plexus: a light and electron microscopic study, J. Neurosurg. **33:**506, 1970.

Eisenberg, H.M., McComb, J.G., and Lorenzo, A.V.: Cerebrospinal fluid overproduction and hydrocephalus associated with choroid plexus papilloma, J. Neurosurg. **40**:381, 1974.

Fujii, K., Lenkey, C., and Rhoton, A.L. Jr.: Microsurgical anatomy of the choroidal arteries: fourth ventricle and cerebellopontine angles, J. Neurosurg. **52**:504, 1980. *This and the next article are finely detailed and beautifully illustrated.*

Fujii, K., Lenkey, C., and Rhoton, A.L. Jr.: Microsurgical anatomy of the choroidal arteries: lateral and third ventricles, J. Neurosurg. **52**:165, 1980.

Gudeman, S.K., et al.: Surgical removal of bilateral papillomas of the choroid plexus of the lateral ventricles with resolution of hydrocephalus, J. Neurosurg. **50**:677, 1979.

Gutierrez, Y., Friede, R.L., and Kaliney, W.J.: Agenesis of arachnoid granulations and its relationship to communicating hydrocephalus, J. Neurosurg. **43**:553, 1975.

Hewitt, W.: The median aperture of the fourth ventricle, J. Anat. **94:** 549, 1960.

Kier, E.L.: The cerebral ventricles: a phylogenetic and ontogenetic study. In Newton, T.H., and Potts, D.G., editors: Radiology of the skull and brain, vol. 3: anatomy and pathology, St. Louis, 1977, The C.V. Mosby Co. *A long but fascinating and beautifully illustrated account.*

Lindvall, M., Edvinsson, E., and Owman, C.: Sympathetic nervous control of cerebrospinal fluid production from the choroid plexus, Science **201**:176, 1978.

McRae, D.L., Branch, C.L., and Milner, B.: The occipital horns and cerebral dominance, Neurol. **18**:95, 1968.

Milhorat, T.H.: Choroid plexus and cerebrospinal fluid production, Science **166**:1514, 1969. *An account of the continued production of cerebrospinal fluid in the lateral ventricles of monkeys after removal of the choroid plexus.*

Milhorat, T.H.: Hydrocephalus and the cerebrospinal fluid, Baltimore, 1972, The Williams and Wilkins Co.

Millen, J.W., and Woollam, D.H.M.: The anatomy of the cerebrospinal fluid, New York, 1962, Oxford University Press.

Pollay, M.: Review of spinal fluid physiology: production and absorption in relation to pressure, In Keener, E.B., editor: Clinical neurosurgery. Baltimore, 1977, The Williams and Wilkins Co. *Well written, concise review.*

Pollay, M., and Curl, F.: Secretion of cerebrospinal fluid by the ventricular ependyma of the rabbit, Am. J. Physiol. **213**:1031, 1967. *Technically admirable experiments demonstrating the production of cerebrospinal fluid within the aqueduct and rostral fourth ventricle.*

Rodriguez, E.M.: The cerebrospinal fluid as a pathway in neuroendocrine integration, J. Endocrinol. **71**:407, 1976.

Voetmann, E.: On the structure and surface area of the human choroid plexus, Acta Anat., suppl. 10, 1949.

Welch, K., and Pollay, M.: The spinal arachnoid villi of the monkeys *Cercopithecus aethiops sabaeus* and *Macaca irus*, Anat. Rec. **145:** 43:1963.

Wright, E.M.: Transport processes in the formation of the cerebrospinal fluid, Rev. Physiol. Biochem. Pharmacol. **83**:1, 1978.

CHAPTER 5

BLOOD SUPPLY OF THE BRAIN

The placement of a discussion of the vasculature of the central nervous system presents a problem in any consideration of neuroanatomy. It is reasonably efficient to treat the arterial supply of individual portions of the brain at the same time as the structure and function of that area. This approach requires a prior general overview of the circulatory system, which this chapter attempts to provide.

The arterial supply of the brain is derived from two pairs of vessels, the *internal carotid arteries* and the *vertebral arteries*. The internal carotid system supplies most of the telencephalon and much of the diencephalon. The vertebral system supplies the brainstem and cerebellum, as well as parts of the diencephalon, spinal cord, and occipital and temporal lobes.

Venous drainage occurs by way of a system of *superficial veins* and *deep veins*, which empty into the dural venous sinuses and ultimately into the internal jugular vein.

ARTERIAL SUPPLY
Internal carotid system

We will arbitrarily begin considering the internal carotid artery above the cavernous sinus and adjacent to the optic chiasm, assuming that other aspects of its anatomy, such as the carotid siphon and previous branches like the ophthalmic artery, are discussed in most gross anatomy courses. The internal carotid proceeds superiorly alongside the optic chiasm (Fig. 5-1) and bifurcates into the *middle* and *anterior cerebral arteries*. Before bifurcating it gives rise to two smaller branches, the *anterior choroidal artery* and the *posterior communicating artery*. The anterior choroidal artery is a long, thin artery that can be very significant clinically, since it supplies a number of different structures and is not infrequently involved in cerebrovascular accidents. Along its course (indicated in Fig. 5-1), it supplies the optic tract, the choroid plexus of the inferior horn of the lateral ventricle, part of the cerebral peduncle, and some

deep structures such as portions of the internal capsule, basal ganglia, and hippocampus. The posterior communicating artery passes posteriorly, inferior to the optic tract and toward the cerebral peduncle, and joins the *posterior cerebral artery* (part of the vertebral artery system).

The anterior cerebral artery runs medially, superior to the optic nerve, and enters the longitudinal fissure (Fig. 5-1). It and its branches then arch posteriorly, following the corpus callosum, to supply the medial aspect of the frontal and parietal lobes (Fig. 5-2). Some of the smaller branches extend onto the dorsolateral surface of the hemisphere (Fig. 5-3). Along this course, it divides into two particularly prominent branches, the *pericallosal artery*, which stays immediately adjacent to the corpus callosum, and the *callosomarginal artery*, which follows the cingulate sulcus (Figs. 5-2 and 5-11). The two anterior cerebral arteries, near their entrance into the longitudinal fissure, are connected by the *anterior communicating artery*. Since parts of the precentral and postcentral gyri extend onto the medial surface of the frontal and parietal lobes, the occlusion of an anterior cerebral artery causes restricted contralateral motor and somatosensory deficits.

The large middle cerebral artery proceeds laterally into the lateral sulcus (Fig. 5-1). It divides into a number of branches that supply the insula, emerge from the lateral fissure, and spread out to supply virtually the entire lateral surface of the cerebral hemisphere. Since most of the precentral and postcentral gyri are within this area of supply, the occlusion of a middle cerebral artery causes major motor and somatosensory deficits. In most individuals, if the left hemisphere is the one involved, language deficits will also be found. Although the anterior choroidal artery is usually a branch of the internal carotid, it sometimes arises from the middle cerebral artery.

Along its course toward the lateral fissure, the middle cerebral artery gives rise to many very small branches

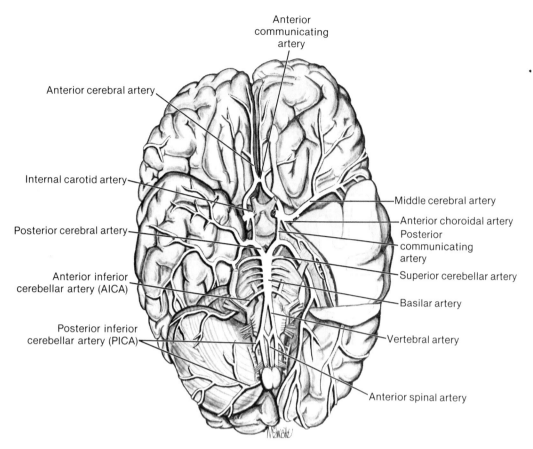

Fig. 5-1. Arteries on the inferior surface of the brain. The left half of the cerebellum and part of the left temporal lobe have been removed. (Modified from Hamilton, W.J., editor: Textbook of human anatomy, ed. 2. St. Louis, 1976, The C.V. Mosby Co.)

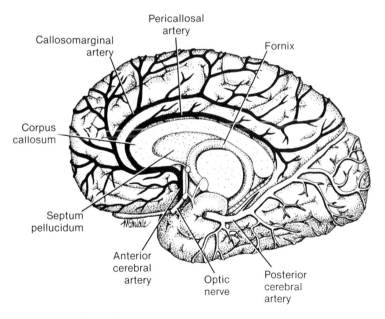

Fig. 5-2. Arteries of the medial surface of the brain. The anterior cerebral artery and its branches are shown in black; the posterior cerebral artery and its branches are shown in white. (Modified from Hamilton, W.J., editor: Textbook of human anatomy, ed. 2. St. Louis, 1976, The C.V. Mosby Co.)

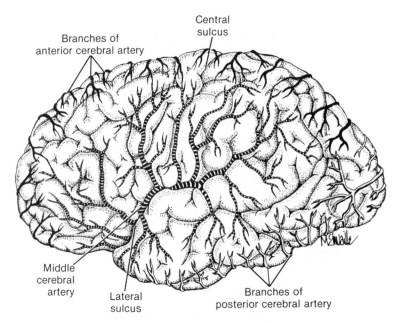

Fig. 5-3. Arteries of the lateral surface of the brain. The middle cerebral artery and its branches are shown striped. The small branches of the anterior cerebral artery reaching around from the medial surface are shown in black, and those of the posterior cerebral artery are shown in white. (Modified from Hamilton, W.J., editor: Textbook of human anatomy, ed. 2. St. Louis, 1976, The C.V. Mosby Co.)

that penetrate the brain near their origin and supply deep structures of the diencephalon and telencephalon. These particular arteries are called the *lateral striate* (or *lenticulostriate*) *arteries*, but similar small branches arise from all the arteries around the base of the brain. They are referred to collectively as *ganglionic* or *penetrating* branches. Ganglionic arteries are particularly numerous in the area adjacent to the optic chiasm and in the area between the cerebral peduncles; these are called the *anterior* and *posterior perforated substances*, respectively. The narrow, thin-walled vessels of those areas are frequently involved in strokes. The deep cerebral structures that they supply are such that damage to these small vessels can cause neurological deficits out of proportion to their size. For example, the somatosensory projection from the thalamus to the postcentral gyrus must pass through the internal capsule; damage to a small part of the internal capsule, from rupture of a penetrating artery, can cause deficits similar to those resulting from damage to a large expanse of cortex.

Vertebral-basilar system

The two vertebral arteries run rostrally alongside the medulla and fuse at the junction between the medulla and pons to form the midline *basilar artery*, which proceeds rostrally along the ventral surface of the pons (Fig. 5-1).

Before joining the basilar artery, each vertebral artery

gives rise to three branches, the *posterior spinal artery, anterior spinal artery,* and *posterior inferior cerebellar artery.* The posterior spinal artery runs caudally along the dorsolateral aspect of the spinal cord and supplies the posterior third of that half of the cord. The anterior spinal artery joins its mate from the opposite side, forming a single anterior spinal artery that runs caudally along the ventral midline of the spinal cord, supplying the anterior two thirds of the cord. These spinal arteries cannot carry enough blood from the vertebral arteries to supply more than the cervical segments of the spinal cord and must be reinforced at various points caudal to this (discussed in Chapter 7). The posterior inferior cerebellar artery (often referred to by the acronym "PICA"), as its name implies, supplies much of the inferior surface of the cerebellar hemisphere (Fig. 5-4); however, it sends branches to other structures on its way to the cerebellum. As it curves around the brainstem, the artery supplies the choroid plexus of the fourth ventricle and much of the lateral medulla. This is a uniform occurrence in the large named branches of the vertebral-basilar system: on their way to their major area of supply, they send branches to brainstem structures.

The basilar artery proceeds rostrally and, at the level of the midbrain, bifurcates into the two *posterior cerebral arteries.* Before this bifurcation, it gives rise to numerous unnamed branches and two named branches, the *anterior inferior cerebellar artery* and the *superior cerebellar artery.*

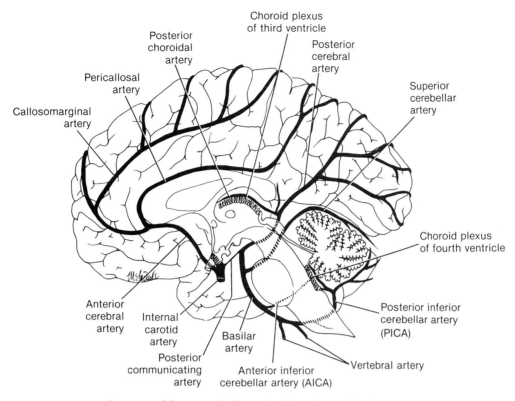

Fig. 5-4. A hemisected brain, with the path of branches of the basilar artery shown.

The anterior inferior cerebellar artery (often referred to by the acronym "AICA") arises just rostral to the point of formation of the basilar artery and supplies the more anterior portions of the inferior surface of the cerebellum (for example, the flocculus), as well as parts of the caudal pons. The superior cerebellar artery arises just caudal to the bifurcation of the basilar artery and supplies the superior surface of the cerebellum and much of the caudal midbrain and rostral pons. The many smaller branches of the basilar artery, collectively called *pontine arteries,* supply the remainder of the pons. One of these, the *internal auditory* (or *labyrinthine*) *artery* (which may also be a branch of the AICA), though hard to distinguish from the others by appearance, is functionally very important because it also supplies the inner ear. Its occlusion can lead to vertigo and ipsilateral deafness.

The posterior cerebral artery curves around the midbrain and passes through the superior cistern; its branches spread out to supply the medial and inferior surfaces of the occipital and temporal lobes (Figs. 5-1, 5-2, and 5-4). Along the way, it sends branches to the rostral midbrain and caudal diencephalon. It also gives rise to several *posterior choroidal arteries,* which supply the choroid plexus of the third ventricle and of the body of the lateral ventricle. The anterior and posterior choroidal arteries form anastomoses in the vicinity of the glomus. Since primary visual cortex is located in the

occipital lobe, occlusion of a posterior cerebral artery leads to visual field losses in addition to other deficits referable to the midbrain and diencephalon.

Circle of Willis

The posterior cerebral artery is connected to the internal carotid artery by the posterior communicating artery. This completes an arterial loop, called the *circle of Willis,* through which the anterior cerebral, internal carotid, and posterior cerebral arteries of both sides are interconnected. Normally there is little or no blood flow around this circle, since the appropriate pressure differentials are not present. The arterial pressure in the right internal carotid artery is about the same as that in the right posterior cerebral artery, so little or no blood flows through the right posterior communicating artery. However, in cases where one major vessel is slowly occluded, either within the circle of Willis or proximal to it, the normally small communicating arteries may slowly enlarge and allow anastomotic flow to compensate for the occlusion. By such a mechanism, it would theoretically be possible (though highly unlikely) for the entire brain to be perfused by just one of the four major arteries that normally supply it. Note, however, that the communicating arteries are normally quite small and are generally inadequate to compensate for sudden occlusion of a major vessel.

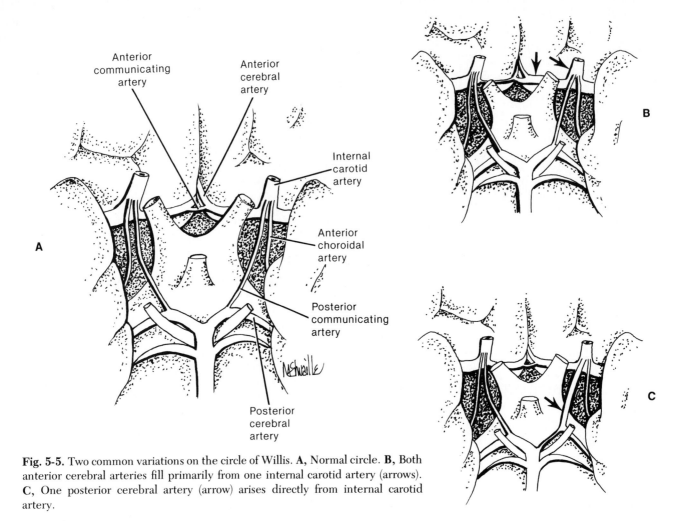

Fig. 5-5. Two common variations on the circle of Willis. **A,** Normal circle. **B,** Both anterior cerebral arteries fill primarily from one internal carotid artery (arrows). **C,** One posterior cerebral artery (arrow) arises directly from internal carotid artery.

There are fairly frequent variations of the "normal" configuration of the circle of Willis. In many brains the posterior cerebral artery on one side is a branch of the internal carotid artery rather than of the basilar artery (Fig. 5-5). Both anterior cerebral arteries may arise from a single internal carotid artery; there are also intermediate conditions in which the anterior cerebral artery on one side receives some blood from the ipsilateral internal carotid artery and the rest from the contralateral internal carotid artery via the anterior communicating artery. Finally, the circle of Willis may not be a complete circle; an interruption may occur at a number of sites. For example, it may occur anteriorly if both anterior cerebral arteries arise from one internal carotid artery.

Other routes of collateral circulation are available, although the circle of Willis is likely to be the most important. There are anastomoses, at the arteriolar and capillary levels, between terminal branches of the cerebral arteries. These are usually inadequate in the adult to maintain the entire territory of a major cerebral artery if it becomes occluded, but occasionally they may be sufficient to maintain a large part of this territory. In addition, well-defined arterial anastomoses may enlarge to a remarkable degree to compensate for slowly developing occlusions. For example, there have been documented cases in which the territory of one posterior cerebral artery was supplied by the internal carotid artery of that side by means of flow through the anterior choroidal artery and from there through a posterior choroidal artery and into the posterior cerebral.

Control of cerebral blood flow

The brain is very active metabolically but has no effective way to store oxygen or glucose. A stable and copious blood supply is therefore required, and the brain, which represents only 2% of the total body weight, uses about 15% of the normal cardiac output and accounts for nearly 25% of the body's oxygen consumption. The overall flow rate is maintained at a very constant level, but this rate may increase or decrease in particular regions of the brain, in a pattern correlated with neural activity.

The mechanisms that control cerebral blood flow are

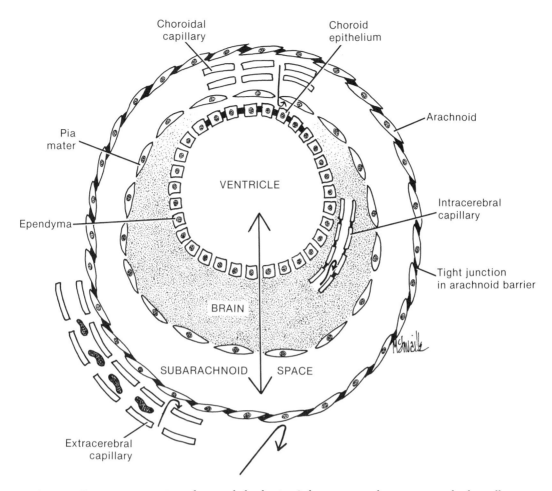

Fig. 5-6. Barrier systems in and around the brain. Substances can leave extracerebral capillaries but are then blocked by the arachnoid barrier. They can also leave choroidal capillaries but are then blocked by the choroid epithelium. They cannot leave any other capillaries that are inside the arachnoid barrier. The ventricular and subarachnoid spaces are in free communication with each other, and both communicate with the extracellular space of the brain.

not well understood, but at least three factors seem to be involved. The first is a process termed *autoregulation,* by which cerebral blood vessels themselves act to maintain constant flow; the vessels constrict (thus increasing their resistance) in response to increased blood pressure, and they relax in response to decreased pressure. The second factor may be generally thought of as a response of the cerebral vessels to metabolites, of which carbon dioxide is the best studied. Increases of carbon dioxide tension in brain extracellular fluid cause dilation of the cerebral vessels and increased blood flow; decreases of carbon dioxide tension have opposite effects. Changes in oxygen tension have reciprocal effects to those of carbon dioxide. Local changes in metabolite concentration may be part of the basis for regional variations in blood flow. Finally, cerebral vessels have a definite autonomic innervation. The evidence concerning the role of this innervation is somewhat conflicting,

but the consensus is that neural control of cerebral blood flow is of relatively minor importance.

Blood-brain barrier

The concept of a *blood-brain barrier* arose from the early observation that many substances, when injected into the bloodstream, could not gain access to the brain. Such a barrier must consist of more than just an impediment at the junction between blood vessels and brain, since this alone would not prevent substances in tissues around the brain from diffusing into it. The term "blood-brain barrier" is therefore commonly used in a more general sense to refer to the anatomical and physiological complex that controls the movement of substances from the general extracellular fluid of the body to the extracellular fluid of the brain. Used in this way, the barrier includes the arachnoid barrier layer and the blood–cerebrospinal fluid barrier (Fig. 5-6). It also includes a true

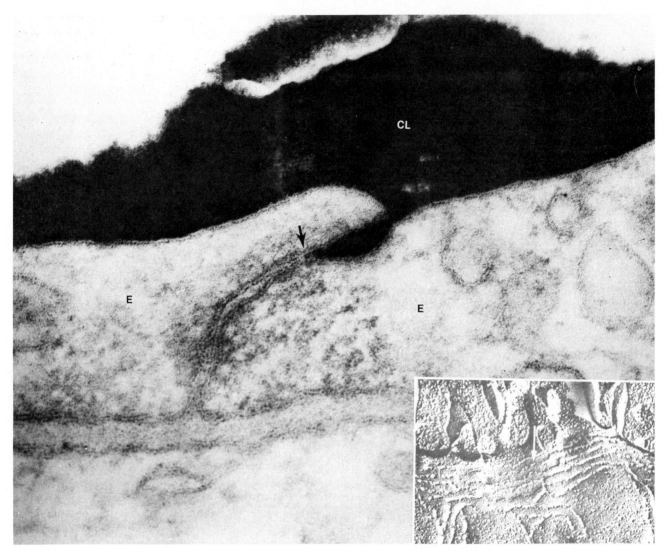

Fig. 5-7. Endothelial wall of a mouse cerebral capillary. An electron-dense marker (lanthanum hydroxide) that had been injected into the mouse's aorta begins to leave the capillary lumen *(CL)* but is stopped by a tight junction (arrow) between two endothelial cells *(E)*. Inset: bands of equivalent tight junctions (arrow) between adjacent choroid epithelial cells, revealed by freeze-fracturing. In this technique, the tissue is frozen and then split; the exposed surfaces are then coated with gold or platinum and examined in a scanning electron microscope. (Courtesy of Dr. Milton Brightman, National Institutes of Health.)

blood-brain barrier, which consists of rows of tight junctions between adjacent endothelial cells of cerebral capillaries (Fig. 5-7). As in the case of the blood–cerebrospinal fluid barrier, this barrier is selective; glucose can cross it by a process of facilitated diffusion, but other molecules of similar size cannot. In addition, it appears that various substances can be actively transported in both directions across this endothelial wall.

This complex barrier system can be a mixed blessing. It is rather efficient at keeping microorganisms out of the brain, but it is equally efficient at keeping most antibiotics out. An intracranial infection can therefore be

difficult to treat. The development of techniques for reversibly opening the blood-brain barrier and the synthesis of therapeutic agents that can cross an intact blood-brain barrier are both active areas of research.

As discussed in Chapter 4, the capillaries of the choroid plexus are fenestrated, and substances can leave them, only to be stopped by the arrays of tight junctions between adjacent choroid epithelial cells. There are several other locations where the cerebral capillaries are fenestrated and allow free communication between the blood and the brain's extracellular fluid. These additional sites are in contact with the walls of the ventricular

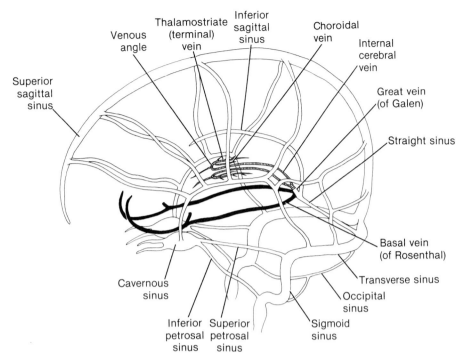

Fig. 5-8. Venous system of the brain. Dural sinuses and superficial veins are white, deep veins are striped, and the basal vein and its tributaries are black. (Modified from Warwick, R., and Williams, P.L., editors: Gray's anatomy, Br. ed. 35. Philadelphia, 1973, W.B. Saunders.)

system and are collectively termed the *circumventricular organs.* They include the pineal gland, portions of the hypothalamus, and a few other structures. Each circumventricular organ probably has either a secretory function or a role in monitoring the composition of the general extracellular fluid; in both cases, free access to the bloodstream seems reasonable in terms of efficient operation. No particular barrier system surrounding the circumventricular organs has been described, and at the present time, they appear to be small "holes" in the blood-brain barrier.

VENOUS DRAINAGE

The principal route of venous drainage of the brain is through a system of cerebral veins that empty into the dural venous sinuses and ultimately into the internal jugular vein (Fig. 5-8). There are also a collection of *emissary veins* connecting extracranial veins with dural sinuses and a *basilar venous plexus* around the base of the brain that communicates with the *epidural venous plexus* of the spinal cord. These play a relatively minor role in the normal circulatory pattern of the brain, but emissary veins can be very important clinically as a path for the spread of infection into the cranial cavity.

Cerebral veins are conventionally divided into *superficial* and *deep* groups. In general, the superficial veins lie on the surface of the cerebral hemispheres and empty

into the superior sagittal sinus, while the deep veins drain internal structures and eventually empty into the straight sinus. The *basal vein,* described shortly, does not fit comfortably into this scheme; some consider it a superficial vein because it drains some cortical areas, but others consider it a deep vein because it also drains some deep structures and eventually empties into the straight sinus.

Cerebral veins are valveless and, in contrast to cerebral arteries, are interconnected by numerous functional anastomoses, both within a group and between superficial and deep groups.

Superficial veins

The superficial veins are quite variable and consist of a superior group that empties into the superior and inferior sagittal sinuses and an inferior group that empties into the transverse and cavernous sinuses (Fig. 5-9). Only three of these veins are reasonably constant from one brain to another. These are (1) the *superficial middle cerebral vein,* which runs anteriorly and inferiorly along the lateral sulcus, draining most of the temporal lobe into the cavernous sinus or into the nearby sphenoparietal sinus; (2) the *superior anastomotic vein (or vein of Trolard),* which typically travels across the parietal lobe and connects the superficial middle cerebral vein with the superior sagittal sinus; and (3) the *inferior anasto-*

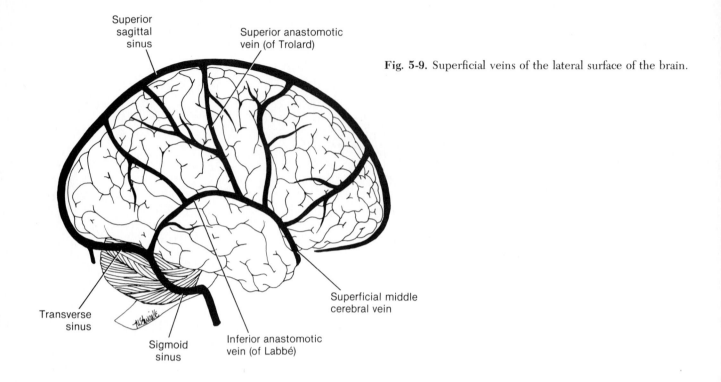

Fig. 5-9. Superficial veins of the lateral surface of the brain.

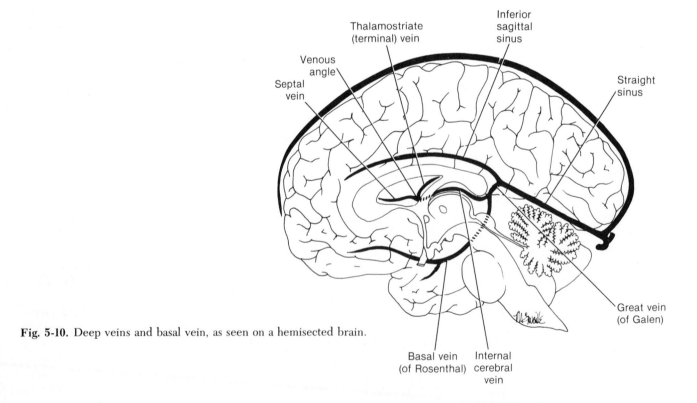

Fig. 5-10. Deep veins and basal vein, as seen on a hemisected brain.

motic vein (or *vein of Labbé*), which travels posteriorly and inferiorly across the temporal and/or occipital lobes and connects the superficial middle cerebral vein with the transverse sinus.

Deep veins

The deep veins (Fig. 5-10) are more constant in configuration than are the superficial veins. Since they are found deep in the brain in locations where arteries are small, they form clinically useful radiological landmarks.

The major deep vein is the *internal cerebral vein*, which is formed at the interventricular foramen by the confluence of two smaller veins, the *septal vein* (which runs posteriorly across the septum pellucidum) and the *thalamostriate* (or *terminal*) *vein* (which travels in the groove between the thalamus and the caudate nucleus, draining much of both these structures). Near the interventricular foramen, the thalamostriate vein receives the *choroidal vein*, a tortuous vessel that drains the choroid plexus of the lateral ventricle.

Immediately after forming, the internal cerebral vein bends sharply in a posterior direction. This bend is called the *venous angle* and is used in x-ray studies as an indication of the interventricular foramen (Fig. 5-13). The paired internal cerebral veins proceed posteriorly through the transverse cerebral fissure and fuse in the superior cistern to form the unpaired *great cerebral vein* (or *vein of Galen*). The great vein turns superiorly and joins the inferior sagittal sinus to form the straight sinus.

Along its short course, the great vein receives the basal veins (or *veins of Rosenthal*). On each side the basal vein is formed near the optic chiasm by the *deep middle cerebral vein*, which drains the insula, and several other tributaries that drain inferior portions of the basal ganglia and the orbital surface of the frontal lobe. It then proceeds along the medial surface of the temporal lobe, curves around the cerebral peduncle, and enters the great vein.

In addition to the superficial and deep veins already described, there is a separate, complex collection of veins that serves the cerebellum and brainstem. These drain into the great vein and into the straight, transverse, and petrosal sinuses.

SOME FUNCTIONAL ASPECTS OF THE BLOOD SUPPLY OF THE CNS

Cerebrovascular disease and accidents constitute the most common cause of neurological deficits. Since the brain, compared to other organs, has a very high demand for oxygen and glucose, vascular insufficiency lasting more than a few minutes results in necrosis of the involved brain tissue. A necrotic region of tissue is called an *infarct*. An abrupt incident of vascular insufficiency or of bleeding into, or immediately adjacent to, the brain is called a *stroke*.

Ischemic strokes (those due to sudden vascular insufficiency) are most commonly caused by a *thrombus* (a blood clot formed within a vessel) or an *embolus* (a bit of foreign matter, such as part of a blood clot, that is carried along in the bloodstream). Either can cause occlusion of an artery supplying the brain, and both are highly correlated with atherosclerosis (although this is by no means the only cause). If the occlusion occurs within or proximal to the circle of Willis, there is some possibility of adequate collateral circulation, particularly if the involved artery had slowly become occluded prior to the stroke. On the other hand, anastomoses between arteries distal to the circle of Willis are variable and collateral circulation less likely to be adequate, so occlusion of one of these vessels typically results in an infarct. The size of the infarct will obviously be related to the size of the occluded vessel and to the degree of collateral circulation available. However, as pointed out earlier in this chapter, the magnitude of a neurological deficit is not necessarily related to the size of the infarct causing it. A very small lesion in the brainstem or internal capsule can have a much more devastating effect than damage to certain relatively large areas of the cerebellum or cerebral hemispheres.

Another vascular problem with symptoms somewhat similar to an ischemic stroke is the *transient ischemic attack* (TIA). The crucial difference between a transient ischemic attack and an ischemic stroke is that the deficits associated with a transient ischemic attack (as the name implies) persist for only a few minutes to a few hours and are followed by an essentially complete recovery. It is thought that transient ischemic attacks are usually caused by minute emboli that originate from atherosclerotic plaques or thrombi, partially occlude brain arteries, and are then broken down by normal body mechanisms.

Hemorrhagic strokes most commonly result from the rupture of small ganglionic arteries or the rupture of an aneurysm (see next paragraph). The lateral striate (lenticulostriate) arteries are the most frequent site of the former type of hemorrhage. These are particularly thin-walled vessels, and the likelihood of their spontaneous rupture is greatly increased in individuals suffering from hypertension. The lateral striate arteries supply some important deep cerebral structures, and hemorrhage here can be rapidly fatal.

Aneurysms are balloon-like swellings of arterial walls. They occur most frequently at or near the place where an artery bifurcates. Those close to the brain usually occur in or near the anterior half of the circle of Willis, although they are also found at other locations. An aneurysm can cause neurological deficits in two ways: as it grows (and some become huge), it can push against and compress brain structures, much as a growing tumor would. It can also rupture and, depending on its size and

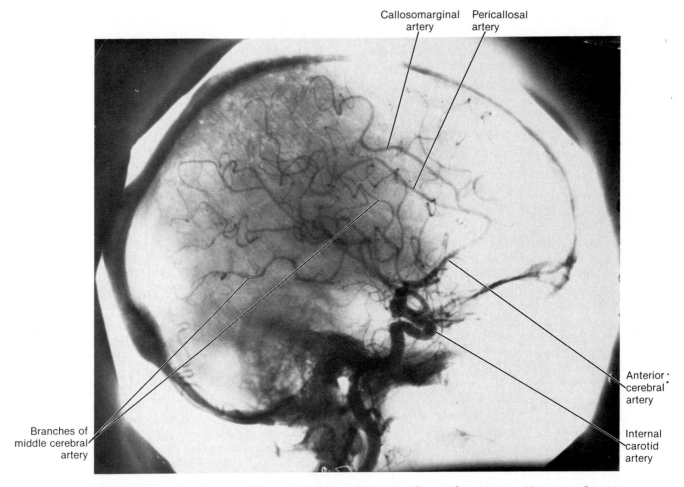

Fig. 5-11. Lateral projection of the arterial phase of an internal carotid angiogram. (Courtesy of Dr. Michael Earnest, Denver General Hospital and University of Colorado Medical Center.)

Branches of middle cerebral artery

Branches of anterior cerebral artery

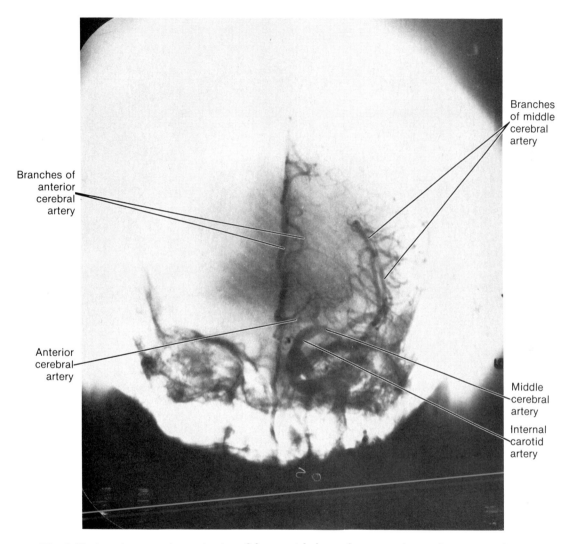

Anterior cerebral artery

Middle cerebral artery

Internal carotid artery

Fig. 5-12. Anterior-posterior projection of the arterial phase of an internal carotid angiogram. (Courtesy of Dr. Michael Earnest, Denver General Hospital and University of Colorado Medical Center.)

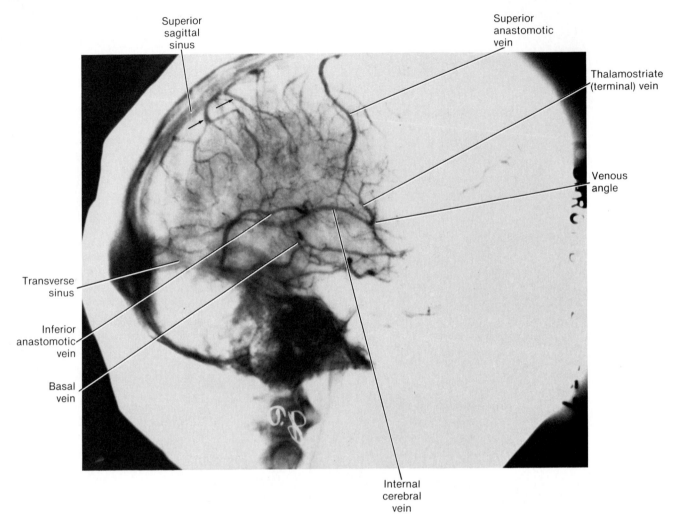

Fig. 5-13. Lateral projection of the venous phase of an internal carotid angiogram demonstrating the venous angle. Superior superficial veins (arrows) can be seen draining into the superior sagittal sinus. The images of the internal cerebral and inferior anastomotic veins overlap in this picture, but these two veins do not communicate with each other. (Courtesy of Dr. John Stears, University of Colorado Medical Center.)

location, have disastrous consequences. Many aneurysms, particularly if they are detected before they become too large, can be corrected surgically.

Another type of vascular problem is an *arteriovenous malformation* (AVM). This is a congenital malformation in which large anastomoses exist between arteries and veins in a relatively circumscribed area. These malformations may become larger with age and can cause neurological problems, either by "stealing" blood from adjacent normal brain tissue as a result of their low resistance or by hemorrhaging.

Vascular problems involving the venous system are not seen nearly as often as those involving the arterial supply. This is partly because occlusions and hemorrhages occur less often in the venous system and partly

because of the large number of functional anastomoses. Thus a slowly developing occlusion of the anterior portion of the superior sagittal sinus would probably be asymptomatic. Even if such an occlusion developed rapidly, the symptoms might be no more than a transient headache. However, if the occlusion were in a more critical location, such as the posterior portion of the superior sagittal sinus, the consequences would be much more serious and might include seizures, motor problems, and even coma and death.

Conditions such as thrombosed arteries, aneurysms, and arteriovenous malformations can be detected by a technique called *cerebral angiography*. This involves injecting a radiopaque dye into the carotid or vertebral circulation and then taking a rapid series of x-ray photo-

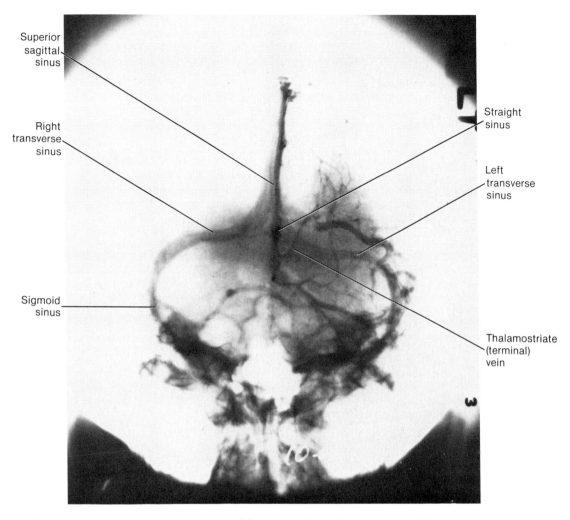

Superior sagittal sinus

Right transverse sinus

Sigmoid sinus

Straight sinus

Left transverse sinus

Thalamostriate (terminal) vein

Fig. 5-14. Anterior-posterior projection of the venous phase of an angiogram. The superior sagittal sinus drains into the right transverse sinus. The straight sinus, seen end-on, drains into the left transverse sinus. (Courtesy of Dr. John Stears, University of Colorado Medical Center.)

graphs. Early photographs demonstrate the arterial circulation (Figs. 5-11 and 5-12), and later ones show the venous circulation (Figs. 5-13 and 5-14).

ADDITIONAL READING

Bradbury, M.: The concept of a blood-brain barrier, New York, 1979, John Wiley & Sons, Inc.

Brightman, M.W., and Reese, T.S.: Junctions between intimately apposed cell membranes in the vertebrate brain, J. Cell Biol. **40:** 648, 1969.

Broadwell, R.D., and Brightman, M.W.: Entry of peroxidase into neurons of the central and peripheral nervous systems from extracerebral and cerebral blood, J. Comp. Neurol. 166:257, 1976. *Detailed description of the movement of tracer protein into the circumventricular organs.*

Chorobski, J., and Penfield, W.: Cerebral vasodilator nerves and their pathway from the medulla oblongata: with observations on the pial and intracerebral vascular plexus, Arch. Neurol. Psychiatr. 28:1257, 1932.

Cobb, S., and Finesinger, J.E.: Cerebral circulation. XIX. The vagal pathway of the vasodilator impulses, Arch. Neurol. Psychiatr. **28:** 1243, 1932. *While not all subsequent investigators agree with the findings, this paper provides a straightforward and convincing demonstration of a pathway through the vagus nerve into the brainstem and out through the facial nerve, causing dilation of cortical vessels.*

Duvernoy, H.M.: Human brainstem vessels, New York, 1978, Springer-Verlag, Inc. *A painstakingly detailed, magnificently illustrated, fabulously expensive book.*

Galatius-Jensen, F., and Ringberg, V.: Anastomosis between the anterior choroidal artery and the posterior cerebral artery demonstrated by angiography, Radiol. 81:942, 1963.

Gunning, A.J., et al.: Mural thrombosis of the internal carotid artery and subsequent embolism, Quart. J. Med. 33:155, 1964. *Presents a case for small unstable emboli as a cause of transient ischemic attacks.*

Lassen, N.A., Ingvar, D.H., and Skinhøj, E.: Brain function and blood flow, Sci. Am. **239**(4):62, 1978. *An exciting new technique for studying the activity of different areas of the brain by measuring, with an external gamma-ray camera, the amounts of radioactive isotope delivered to different areas through the arterial circulation.*

Levy, L., and Wicke, J.D.: The effect of alpha-adrenergic innervation on caudate blood flow, Ann. Neurol. **7**:150, 1980.

Millen, J.W., and Woollam, D.H.M.: Vascular patterns in the choroid plexus, J. Anat. **87**:114, 1953.

Nelson, E., and Rennels, M.: Innervation of intracranial arteries, Brain **93**:475, 1970.

Oldendorf, W.H.: Permeability of the blood-brain barrier. In Tower, D.B., editor: The nervous system, vol. 1, New York, 1975, Raven Press. *A concise, provocative review of the properties of the normal blood-brain barrier and the ways in which it may be penetrated.*

Owman, C., and Edvinsson, L., editors: Neurogenic control of the brain circulation, Wenner-Gren Symposium, vol. 30, Elmsford, N.Y., 1977, Pergamon Press, Inc.

Pia, H.W., Langmaid, C., and Zierski, J.: Cerebral aneurysms: advances in diagnosis and therapy, New York, 1979, Springer-Verlag, Inc.

Purves, M.: The physiology of the cerebral circulation, New York, 1972, Cambridge University Press.

Purves, M.J.: Control of cerebral blood vessels: present state of the art, Ann. Neurol. **3**:377, 1978. *A brief but comprehensive overview of current knowledge and conflicting evidence about control of cerebral circulation.*

Reese, T.S., and Karnovsky, M.J.: Fine structural demonstration of a blood-brain barrier to exogenous peroxidase, J. Cell Biol. **34**:207, 1967.

Reivich, M.: Embryology, anatomy and pathophysiology of the cerebral circulation. In Goldensohn, E.S., and Appel, S.H., editors: Scientific approaches to clinical neurology, Philadelphia, 1977, Lea & Febiger. *A nice review with a good bibliography covering the clinical manifestations of various vascular problems.*

Rhoton, A.L., Jr., Fujii, K., and Fradd, B.: Microsurgical anatomy of the anterior choroidal artery, Surg. Neurol. **12**:171, 1979. *Finely detailed and beautifully illustrated.*

Riggs, H.E., and Rupp, C.: Variation in form of circle of Willis. Arch. Neurol. **8**:8, 1963.

Scheinberg, P.: Cerebral blood flow. In Tower, D.B., editor: The Nervous System, vol. 2, New York, 1975, Raven Press.

Stephens, R.B., and Stilwell, D.L.: Arteries and veins of the human brain, Springfield, Ill., 1969, Charles C Thomas, Publisher. *A well-photographed series of dissections of brains in which the arteries or veins had been injected.*

Van den Bergh, R., and Vander Eecken, H.: Anatomy and embryology of cerebral circulation. Progr. Brain Res. **30**:1, 1968.

Vander Eecken, H.M., and Adams, R.D.: The anatomy and functional significance of the meningeal arterial anastomoses of the human brain, J. Neuropathol. Exp. Neurol. **12**:132, 1953.

Wackenheim, A., and Braun, J.P.: The veins of the posterior fossa, New York, 1978, Springer-Verlag, Inc.

Weindl, A.: Neuroendocrine aspects of circumventricular organs. In Ganong, W.F., and Martini, L., editors: Frontiers of neuroendocrinology, vol. 3, New York, 1973, Oxford University Press.

Welch, K., et al.: The collateral circulation following middle cerebral branch occlusion, J. Neurosurg. **12**:361, 1955. *Discussion of two cases in which much of the middle cerebral artery filled through the anterior cerebral artery.*

Wilson, M.: The anatomic foundation of neuroradiology of the brain, ed. 2, Boston, 1972, Little, Brown and Co.

CHAPTER 6

SENSORY RECEPTORS AND PERIPHERAL NERVOUS SYSTEM

The ongoing activity and output of the central nervous system are greatly influenced, and sometimes more or less determined, by incoming sensory information. An example is our constant awareness of the position of our limbs in space and the use of this awareness in guiding our movements. This chapter considers the functional organization of the general receptors of the body as a prelude to the discussion of how sensory information is routed and processed within the nervous system. Specialized receptors, such as those of the eye and the ear, are described in later chapters.

RECEPTORS
Classification

There are many types of receptors on and within the human body and several different systems for classifying them. One system subdivides them into *interoceptors*, *proprioceptors*, and *exteroceptors*. Interoceptors monitor events within the body, such as distention of the stomach or changes in the pH of the blood. Proprioceptors respond to changes in the position of the body or its parts; examples are the receptors in muscles and in joint capsules. Vestibular receptors of the inner ear are commonly classified as proprioceptors, since they signal movement and changes in the orientation of the head in space. Exteroceptors respond to stimuli that arise outside the body, such as the receptors involved in touch, hearing, and vision. Exteroceptors are sometimes subdivided into *teloreceptors,* which respond to stimuli or objects separated from the body (for example, visual receptors and auditory receptors), and *contact receptors* (for example, tactile receptors and pain receptors). Interoceptor-proprioceptor-exteroceptor terminology is not used as commonly today as it was in the past, partly because some receptors do not fit neatly and uniquely into one of these categories. For example, heat-sensitive

receptors respond to both radiant heat and to contact with a warm object, so to classify them as either teloreceptors or contact exteroceptors is somewhat arbitrary. Also, some vestibular receptors respond to gravity, an external force, but are classified as proprioceptors; on the other hand, the visual system is very much involved in our perception of motion and body position, but visual receptors are considered exteroceptors.

A more commonly used classification system subdivides receptors on the basis of the type of stimulus to which they are most sensitive (called the *adequate stimulus*). *Chemoreceptors* include those for smell, taste, and many internal stimuli such as pH and metabolite concentrations. *Photoreceptors* are the visual receptors of the retina. *Thermoreceptors* respond to temperature and its changes. *Mechanoreceptors*, the most varied group, respond to physical deformation. They include cutaneous receptors for touch, receptors that monitor muscle tension, auditory and vestibular receptors, and others. Pain receptors are a bit difficult to classify, since the physical mechanism by which they are actually stimulated is not understood. This problem is commonly finessed by classifying them separately as *nociceptors* (Latin, noci = hurt, as in noxious or obnoxious).

General organization

The basic task of a receptor is to monitor some aspect of its environment by converting and amplifying part of the stimulus energy into an electrical signal that is meaningful to the nervous system. This process is called *transduction*. Receptors do this by producing relatively slow potential changes called *receptor potentials* in response to an appropriate stimulus. The magnitude of the receptor potential is related in a systematic way to the magnitude of the stimulus. The duration of the receptor potential is typically (but not always) the same as that of the

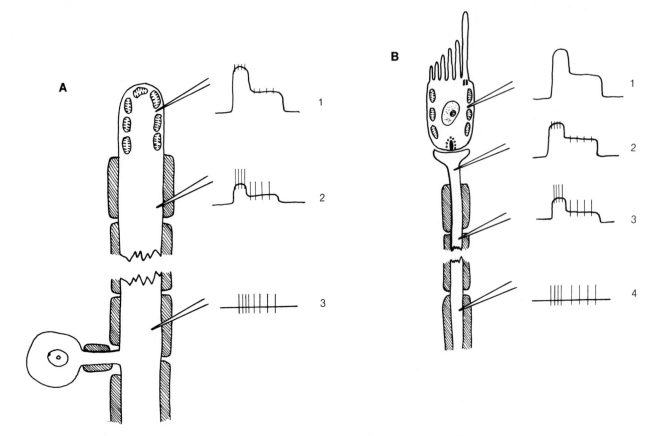

Fig. 6-1. Organization of long and short receptors. **A,** A long receptor, such as a mechanoreceptor with its cell body in a dorsal root ganglion. Stimulation of the sensory ending causes a generator potential, recorded at *1,* with small passively conducted action potentials superimposed on it. The generator potential decays with distance from the ending *(2),* until at distances of more than a few millimeters from the ending, it has died out completely *(3).* Action potentials, however, are conducted without decrement from a point near the ending all the way to the CNS *(2* and *3).* **B,** A short receptor, such as a hair cell in a semicircular canal. Stimulation of the hair cell causes a receptor potential *(1).* This in turn causes a postsynaptic potential in an eighth nerve fiber *(2).* Subsequent events are similar to those in the long receptor: the postsynaptic potential decays, but action potentials are conducted to the CNS *(3* and *4).*

stimulus; in some cases, the receptor potential is a transient event at the beginning of the stimulus (and sometimes at the end of the stimulus as well). If a particular receptor (a *short receptor*) contacts the next cell in its neuronal pathway close to the site of transduction, then the receptor potential itself can adequately modulate the receptor's rate of transmitter release and thereby cause either changes in spike frequency or slow potential changes in the second cell (Fig. 6-1). However, some receptors *(long receptors)* must convey information over long distances (for example, from a big toe to the spinal cord), and the receptor potential dies out in a relatively short distance. In such cases, most of the receptor, beginning near the site of transduction, is capable of propagating action potentials. The spike frequency is then modulated by the receptor potential (Fig. 6-1). Receptor

potentials that directly cause changes in spike frequency are also called *generator potentials.* All general receptors of the body are long receptors. Short receptors are found in some special sense organs of the head, such as the eye and ear.

Although their morphology varies widely, all receptors seem to have three general parts: a receptive area, an area rich in mitochondira (near the receptive area), and a synaptic area (Fig. 6-2). The receptive area may have specializations suited to the adequate stimulus, as in the case of photoreceptors, which have an elaborately folded array of photopigment-bearing membrane; in other cases, there are no obvious specializations in this area. The area rich in mitochondria is either immediately adjacent to the receptive membrane or nearby and is presumed to supply the energy needs of the trans-

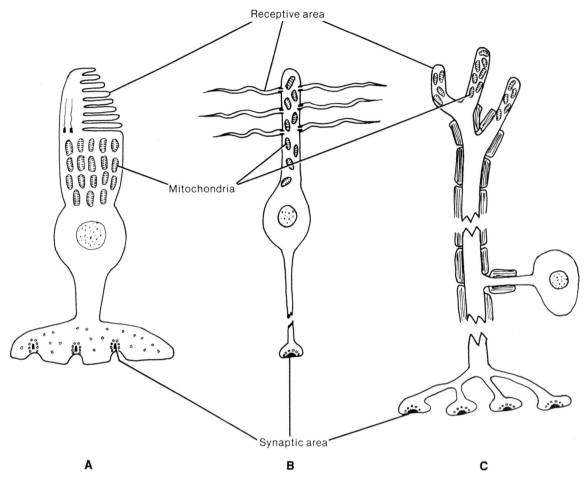

Fig. 6-2. General features of receptor anatomy. **A,** A retinal cone (photoreceptor). **B,** An olfactory receptor cell (chemoreceptor). **C,** A mechanoreceptor or pain receptor from skin. All have a specialized area for the reception of stimuli, a nearby area rich in mitochondria, and a synaptic area that may be some distance away.

duction process. In long receptors, the synaptic area may be far removed from the other two.

All receptors show some *adaptation*, which means they become less sensitive during the course of a maintained stimulus. Those that adapt relatively little are called *slowly adapting* and are suitable receptors for such things as static position. Those that adapt a great deal are called *rapidly adapting* and can only indicate change and movement of stimuli (Fig. 6-3). Adaptation is generally a property of one or more parts of the receptor's membrane: a maintained stimulus may cause less and less receptor potential with time, or (in long receptors) a given value of the receptor potential may generate fewer action potentials. In addition, accessory structures such as cellular capsules may modify the physical stimulus before it reaches the sensory ending.

Cutaneous receptors

The skin and adjacent subcutaneous tissues are richly innervated by a wide variety of sensory endings. These endings may conveniently be divided into *encapsulated* and *nonencapsulated* receptors, depending on whether an accessory structure surrounds the ending. A bewildering variety of encapsulated receptors have been described in the past, and a bewildering variety of mostly eponymous names have been attached to them. These classifications seem to be merely variations on two common themes: receptors with lamellated capsules and receptors with thin capsules. This chapter will describe only the best known of these. The function of the capsule is not known for all encapsulated receptors, but in at least some instances it serves as a mechanical filter, modifying mechanical stimuli before they reach the sensory ending. For example, receptors with lamellated capsules are rapidly adapting, due in large part to these mechanical properties of the capsules. The capsules also have barrier properties (discussed later in this chapter) that may be important in regulating the composition of the fluid surrounding the sensory endings contained within them.

Fig. 6-3. Slowly adapting versus rapidly adapting receptors. **A,** A tendon receptor (Golgi tendon organ) continues to fire action potentials as long as tension is maintained on the tendon. **B,** Most hair receptors fire a short burst of action potentials and are then silent, even if bending of the hair is maintained.

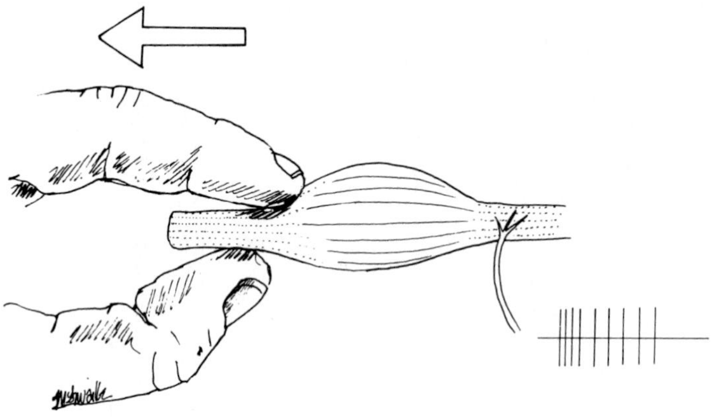

A

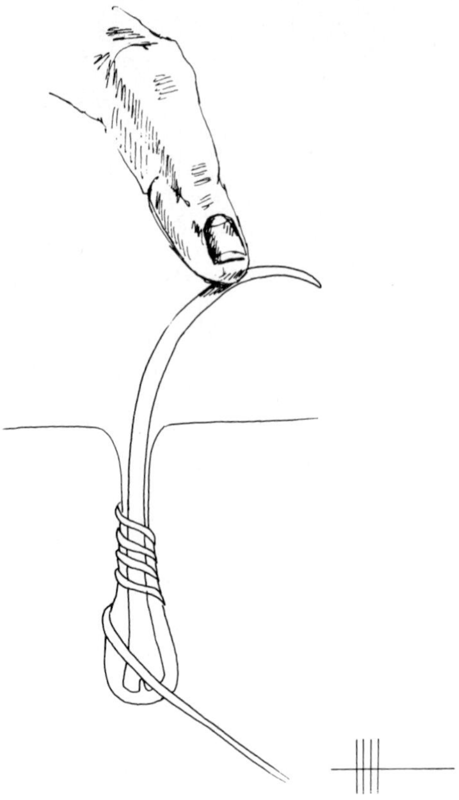

B

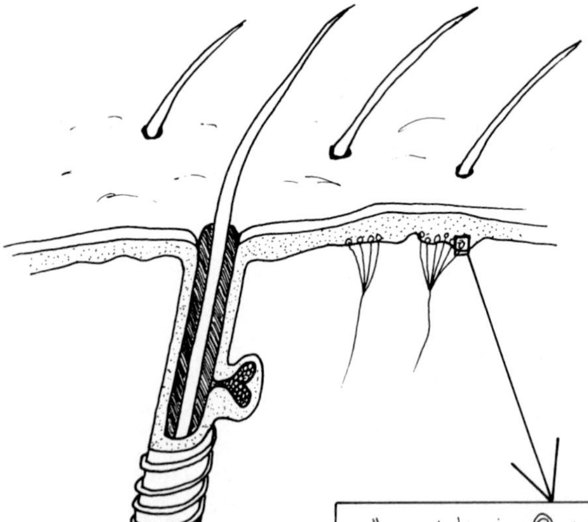

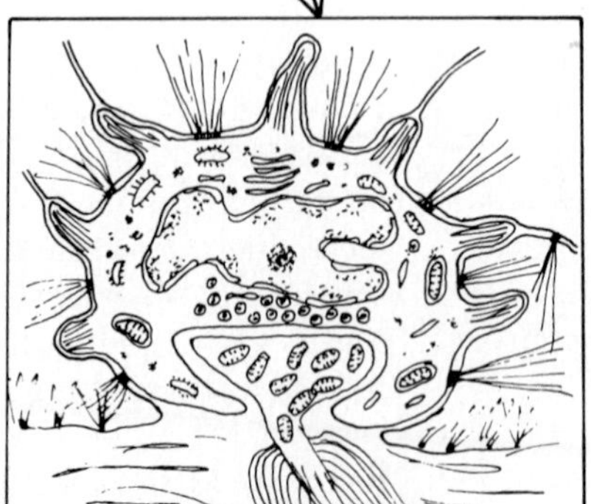

Fig. 6-4. Two receptor types from hairy skin. Receptor endings wrap around hairs in a wide variety of configurations; a simple helical winding is shown. The inset is an enlarged drawing of a Merkel cell–neurite complex in the basal layer of the epidermis. (Inset modified from Bannister, L.H.: Sensory terminals of peripheral nerves. In Landon, D.N., editor: The peripheral nerve, London, 1976, Chapman & Hall Ltd.)

Unencapsulated receptors may be divided into *free nerve endings* and endings with *accessory structures* that do not surround the ending. Free nerve endings, as the name implies, are formed by branching terminations of sensory fibers in the skin, with no obvious specialization around them. Such endings are not restricted to the skin but are found throughout the body. Even though microscopically they look similar to one another, some are thought to be mechanoreceptors, others thermoreceptors, and still others nociceptors.

Cutaneous mechanoreceptors. In addition to mechanoreceptive free nerve endings, there are five other prominent types of mechanoreceptors found in the skin and adjacent subcutaneous tissue. Two are nonencapsulated endings with accessory structures, and three are encapsulated.

Endings around hairs vary in their degrees of com-

plexity. Those around the base of a cat's whiskers are very elaborate, but those around most ordinary human body hairs are longitudinal neural processes and spiral endings that wrap around the base of the hair (Fig. 6-4). Bending the hair is presumed to deform the sensory ending somehow and lead to the production of a generator potential. The events coupling the stimulus at the receptor membrane to the receptor potential are not known for this or for any other receptor. Most hair receptors are rapidly adapting; they respond well to something brushing across the skin but not to a steady pressure.*

The second type of nonencapsulated receptor, found

---

*You can easily demonstrate this on yourself: bend a single hair on the back of your hand (or have someone else do it), then hold it in the bent position. You will feel it bending but will almost immediately lose awareness of its new position.

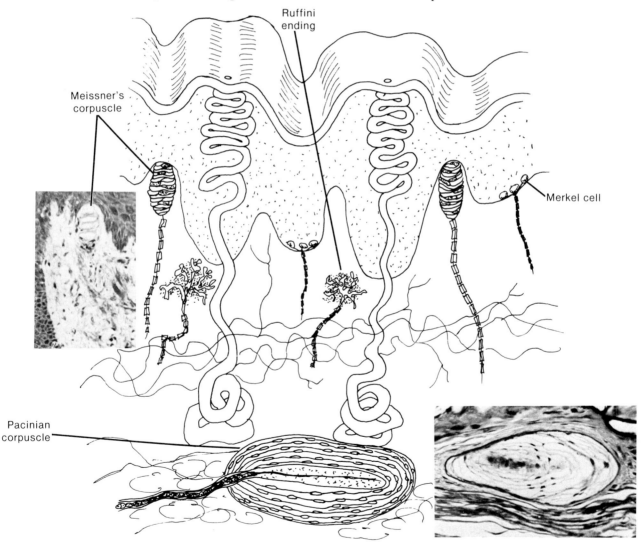

Fig. 6-5. Some of the sensory endings found in glabrous skin. Lower inset is a photomicrograph of a pacinian corpuscle cut at an oblique angle; upper inset is a photomicrograph of a Meissner corpuscle. Both micrographs are at the same magnification. (Courtesy of Pamela Eller, University of Colorado Medical Center.)

in both hairy and glabrous skin, is currently known by the unwieldy name of *Merkel cell–neurite complex* (Fig. 6-4). The ending is a disc-shaped expansion of the terminal of a sensory fiber, which is inserted into the base of a specialized cell called a Merkel cell. The Merkel cell is situated in the basal layer of the epidermis and contains dense-cored vesicles in what looks like a synaptic ending onto the sensory terminal. What the Merkel cell has to do with the transduction process and whether the apparent synapse is functional are largely unknown at this time. However, recordings from the sensory fiber have shown that the Merkel cell–neurite complex is a slowly adapting mechanoreceptor. A single fiber branches to innervate several Merkel cells, which tend to occur in groups.

Meissner's corpuscles are elongated encapsulated endings in the dermal papillae of hairless skin just beneath the epidermis and are oriented with their long axis perpendicular to the surface of the skin (Fig. 6-5). The accessory structures consist of a thin outer capsule and a lamellated stack of epithelial cells within the capsule, each oriented perpendicular to its long axis. One or more myelinated fibers approach the base of the corpuscle, lose their myelin, and wind back and forth between the stacked cells within the capsule. These are rapidly adapting receptors, and it is assumed that the capsule is important in determining the degree of adaptation. Vertical pressure on a dermal papilla compresses the nerve endings between the stacked capsular cells of a Meissner corpuscle, while pressure on a neighboring papilla is not nearly so effective. Meissner's corpuscles are quite numerous in the skin of fingertips, and it is thought that they are largely responsible for our ability to perform fine tactile discriminations with our fingertips.

Pacinian corpuscles are almost as widespread as free nerve endings. They are found subcutaneously over the entire body and in numerous other connective tissue sites. They are wrapped in the ultimate expression of a lamellated capsule and look like an onion in cross section (Fig. 6-5). The capsule consists of many concentric layers of very thin epithelial cells, with fluid spaces between adjacent layers. Pacinian corpuscles are also rapidly adapting, and in this case the role of the capsule is understood. Quickly applied forces are transmitted through the interior of the capsule and reach the ending, but maintained forces are not, as a result of the elastic properties of the capsular lamellae. During maintained pressure, each successive lamella is slightly less deformed than its outer neighbor, and the ending itself is not deformed at all. These corpuscles are amazingly sensitive and they, like the Merkel endings, can respond to skin indentations as small as 1 μm.

Because pacinian corpuscles are probably the most rapidly adapting receptors we have, they are poor receptors for pressure but good ones for vibration. A vibratory stimulus causes a steady train of impulses from such an ending, so that in this sense the receptor is "slowly adapting." It is important to understand that slowly adapting receptors, as they are conventionally defined, are simply receptors that respond best to unchanging stimuli. Rapidly adapting receptors, on the other hand, respond best to changing stimuli, giving a constant output to a stimulus with constant velocity, constant acceleration, or some other temporal property.

The fifth type of cutaneous mechanoreceptor is an encapsulated receptor called a *Ruffini ending*, which is widespread in the dermis and in subcutaneous and other connective tissue sites. It consists of a thin, cigar-shaped capsule traversed longitudinally by strands of collagenous connective tissue. A sensory fiber enters the capsule and branches profusely, so that many small processes are interspersed among the collagenous strands. This is a slowly adapting receptor and is thought to work by the squeezing of sensory terminals between strands of connective tissue when tension is applied to one or both ends of the capsule. Since collagen is not very elastic, the deformation of the endings is maintained as long as the tension is maintained, so adaptation is slow.

Other cutaneous receptors. Thermoreceptors, nociceptors, and some mechanoreceptors are probably all free nerve endings; no pronounced morphological differences can be seen among them with presently available techniques. Electrophysiological studies, however, have clearly shown that all exist. Some individual fibers respond selectively to cooling the skin, others to warming it, and still others to stimuli that would be perceived by a conscious animal as touch or as pain.

Patterns of innervation. The skin is often thought of as a uniform sensory surface varying in hairiness but basically uniform in sensitivity. This is far from true, however; some areas (such as the lips and fingertips) are much more densely innervated than other areas (such as the back). More densely innervated areas can subserve subtler tactile discriminations than can less densely innervated areas because of the close packing of receptors. One way this capability can be measured is in terms of *two-point discrimination*, which refers to the minimum distance by which two stimuli can be separated and still be perceived as two stimuli. This minimum distance is only about 2 mm for the fingertips but is several centimeters for the back. Corresponding to this two-point discrimination ability is the capacity to accurately localize single stimuli. We can easily detect the movement of a stimulus from one ridge to the next on a fingertip, but we are not nearly so accurate for stimuli delivered to the back of the thigh.

Granted that acuity is better in some areas than in others, many of us still tend to consider the skin a uniform sensory surface, because we think we can detect the occurrence of a stimulus anywhere on it. This too is inaccurate, because receptors are discrete entities whose zones of termination in the skin may not overlap with each other. For example, temperature sensitivity is distributed like polka dots across the skin (more densely in some areas than in others). A fine, cold probe touched to an appropriate spot on the skin elicits a sensation of coolness. The same probe touched to the skin between cold-sensitive spots may elicit only a sensation of touch. Because the skin is more or less densely innervated everywhere, there are probably no places that are insensitive to all stimuli, but a given small location is likely to be most sensitive to a particular *type* of stimulus. In real life, we are usually not stimulated by fine probes, so we are not aware that sensitivity is distributed across the skin in small, selective spots.

Muscle receptors

Muscle, like other tissues, receives an abundant supply of free nerve endings. The function of these endings is largely unknown, but some are assumed to be involved in muscle pain, while others may be chemoreceptors responsive to changes in extracellular fluid composition during muscle activity.

Muscles are also supplied with two important types of encapsulated receptors: the *muscle spindle*, which is unique to muscle, and the *Golgi tendon organ*, which is similar to a Ruffini ending.

Muscle spindles. Scattered throughout virtually every muscle in the body are long, thin, stretch receptors called muscle spindles (Fig. 6-6). They are quite simple in principle, consisting of a few small muscle fibers with a capsule surrounding the middle third of the fibers. These fibers are called *intrafusal muscle fibers* (Latin,

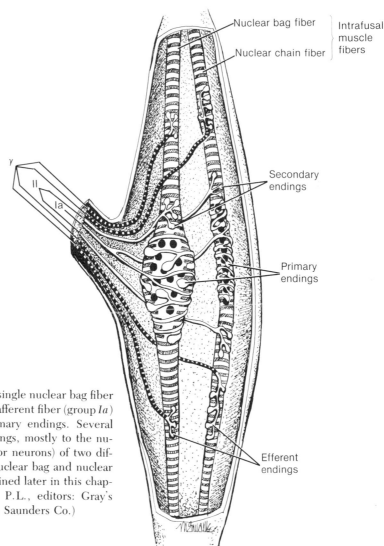

Fig. 6-6. Simplified diagram of a muscle spindle. A single nuclear bag fiber and a single nuclear chain fiber are shown. A single afferent fiber (group *Ia*) supplies all the intrafusal muscle fibers with primary endings. Several smaller afferents (group *II*) provide secondary endings, mostly to the nuclear chain fibers. Small motor axons (*gamma* motor neurons) of two different types innervate the contractile portions of nuclear bag and nuclear chain fibers. (The Ia-II-gamma terminology is explained later in this chapter.) (Modified from Warwick, R., and Williams, P.L., editors: Gray's anatomy, Br. ed. 35, Philadelphia, 1975, The W.B. Saunders Co.)

intra = within; fusus = spindle), in contrast to the ordinary *extrafusal muscle fibers* (Latin, extra = outside). The ends of the intrafusal fibers are attached to extrafusal fibers, so whenever the muscle is stretched, the intrafusal fibers are also stretched. The central region of each intrafusal fiber has few myofilaments and is noncontractile, but it does have one or more sensory endings applied to it. When the muscle is stretched, the central part of the intrafusal fiber is stretched, and each sensory ending fires impulses.

Numerous specializations occur in this simple basic organization, so that in fact the muscle spindle is one of

the most complex receptor organs in the body. Only three of these specializations are described here; their overall effect is to give the muscle spindle a dual function, part of it being particularly sensitive to the length of the muscle in a static sense and part of it particularly sensitive to the rate at which this length changes:

1. Intrafusal muscle fibers are of two types. All are multinucleated, and the central, noncontractile region contains the nuclei. In one type of intrafusal fiber, the nuclei are lined up single file; these are called *nuclear chain fibers*. In the other type, the nuclear region is broader, and the nuclei are arranged several abreast;

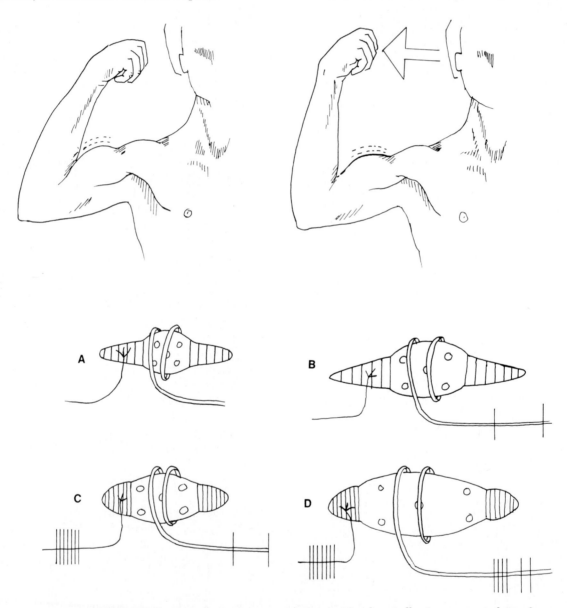

Fig. 6-7. Mechanism of action of gamma motor neurons. **A,** Muscle spindles in a contracted muscle (in this case the biceps) are unstretched and thus electrically silent. As a result, slight extension of the muscle causes few action potentials (**B**). However, activity of gamma motor neurons "prestretches" the central receptive region of the muscle spindle, causing a few action potentials when the biceps is contracted (**C**) and many more when it is slightly extended (**D**).

these are called *nuclear bag fibers*. There are typically 2 or 3 nuclear bag fibers per spindle and about twice that many chain fibers, but these numbers are variable.

2. There are also two types of sensory endings in the muscle spindle. The first type, called the *primary ending*, is formed by a single very large nerve fiber that enters the capsule and then branches, supplying every intrafusal fiber in a given spindle (although it innervates the bag fibers more heavily than the chain fibers). Each branch wraps around the central region of an intrafusal fiber, frequently in a spiral fashion, so these are some-

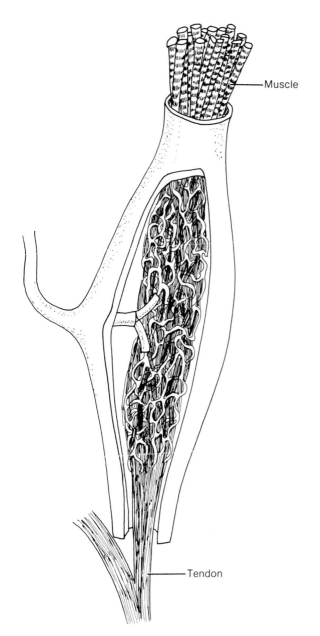

Fig. 6-8. Golgi tendon organ. A large afferent fiber enters a capsule around part of the myotendinous junction and then breaks up into many branches that interweave with bundles of collagen.

times called *annulospiral endings*. The second type of ending is formed by a few smaller nerve fibers that branch and primarily innervate nuclear chain fibers on both sides of the primary ending. These are the *secondary endings*, which are sometimes referred to as *flower-spray endings* because of their appearance. Primary endings are selectively sensitive to the onset of muscle stretch but discharge at a slower rate while the stretch is maintained. Secondary endings are less sensitive to the onset of stretch, but their discharge rate does not decline very much while the stretch is maintained.

3. Muscle spindles also receive a motor innervation. The large motor neurons that supply extrafusal muscle fibers are called *alpha motor neurons*, while the smaller ones supplying the contractile portions of intrafusal fibers are called *gamma motor neurons* (or *fusimotor neurons*). Intrafusal fibers are too small and too few to contribute to the strength of a muscle, and firing all the gamma motor neurons to a muscle does not generate significant tension. The function of this motor innervation will be discussed in conjunction with motor control systems (Chapter 12), but a simple example will indicate one of the possibilities (Fig. 6-7). Consider a muscle spindle in the biceps, and suppose that this muscle is contracted. This will relieve most or all of the tension on the nuclear region of the intrafusal fibers, so the sensory endings will be quite insensitive to muscle stretch that starts from this contracted state. Suppose that, at the same time, the gamma motor neurons to that spindle fire. This will cause the parts of each intrafusal fiber on both sides of the nuclear region to contract. This in turn will generate some tension on the nuclear region and restore its sensitivity. Thus gamma motor neurons can regulate the sensitivity of a muscle spindle so that this sensitivity can be maintained at any given muscle length. Not surprisingly, there are two types of gamma motor neurons, one of which preferentially ends on bag fibers, the other on chain fibers.

This is just one example of feedback control by the nervous system over its sensory pathways. Such control is very common; sometimes it occurs at the level of the receptor (as in this instance), and sometimes it occurs at relay nuclei, but it seems to occur at one or more locations in every sensory pathway.

Golgi tendon organs. Spindle-shaped receptors called Golgi tendon organs are found at the junctions between muscles and tendons. They are similar to Ruffini endings in their basic organization, consisting of interwoven collagen bundles surrounded by a thin capsule (Fig. 6-8). A large sensory fiber enters the capsule and branches into fine processes that are inserted among the collagen bundles. It is thought that tension on the capsule along its long axis squeezes these fine processes, and the resulting distortion stimulates them. As in the case of Ruffini endings, these are slowly adapting receptors, since the collagen is nonelastic and the squeezing action is maintained as long as the tension is maintained.

For many years, Golgi tendon organs were studied physiologically by pulling on a tendon while recording from the sensory axon. When they are stimulated in this way, considerable tension must be applied to the tendon before a response is obtained, and so it was thought that these were high-threshold receptors designed to inform the nervous system when muscle tension was reaching dangerous levels. However, the amount of tension actually applied to a tendon organ by such a stimulus is quite small: the muscle acts rather like a rubber band attached to a piece of string, absorbing most of the tension. However, if tension is generated in a tendon by making its attached muscle contract, the tendon organ is found to be much more sensitive and can actually respond to the contraction of just a few muscle fibers. Thus the Golgi tendon organ very specifically monitors the tension generated by muscle contraction and is now considered to play an active role in the process by which the nervous system controls motor activity.

Thus the mode of action of the Golgi tendon organ is quite different from that of the muscle spindle. If a muscle contracts isometrically, tension will be generated across its tendons, and the tendon organs will signal this; however, the muscle spindles will signal nothing since muscle length has not changed (assuming that the activity of the gamma motor neurons remains unchanged). On the other hand, a relaxed muscle can be stretched easily, and the muscle spindles will fire; the tendon organs, in contrast, will experience little tension and will remain silent. A muscle, by virtue of these two types of receptors, can simultaneously monitor its own length and tension.

Other receptors

Joint receptors. The receptors found in joints and their capsules are similar to some of those found in skin and muscle. In addition to the usual free nerve endings, there are endings equivalent to Golgi tendon organs in the ligaments and Ruffini endings and a few pacinian corpuscles in joint capsules (Table 2). As might be ex-

pected from their morphology, a few joint receptors (presumably the pacinian corpuscles) are rapidly adapting, but most are slowly adapting and respond to joint position and movement.

Visceral receptors. Much less is known about visceral receptors than about the other types discussed in this chapter; they have been studied mostly in terms of their physiology and their reflex effects. They tend to be supplied by thin, often unmyelinated fibers that terminate as free nerve endings, sometimes with complex branching patterns. Functionally most of these receptors act at a subconscious level through visceral reflexes. They include (1) mechanoreceptors in the walls of hollow organs (such as the endings in the aortic arch and carotid sinus, which, when stimulated by increased arterial pressure, reflexly cause vasodilation and decreased heart rate), (2) chemoreceptors (such as those of the carotid body, which, when stimulated by changes in blood gases or pH, reflexly cause compensating cardiovascular and respiratory changes), and (3) numerous nociceptors in the viscera (which can cause severe pain when stimulated, as by distention of an organ or its capsule).

PERIPHERAL NERVES

The nerve fibers innervating the receptors described thus far have their cell bodies in dorsal root ganglia adjacent to the spinal cord or, in the case of those serving the head, in various cranial nerve ganglia near the brainstem. The central process of each of these ganglion cells enters the CNS. The peripheral processes join motor axons emerging from the spinal cord (or brainstem) and form spinal nerves (or cranial nerves). The formal boundary between the central and peripheral nervous systems occurs between the sensory ganglia and the spinal cord/brainstem, at the point where the myelinating cells change from oligodendrocytes to Schwann cells. However, it is more convenient in the present discussion to consider only those portions peripheral to the sensory ganglia (that is, the wrappings and contents of spinal and cranial nerves). Aspects of the sensory ganglia and of the sensory and motor roots of

TABLE 2

Principal types of somatic receptors found in various tissues*

	Free nerve endings with accessory structures	Receptors with lamellated capsules	Receptors with thin capsules
Hairy skin	Endings around hairs (R); Merkel endings	Pacinian corpuscles (R)	Ruffini endings
Glabrous skin	Merkel endings	Pacinian corpuscles (R) Meissner's corpuscles (R)	Ruffini endings
Muscle/tendon			Muscle spindle; Golgi tendon organ
Joints		Pacinian corpuscles (R)	Ruffini endings; Golgi endings

*Free nerve endings are not included, since they are ubiquitous. (R) indicates that the receptor adapts rapidly to a maintained stimulus.

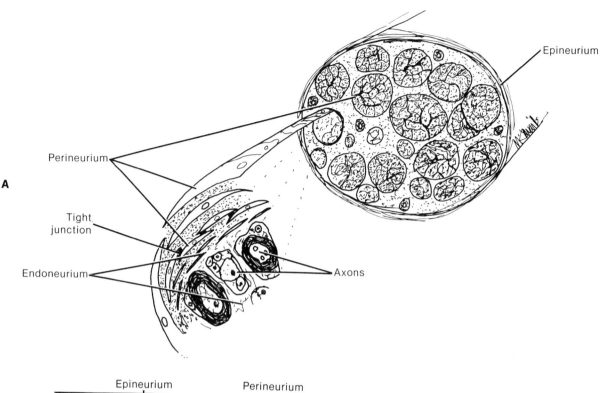

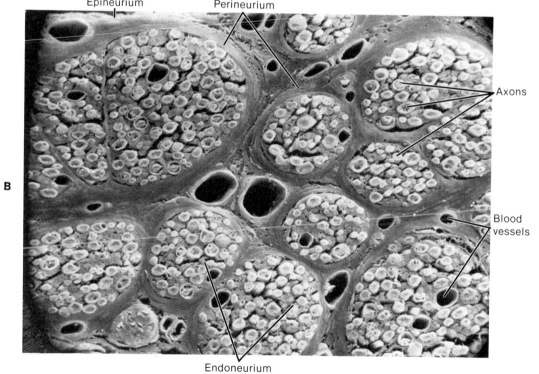

Fig. 6-9. A, Schematic illustration of a peripheral nerve and its connective tissue sheaths. Note the junctions connecting certain adjacent perineurial cells; these are responsible for the barrier properties of the perineurium. **B,** Scanning electron micrograph of a freeze-fractured preparation of peripheral nerve. (From Tissues and organs: a text-atlas of scanning electron microscopy by Richard G. Kessel and Randy H. Kardon. W.H. Freeman and Company. Copyright © 1979.)

the spinal and cranial nerves will be discussed in subsequent chapters.

Wrappings

Peripheral nerves have three connective tissue coverings, each with a different function. From the outside layer in, these are the *epineurium*, the *perineurium*, and the *endoneurium* (Fig. 6-9).

The epineurium is a loose connective tissue sheath surrounding each peripheral nerve. Composed mainly of collagen and fibroblasts, it forms a substantial covering over nerve trunks, then thins to an incomplete layer around smaller branches near their terminations. The abundant longitudinally and spirally arranged collagen fibers of the epineurium are largely responsible for the considerable tensile strength of peripheral nerves. The epineurium is continuous centrally with the dura. Peripherally it usually ends near the termination of a nerve fiber, but it may continue as the capsule of Meissner's corpuscles and a few other encapsulated endings.

The perineurium, lying within the epineurium, is a layer of thin, concentrically arranged cells with interspersed collagen. Adjacent perineurial cells are connected to one another by tight junctions that effectively isolate the epineurial spaces from the endoneurial spaces around peripheral nerve fibers. In addition, the endothelial cells of capillaries within the perineurium are connected to one another by tight junctions. Thus functional equivalents of the arachnoid barrier and the blood-brain barrier persist in the peripheral nervous system. The perineurium continues as the capsule of some endings, such as pacinian corpuscles, muscle spindles, and Golgi tendon organs. However, at other places, such as near neuromuscular junctions, the perineurium is open ended, allowing the endoneurial space around nerve fibers to communicate with the general extracellular space of the body. This may be of clinical importance, since some evidence indicates that certain toxins and viruses may gain access to the nervous system at these sites.

The endoneurium is the loose connective tissue within the perineurium that continues into nerve fascicles and surrounds individual fibers. In at least some species, these individual endoneurial sheaths are compact enough that they may help to direct the regrowth of nerve fibers after injury.

Contents

Peripheral nerve fibers come in a wide range of diameters; some are myelinated, while others are not. There is some correlation between the size of a fiber and its function, so it has proven useful to subdivide them. Unfortunately there are two major classification systems, and neither is used universally for all fibers.

The first system is based on conduction velocity. Larger fibers conduct action potentials faster than do smaller fibers. If the compound action potential of a peripheral nerve is recorded at some distance from the site at which the nerve was stimulated electrically, the fast impulses will reach the recording electrode before the slower ones. Conduction velocities (and axonal diameters) are not distributed in a bell-shaped curve but rather in a curve with several peaks. Therefore the remotely recorded compound action potential will have several peaks corresponding to these favored conduction velocities. Three deflections can be easily demonstrated; they are named *A*, *B*, and *C*. The fibers responsible for the A deflection (the A fibers) are the myelinated sensory and motor fibers. B fibers are myelinated visceral fibers, both visceral afferents and preganglionic autonomic fibers. C fibers are unmyelinated. The A deflection is complex and was subdivided into α, β, γ, and δ peaks (α being the fastest). Although the β and γ peaks as originally described were probably recording artifacts, the terminology has become established in the literature and is still commonly used. Thus Aα fibers are the largest and most rapidly conducting myelinated fibers, and Aδ are the smallest and slowest of the A group.

The second classification system is based on direct microscopic measurement of axonal diameters. In this system myelinated fibers are placed into group *I*, *II*, or *III* in order of decreasing size. Unmyelinated fibers are group *IV*.

Portions of both systems are commonly used. In general, the letter system is used for myelinated efferent fibers and the roman numeral system for myelinated afferents. Unmyelinated fibers are interchangeably referred to as C fibers or group IV. The sizes, conduction velocities, and functional correlates involved in both systems are listed in Table 3 for reference purposes.

The commonly used terminology for efferent fibers is fairly simple. The large axons innervating the extrafusal fibers of skeletal muscle are in the Aα category, and the smaller axons innervating intrafusal muscle fibers are in the Aγ category. The "A" is commonly dropped, and these are simply called α and γ motor neurons. Preganglionic autonomic axons are usually called just that but may also be referred to as B fibers.

Myelinated afferents are slightly more complicated. The largest fibers, group I, are found only in muscle nerves; they form the primary endings of muscle spindles and innervate Golgi tendon organs. In order to distinguish between them, spindle primary fibers are called *Ia* and tendon organ fibers are called *Ib*. Group II is quite diverse and includes the fibers that form the secondary endings of muscle spindles and those that form all the encapsulated receptors of skin and joints. Group III consists of small myelinated afferents that form free nerve endings and includes mechanoreceptors, cold-sensitive thermoreceptors, and some nociceptors.

TABLE 3

Classification of peripheral nerve fibers

Roman numeral classification	Diameter	Letter classification	Conduction velocity	Myelinated	Types of structures innervated
Ia	12-20 μm	Not used	70-120 m/sec	Yes	Muscle spindle primary endings
Ib	12-20 μm	Not used	70-120 m/sec	Yes	Golgi tendon organs
Not used	12-20 μm	α	70-120 m/sec	Yes	Efferents to extrafusal muscle fibers
II	6-12+ μm	Aα*	30-70 m/sec	Yes	Other encapsulated endings and endings with accessory structures: Meissner's corpuscles, Merkel endings, muscle spindle secondary endings, etc.
Not used	2-10 μm	γ	10-50 m/sec	Yes	Efferents to intrafusal muscle fibers
III	1-6 μm	Aδ	5-30 m/sec	Yes	Some nociceptors Some cold receptors Some hair receptors
Not used	<3 μm	B	3-15 m/sec	Yes	Preganglionic autonomic efferents
IV	<1.5 μm	C	0.5-2 m/sec	No	Most nociceptors Some cold receptors Warmth receptors Some mechanoreceptors Postganglionic autonomic efferents

*Some afferents in nonmuscle nerves, particularly joint afferents, range up to 17 μm in diameter. Some investigators refer to these larger fibers, in the 12-17 μm range, as Aα and call those in the 6-12 μm range Aβ. Others refer to all nonmuscle afferents larger than 6 μm as Aα.

Group III corresponds to Aδ, and so these fibers are sometimes referred to as δ fibers.

SOME FUNCTIONAL ASPECTS OF THE PERIPHERAL NERVOUS SYSTEM
Receptors and sensation

Since we have so many different types of receptors, it was widely assumed in the past that different types are uniquely responsible for particular sensations. While this is true in a very general sense, the actual situation is somewhat more complicated. First, few situations dealing with mechanical stimuli (such as touch and movement) involve only one receptor type; it seems likely that under ordinary circumstances the overall pattern of activity in an array of receptors is important in determining the resulting sensation. This applies mainly to receptors that signal touch, position, and movement. Other types, such as photoreceptors and auditory receptors, are ordinarily stimulated selectively. Second, it is not possible, even with very small and carefully controlled stimuli, to demonstrate a one-to-one correlation of types of receptors and varieties of sensation. This is so at least partly because morphologically identical receptors can cause distinctly different sensations. For example, Ruffini endings in the skin signal touch, while those in joint capsules signal limb position and/or movement. Another example involves free nerve endings. It was long thought that stimulation of the cornea, which contains only free nerve endings, elicited only pain, thus

demonstrating that free nerve endings are nociceptors. However, careful study of trusting and courageous volunteers has shown that very gentle touches are recognized as such and are not painful, and that warm and cool stimuli can be correctly identified. This, along with abundant data from experimental animals, leads to the conclusion that some free nerve endings are nociceptors, but others are mechanoreceptors, and still others are thermoreceptors. All long receptors that are not free nerve endings are now thought to be mechanoreceptors of one sort or another.

Despite the fact that cutaneous receptors are usually stimulated in groups, threshold stimulation of single receptors can also give rise to sensation. This has been shown most elegantly in experiments on human volunteers. Recording from a single nerve fiber innervating a mechanoreceptor of the fingertip (almost certainly a Meissner's corpuscle), it was found that a tiny mechanical indentation of a few micrometers, just enough to cause a single action potential in the nerve fiber, gave rise to perception of the touch.

Pain

There are free nerve endings, some of whose axons are classified as group III and others as C fibers, and there are also some nociceptors in each group. Corresponding to this, pain is perceived in two different stages. If a painful stimulus is applied abruptly, there is an initial sensation of sharp, pricking, well-localized pain. This is followed by an aching, longer-lasting pain. The initial sharp pain is carried by the more rapidly conducting group III fibers, and since group III is the same as Aδ, it is sometimes referred to as *delta pain*. The aching pain that follows is carried by the more slowly conducting C fibers. This has been verified experimentally on human volunteers, since it is possible to block different classes of nerve fibers selectively. Local anesthetics applied to peripheral nerves block C fibers before myelinated fibers; during the period when only C fibers are blocked, a pinprick is felt only as a sharp, brief pain. Externally applied pressure, however, blocks axons in order of size, so that myelinated fibers can be blocked while C fibers continue to conduct. In this situation, most forms of tactile sensation disappear, and a pinprick is felt only as a dull, aching pain even more unpleasant than usual.

The two forms of pain apparently are processed differently within the CNS, so they may be dissociated at sites other than peripheral nerves. This is potentially of major clinical importance and will be discussed further in subsequent chapters.

Muscle receptors

The identity of the receptors involved in position sense and kinesthesia (conscious awareness of movement) has long been a topic of debate. It was generally assumed in the past that joint receptors are primarily responsible, and that the output of muscle spindles and Golgi tendon organs does not reach consciousness, being utilized in subconscious motor feedback circuits and in reflexes. While it is true that joint receptors are of major importance, the role of muscle spindles has recently been reexamined, and new evidence indicates that they are probably involved as well. If tendons of human volunteers are vibrated (through the skin), illusions of movement and altered perceptions of position are experienced at the joints where the muscles of these tendons act. A vibrating stimulus of moderate intensity should be ineffective at activating Golgi tendon organs, but it should activate muscle spindles. In particular, it should excite the primary endings, since these are especially sensitive to changing stimuli. The conclusion that muscle receptors are ordinarily involved in kinesthesia and position sense is still somewhat controversial, but the evidence is becoming more and more convincing.

Clinical correlations

Causalgia sometimes follows injury (such as a partial transection) to a peripheral nerve. The patient has episodes of severe burning pain in the area of distribution of the affected nerve. The pain may be triggered by normally trivial stimuli, such as the mere pressure of clothing, or by emotional states. The exact mechanism of causalgia is not known, but it is usually associated with autonomic disturbances in the affected area and is frequently relieved by sympathetic blockade. This has led to the conjecture that efferent sympathetic activity somehow stimulates C fibers at the site of injury, and the subsequent activity is then perceived as pain. Another explanation relies on the phenomenon, noted previously, that activity restricted to C fibers (during blockade of the myelinated fibers) causes particularly intense pain. This led some investigators to reason that if myelinated fibers were selectively stimulated in patients with causalgia, then the normal "balance" of activity between large and small fibers would be restored, and the pain would be relieved. Amazingly enough, this works in many patients. Small electrodes placed on the skin over the affected nerve (proximal to the lesion), if adjusted to stimulate only myelinated fibers, can provide dramatic relief from pain. The relief can outlast the electrical stimulus by minutes or even hours.

Most people think that freedom from pain would be a terrific condition. However, pain has a useful function, which is to warn us of damage; its absence is actually a handicap. Some rare individuals are born without the capability to feel pain. They characteristically have many injuries that heal poorly or remain unhealed. They may fracture bones without ever realizing it, have mutilated fingers and toes, or incur serious burns. The deficit may involve only the sensation of pain, but sometimes other forms of sensation are involved as well. The condition takes several different forms. Some patients have a selective loss of C fibers in their peripheral nerves; others have apparently normal nerves, so in these cases the disorder is probably within the CNS.

ADDITIONAL READING

Andres, K.H., and Düring, M.V.: Morphology of cutaneous receptors. In Iggo, A., editor: Handbook of sensory physiology, vol. II: Somatosensory system, New York, 1973, Springer-Verlag, Inc.

Bannister, L.H.: Sensory terminals of peripheral nerves. In Landon, D.N., editor: The peripheral nerve, London, 1976, Chapman & Hall Ltd. *A nicely written overview of the anatomy and physiology of somatic, olfactory, and gustatory receptors.*

Burgess, P.R., and Perl, E.R.: Cutaneous mechanoreceptors and nociceptors. In Iggo, A., editor: Handbook of sensory physiology, vol II: Somatosensory system, New York, 1973, Springer-Verlag, Inc.

Burkel, W.E.: The histological fine structure of perineurium, Anat. Rec. **158:**177, 1967

Chambers, M.R., et al.: The structure and function of the slowly adapting type II mechanoreceptor in hairy skin, Quart. J. Exp. Physiol. **57:**417, 1972. *The anatomy and physiology of the Ruffini ending of the cat.*

Craske, B.: Perception of impossible limb position induced by tendon vibration, Science **196:**71, 1977.

Dyson, C., and Brindley, G.S.: Strength-duration curves for the production of cutaneous pain by electrical stimuli, Clin. Sci. **30:**237, 1966. *Direct production of both sharp, pricking pain and slow, burning pain by small electrical stimuli.*

Gandevia, S.C., and McCloskey, D.I.: Joint sense, muscle sense, and their combination as position sense, measured at the distal interphalangeal joint of the middle finger, J. Physiol. 260:387, 1976. *Clever experiments taking advantage of an anatomical quirk of the middle finger. This finger can be positioned in such a way that muscles and their receptors are functionally disengaged from its terminal phalanx, so the position sense of the distal interphalangeal joint can be measured both with and without a contribution from muscle receptors.*

Goodwin, G.M., McCloskey, D.I., and Matthews, P.B.C.: The contribution of muscle afferents to kinaesthesia shown by vibration induced illusions of movement and by the effects of paralysing joint afferents, Brain 95:705, 1972. *This paper sparked the recent reinvestigation of the role of muscle spindles in our sense of position and movement. It contains a skeptical review of the earlier literature on this topic as well as several simple but interesting experiments.*

Hallin, R.G., and Torebjörk, H.E.: Studies on cutaneous A and C fibre afferents, skin nerve blocks and perception. In Zotterman, Y., editor: Sensory functions of the skin of primates, Elmsford, N.Y., 1976, Pergamon Press. *A description of experiments involving recordings from the radial nerve; the experimenter notes afferent fiber activity in response to stimulation, and the experimentee reports his sensations, all during selective block of A fibers by pressure or of C fibers by a local anesthetic.*

Hensel, H.: Cutaneous thermoreceptors. In Iggo, A., editor: Handbook of sensory physiology, vol. II: Somatosensory system, New York, 1973, Springer-Verlag, Inc.

Houk, J., and Henneman, E.: Responses of Golgi tendon organs to active contraction of the soleus muscle of the cat, J. Neurophysiol. 30:466, 1967. *The experiments that demonstrated that tendon organs are really highly sensitive receptors when responding to muscle contraction.*

Iggo, A.: Cutaneous receptors. In Hubbard, J.I., editor: The peripheral nervous system, New York, 1974, Plenum Press. *A nice, detailed review of the anatomy and physiology of cutaneous receptors.*

Iggo, A., and Muir, A.R.: The structure and function of a slowly adapting touch corpuscle in hairy skin, J. Physiol. 200:763, 1969. *The slowly adapting receptor of this paper is the Merkel cell–neurite complex of the cat.*

Kenshalo, D.R., and Gallegos, E.S.: Multiple temperature-sensitive spots innervated by single nerve fibers, Science 158:1064, 1967.

Landau, W., and Bishop, G.H.: Pain from dermal, periosteal, and fascial endings and from inflammation: electrophysiological study employing differential nerve block, Arch. Neurol. Psychiatr. 69:490, 1953. *The volunteers in this case were the authors themselves who,*

with admirable fortitude, studied the effects of pressure blocks and local anesthetics on the pain caused by needles, bee stings, and other methods.

Lele, P.P., and Weddell, G.: The relationship between neurohistology and corneal sensibility, Brain 79:119, 1956. *Experiments on brave subjects who sat still while their corneas were touched with nylon sutures of various sizes and with warm and cool copper rods.*

Low, F.N.: The perineurium and connective tissue of peripheral nerve. In Landon, D.N., editor: The peripheral nerve, London, 1976, Chapman & Hall Ltd.

Matthews, P.B.C.: Mammalian muscle receptors and their central actions, London, 1973, Edward Arnold (Publishers) Ltd.

McCloskey, D.I.: Kinesthetic sensibility, Physiol. Rev. 58:763, 1978.

Murthy, K.S.K.: Vertebrate fusimotor neurones and their influences on motor behavior, Prog. Neurobiol. 11:249, 1978.

Olsson, Y., and Reese, T.S.: Inaccessibility of the endoneurium of mouse sciatic nerve to exogenous proteins, Anat. Rec. 163:318, 1969.

Pease, D.C.: and Quilliam, T.A.: Electron microscopy of the Pacinian corpuscle, J. Biophys. Biochem. Cytol. 3:331, 1957.

Schoultz, T.W., and Swett, J.E.: The fine structure of the Golgi tendon organ, J. Neurocytol. 1:1, 1972.

Shanthaveerappa, T.R., and Bourne, G.H.: Perineural epithelium: a new concept of its role in the integrity of the peripheral nervous system, Science 154:1464, 1966.

Skoglund, S.: Joint receptors and kinaesthesis. In Iggo, A., editor: Handbook of sensory physiology, vol. II: Somatosensory system, New York, 1973, Springer-Verlag, Inc.

Swash, M., and Fox, K.P.: Muscle spindle innervation in man, J. Anat. 112:61, 1972.

Thrush, D.C.: Congenital insensitivity to pain: a clinical genetic and neurophysiological study of four children from the same family, Brain. 96:369, 1973.

Vallbo, Å.B., et al.: Somatosensory, proprioceptive, and sympathetic activity in human peripheral nerves, Physiol. Rev. 59:919, 1979.

Vallbo, Å.B., and Johansson, R.: Skin mechanoreceptors in the human hand: neural and psychophysical thresholds. In Zotterman, Y., editor: Sensory functions of the skin of primates, Elmsford, N.Y., 1976, Pergamon Press. *A fascinating study providing evidence that a single impulse in a fiber innervating a Meissner corpuscle in the fingertip leads to the perception of touch.*

Widdicombe, J.G.: Enteroceptors. In Hubbard, J.I., editor: The peripheral nervous system, New York, 1974, Plenum Press.

Winkelmann, R.K., Lambert, E.H., and Hayles, A.B.: Congenital absence of pain, Arch. Derm. 85:325, 1962.

CHAPTER 7

SPINAL CORD

The spinal cord is the traditional starting point for a detailed consideration of the central nervous system. It is a very uniformly organized part of the CNS and also one of the simplest (in a relative sense), but many principles of cord function apply to other levels of the nervous system. It is, at the same time, extraordinarily important in the day-to-day activities we tend not to think about: it gives rise to all the motor neurons to the muscles we use to move our bodies around and to many autonomic efferents; it also receives all the sensory input from the body and part of the head and performs the initial processing operations on most of this input.

GROSS ANATOMY

The adult human spinal cord appears surprisingly small on first inspection, being only about 42 to 45 cm long and about 1 cm in diameter at its widest point. It weighs about 35 g, so one could be mailed for just two stamps. It is anatomically segmented—not obviously like an earthworm but in terms of the nerve roots attached to it (Fig. 7-1). A continuous series of dorsal rootlets enter the cord in a shallow longitudinal groove (the *posterolateral sulcus*) on its posterolateral surface, and a continuous series of ventral rootlets leave from the poorly defined *anterolateral sulcus*. The dorsal and ventral root-

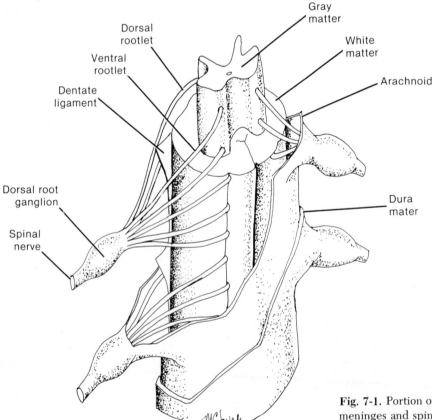

Fig. 7-1. Portion of the spinal cord, showing its relationship to meninges and spinal nerves.

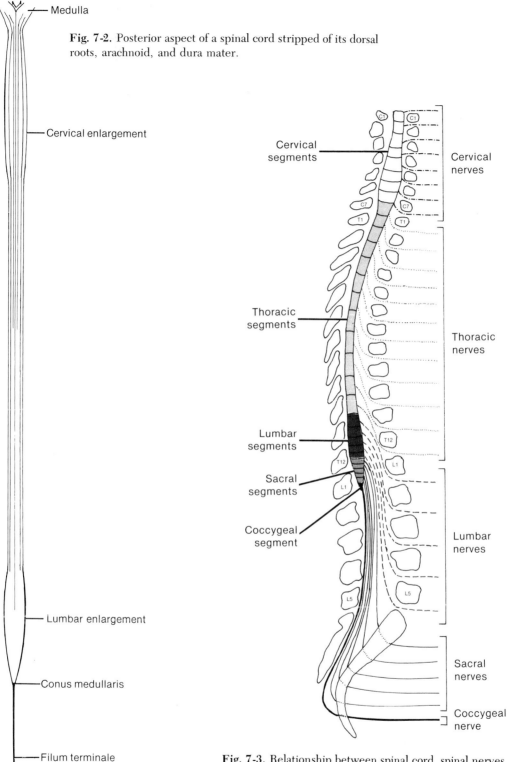

Fig. 7-2. Posterior aspect of a spinal cord stripped of its dorsal roots, arachnoid, and dura mater.

Fig. 7-3. Relationship between spinal cord, spinal nerves, and vertebral column. Note that cervical nerves except C8 emerge *above* the corresponding vertebrae, C8 emerges *between* the C7 and T1 vertebrae, and remaining nerves emerge *below* the corresponding vertebrae. (Modified from Barr, M.L.: The human nervous system, ed. 3, Hagerstown, Md., 1979, Harper and Row, Publishers.)

lets from discrete sections of the cord coalesce to form *dorsal* and *ventral roots*, which in turn join to form *spinal nerves*. Each dorsal root bears a *dorsal root ganglion* just proximal to the junction between dorsal and ventral roots; it contains the cell bodies of virtually all the primary sensory neurons whose processes travel through that particular spinal nerve. A portion of the cord that gives rise to a spinal nerve constitutes a *segment*. There are 31 segments in the human spinal cord: 8 *cervical*, 12 *thoracic*, 5 *lumbar*, 5 *sacral*, and 1 *coccygeal*.

The spinal cord itself, stripped of its dorsal and ventral rootlets, gives no obvious sign of segmentation. Rather, it is a continuous column, with two enlargements, which ends caudally in the pointed *conus medullaris* (Fig. 7-2). The two enlargements occur in those regions of the cord that supply the upper and lower extremities and therefore contain increased numbers of motor neurons and interneurons. The limits of the enlargements are not distinct, but the *cervical enlargement* (which supplies the upper extremities) is conventionally considered to extend from the fifth cervical to the first thoracic segment (C5 to T1), inclusive. The *lumbar* (or *lumbosacral*), enlargement (which supplies the lower extremities) extends from the second lumbar to the third sacral segment (L2 to S3).

The spinal cord approaches its adult length long before the vertebral canal does. Until the third month of fetal life, both grow at about the same rate, and the cord fills the canal. Thereafter the body and the vertebral column grow faster than the spinal cord does, so that at the time of birth the spinal cord ends at the third lumbar vertebra. A small additional amount of differential growth in the vertebral column occurs subsequent to this, and in the adult the cord ends at about the level of the disk between the first and second lumbar vertebrae. However, the spinal nerves still exit through the same intervertebral foramina as they did early in development, and each dorsal root ganglion remains at the level of the appropriate foramen. Proceeding from cervical levels to sacral levels the dorsal and ventral roots become progressively longer, since they have longer and longer distances to travel before reaching their sites of exit from the vertebral canal (Fig. 7-3). The *lumbar cistern*, from the end of the spinal cord at vertebral level L1 to L2 to the end of the dural sheath at vertebral level S2, is filled with this collection of dorsal and ventral roots, collectively referred to as the *cauda equina* (Latin = horse's tail).

Each of the first seven cervical nerves leaves the vertebral canal above the corresponding vertebra: the

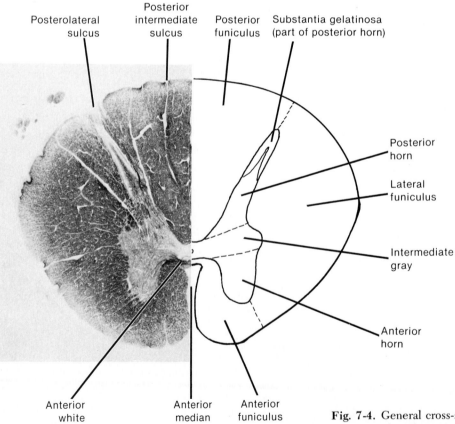

Posterolateral sulcus

Posterior intermediate sulcus

Posterior funiculus

Substantia gelatinosa (part of posterior horn)

Posterior horn

Lateral funiculus

Intermediate gray

Anterior horn

Anterior white commissure

Anterior median fissure

Anterior funiculus

Fig. 7-4. General cross-sectional anatomy of the spinal cord, represented in this case by the second cervical segment.

first cervical nerve leaves between the occiput and the first cervical vertebra (the atlas), the second leaves between the first and second cervical vertebrae (the atlas and the axis), and so on. However, because there are only seven cervical vertebrae, the eighth cervical nerve leaves between the seventh cervical and first thoracic vertebrae, and each of the subsequent nerves leaves *below* the corresponding vertebra (Fig. 7-3).

The meningeal coverings of the spinal cord were described in Chapter 3 (Figs. 3-11 and 7-1). The cord is suspended within an arachnoid-lined dural tube by the dentate ligaments, which are extensions of the pia mater. In addition, the caudal end of the cord is anchored to the end of the dural tube by the *filum terminale,* an extension of the pial covering of the conus medullaris. The filum terminale then acquires a dural outer layer and is in turn anchored to the coccyx.

INTERNAL STRUCTURE

In cross section, the spinal cord consists of a roughly H-shaped area of gray matter than floats like a butterfly in a surround of white matter. The gray matter can be divided into *horns* and the white matter into *funiculi* (Latin, funiculus = string) (Fig. 7-4). Keep in mind that the spinal cord is, to a great extent, a longitudinally organized structure, even though it is most conveniently studied in cross section. For example, the posterior gray horns are continuous cell columns rather than a series of discrete nuclei, and at any given level the posterior horn cells interact with cells from many other levels.

In addition to the posterolateral and anterolateral sulci, several other longitudinal grooves indent the cross-sectional outline of the cord (Fig. 7-4). The deep *anterior median fissure* extends almost to the center of the cord; at the apex of this fissure, only a thin zone of white matter (the *anterior white commissure*) and a thin zone of gray matter separate the central canal from subarachnoid space. The *posterior median sulcus* is much less distinct, but a glial septum extends from it all the way to the gray matter surrounding the central canal. There is therefore only a narrow band of neural tissue through which the two sides of the spinal cord can communicate with each other. Since the fibers of many ascending pathways cross the midline in the spinal cord, this small area where crossing occurs can become very important clinically in diseases affecting the center of the cord. Finally, at cervical and upper thoracic levels, a *posterior intermediate sulcus* is found. Another glial septum projects from this sulcus, partially subdividing each posterior funiculus.

GENERAL ORGANIZATION

The spinal cord is involved in the following three types of activity.

1. *Sensory processing.* Afferent fibers enter the cord via the dorsal roots*; these fibers either ascend directly to relay nuclei in the brainstem or synapse on interneurons and tract cells in the posterior horn and intermediate gray (or both). These tract cells of the spinal gray matter then project their axons through defined sensory pathways of the spinal white matter to more rostral structures. As a general rule, each primary afferent fiber gives rise to many branches and feeds into more than one ascending sensory pathway as well as into local reflex circuits.

2. *Motor outflow.* The motor neurons that innervate skeletal muscle are located in the anterior horns, and many preganglionic autonomic neurons are located in the intermediate gray matter of appropriate segments. The axons of these motor neurons leave the cord in the ventral roots. Activity in these neurons is modulated by pathways that descend through the spinal white matter from the cerebral cortex and from various brainstem structures.

3. *Reflexes.* Certain specified afferent inputs cause stereotyped motor outputs, as in the familiar knee jerk reflex. Many of these involve neural circuitry that is wholly contained within the spinal cord; several examples will be discussed in this chapter.

SPINAL GRAY MATTER
Posterior horn

The posterior horn consists mainly of interneurons whose processes remain within the spinal cord and of tract cells whose axons collect into long ascending sensory pathways. There are three parts to this area of gray matter, two of which are present at all spinal levels and the third only at some levels. These parts are the *substantia gelatinosa, nucleus proprius,* and *Clarke's nucleus.*

The substantia gelatinosa is a distinctive region of gray matter that caps the posterior horn at all spinal levels (Fig. 7-5). In myelin-stained preparations, this region looks very pale compared to the rest of the gray matter, since it mostly deals with the finely myelinated and unmyelinated sensory fibers that carry pain and temperature information. Between the substantia gelatinosa and the surface of the cord is a relatively pale-staining area of white matter called the *dorsolateral fasciculus* (or

---

*The Bell-Magendie law, a long-standing neuroanatomical tenet, states that the dorsal root comprises solely primary afferent fibers and the ventral root solely efferent fibers of various sorts. However, recent evidence indicates that a significant number of the ventral root fibers of the cat are finely myelinated or unmyelinated primary afferents. Preliminary findings indicate that the same may be true for humans and that the ventral root afferents may be at least partially responsible for the persistence or the return of pain after the dorsal roots have been sectioned.

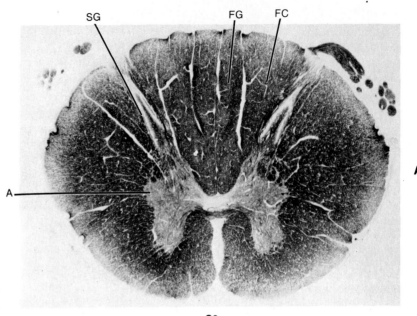

A

C2

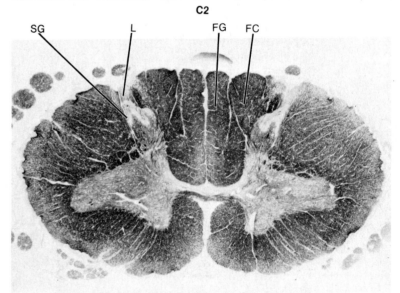

B

C8

Fig. 7-5. Cross sections of the spinal cord at various levels; note the large lateral extensions of the anterior horns in C8 and L2. Scale mark is 5 mm for all sections. *A,* Spinal accessory nucleus; *C,* Clarke's nucleus; *FC,* fasciculus cuneatus; *FG,* fasciculus gracilis; *IL,* intermediolateral cell column; *L,* Lissauer's tract; *SG,* substantia gelatinosa.

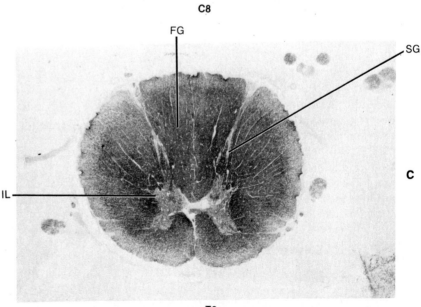

C

T6

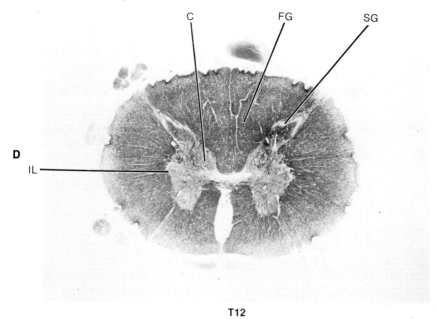

D

C   FG   SG

IL

T12

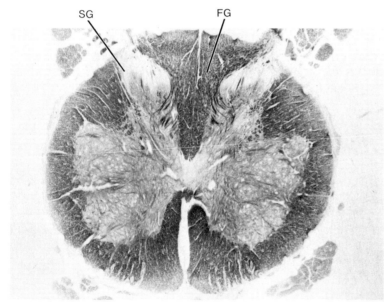

E

SG   FG

L5

Fig. 7-5, cont'd. For legend see opposite page.

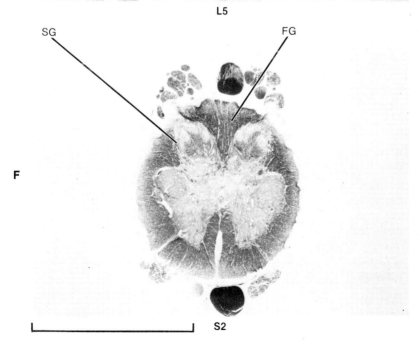

F

SG   FG

S2

Lissauer's tract). This fasciculus stains more lightly than the rest of the white matter, because it contains the finely myelinated and unmyelinated fibers with which the substantia gelatinosa deals.

Nucleus proprius is a general term for the bulk of the posterior horn, consisting mainly of interneurons and tract cells that transmit many types of somatic and visceral sensory information. In this respect, it functionally overlaps parts of the intermediate gray matter.

Clarke's nucleus (or *nucleus dorsalis*) is a rounded collection of large cells located on the medial surface of the base of the posterior horn from about T1 to L2 or L3. It is particularly prominent at lower thoracic levels (Fig. 7-5). This is an important relay nucleus for the transmission of information to the cerebellum.

Anterior horn

The anterior horn contains the cell bodies of the large motor neurons that supply skeletal muscle. These alpha motor neurons, also referred to as *lower motor neurons*, are the only means by which the nervous system can exercise control over body movements, whether voluntary or involuntary; a number of different pathways and parts of the nervous system can influence these lower motor neurons, but they alone can effect muscle contraction. Interruption of the lower motor neurons supplying a muscle therefore causes complete paralysis of that muscle. The paralysis is of a type called *flaccid paralysis*, indicating that the muscle is limp and uncontracted. Reflex contractions can no longer be elicited, and the muscle slowly atrophies (for reasons that are not understood). This occurs, for example, in poliomyelitis, a viral disease that attacks the motor neurons of the anterior horn, and in injuries in which ventral roots are damaged.

Alpha motor neurons occur in groups, separated from each other by areas of interneurons; the groups that innervate axial muscles are medial to those that innervate limb muscles. In the cervical and lumbar enlargements, which contain the limb motor neurons, the anterior horns are enlarged laterally (Fig. 7-5).

Smaller gamma motor neurons are interspersed with alpha motor neurons in all such groups. They innervate the intrafusal muscle fibers of muscle spindles, and so they are also referred to as *fusimotor neurons*.

Two columns of motor neurons in the anterior horn of the cervical cord are recognized as separate entities. The *spinal accessory nucleus* extends from C1 to C5 or C6 and forms a rounded bump on the lateral surface of the ventral horn (Fig. 7-5). The axons of these motor neurons emerge from the lateral surface of the spinal cord just posterior to the dentate ligament as a separate series of rootlets that form the spinal part of the accessory nerve (Fig. 2-12). The *phrenic nucleus*, containing the motor neurons that innervate the diaphragm, is located in the medial portion of the anterior horn in segments C3 to C5. This makes injuries to the upper cervical spinal cord a matter of very grave concern, since destruction of the descending pathways that control the phrenic nucleus and other respiratory motor neurons renders a patient unable to breathe.

Intermediate gray matter

The gray matter that is intermediate to the anterior and posterior horns has some characteristics of both and also contains the spinal preganglionic autonomic neurons. From T1 through L2 or L3, the preganglionic sympathetic neurons for the entire body lie in a column of cells, the *intermediolateral cell column*, which forms a pointy lateral horn on the spinal gray matter (Fig. 7-5). Their axons leave through the ventral roots. Cells in a corresponding location in segments S2 to S4 form the *sacral parasympathetic nucleus* but do not form a distinct lateral horn. Their axons leave through the ventral roots and synapse on the postganglionic parasympathetic neurons for the pelvic viscera.

The remainder of the intermediate gray matter is a collection of various tract cells, sensory interneurons, and interneurons that synapse on motor neurons.

Rexed's laminae

A system was devised by Rexed in 1952 for subdividing the gray matter of the cat's spinal cord into layers, or laminae. The same system has since been applied to the cord of other mammals, including humans (Fig. 7-6). *Lamina I* is a thin layer of gray matter that covers the

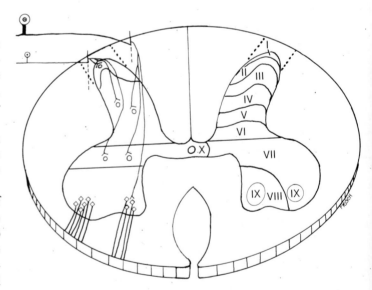

Fig. 7-6. Laminae of Rexed are indicated on the right, and general kinds of cells and connections in these different areas are indicated on the left.

substantia gelatinosa, *lamina II* is the substantia gelatinosa, and *laminae III through VI* are the remainder of the dorsal horn; *lamina VII* roughly corresponds to the intermediate gray matter but also includes Clarke's nucleus and some extensions into the anterior horn; *lamina VIII* comprises most of the interneuronal zones of the anterior horn, while *lamina IX* is the clusters of motor neurons embedded in the anterior horn; *lamina X* is the zone of gray matter surrounding the central canal.

This terminology has proven quite useful for experimental anatomists and physiologists, since the histological differences between the laminae correspond to functional differences. Clinically, however, it has not come into common usage.

REFLEXES

A reflex is an involuntary, stereotyped response to a sensory input. All reflex pathways therefore must involve at least a receptor structure and associated afferent neuron (with its cell body in a dorsal root ganglion or some other sensory ganglion) and an efferent neuron (with its cell body within the CNS). With the exception of the *stretch reflex*, all reflexes involve one or more interneurons as well.

Reflexes range from the very simple ones described in this chapter (which serve as a useful introduction to neural integration and are the basis for common clinical tests) to neural subroutines so complex that calling them "reflexes" seems an oversimplification. For example, a cat with its spinal cord transected at thoracic levels can, under certain conditions, perform coordinated walking movements with its hindlimbs. If its hind feet are placed on a moving treadmill, the gait changes in a predictable fashion with the speed of the treadmill, from alternating stepping movements at low speeds to galloping movements (in which both legs move together in phase) at higher speeds.

Stretch reflex

All skeletal muscles have a tendency, more pronounced in some than others, to contract in response to being stretched. The reflex arc responsible for this contraction is the simplest possible, since it involves only two neurons and a single intervening synapse. It is therefore sometimes referred to as the *monosynaptic reflex* or the *myotatic reflex* (Greek, mys = muscle; tasis = stretch). The afferent limb of the arc is a Ia afferent with its associated muscle spindle primary ending. Central processes of the Ia afferent synapse within the spinal cord directly on the alpha motor neurons that innervate the muscle containing the stimulated spindle (Fig. 7-7).

The stretch reflex is commonly used for clinical testing purposes. Tapping the patellar tendon, as in the familiar *knee jerk reflex*, stretches the quadriceps slightly. Ia endings in quadriceps muscle spindles are excited and in turn excite quadriceps alpha motor neurons; these in turn cause the quadriceps to contract, completing the reflex. Similarly, tapping the Achilles tendon stretches the gastrocnemius slightly, thereby causing a reflex contraction. Since stretch reflexes are usually elicited by tapping a tendon, they are often referred to as *deep tendon reflexes* (sometimes abbreviated DTR). One should remember that even though the reflex is studied in this manner, the responsible receptors are actually in the muscles attached to the tapped tendons.

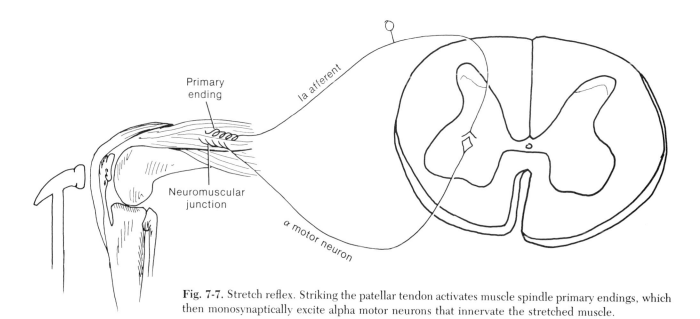

Fig. 7-7. Stretch reflex. Striking the patellar tendon activates muscle spindle primary endings, which then monosynaptically excite alpha motor neurons that innervate the stretched muscle.

Stretch reflexes are important for the constant automatic corrections we perform during movements and postures. As an example, when we stand still and upright, we actually sway to and fro a bit. Each time we sway in one direction, some muscles are stretched and the resulting reflex contraction returns us toward the desired position.

There must, however, be more to the stretch reflex system, or else we would be unable to sit. Sitting should stretch the quadriceps just as tapping the patellar tendon does; reflex contraction of the quadriceps would then be expected to oppose the sitting movement. The answer to this apparent dilemma lies in the gamma motor neurons. During the act of sitting, the gamma motor neurons to quadriceps muscle spindles decrease their firing rate. This decreases the excitability of the quadriceps spindles just enough that they do not respond to the stretch imposed by sitting. The activities of the alpha and gamma motor neuron populations are coordinated generally during movements; this is discussed in more detail in Chapter 12.

Autogenic inhibition

Stimulation of a Ib fiber, from a Golgi tendon organ, has an opposite effect to that of stimulating a Ia fiber: the alpha motor neurons that innervate the muscle connected to that tendon organ are inhibited. This effect is termed *autogenic inhibition* and involves an inhibitory interneuron between the afferent and efferent fibers (Fig. 7-8).

The normal role of this reflex arc is unclear at present. It is frequently stated that it is protective in nature, preventing muscles from developing excess tension. However, in view of the great sensitivity of tendon organs to actively generated tension, it is clear that the reflex should be activated long before hazardous levels are reached. Therefore it seems likely that autogenic inhibition plays an as-yet-unknown role in ordinary motor activities.

Clinically this reflex is manifested in a phenomenon called the *clasp-knife reflex*. In certain pathological conditions following damage to descending motor pathways, the resistance of muscles to manipulation is greatly increased. Thus one would have considerable difficulty flexing the leg of such an individual. If sufficient force is applied, however, the leg slowly flexes until at some point all resistance suddenly disappears and the leg collapses in flexion like a clasp knife snapping shut. This collapse of resistance is commonly attributed to autogenic inhibition initiated by Golgi tendon organs.

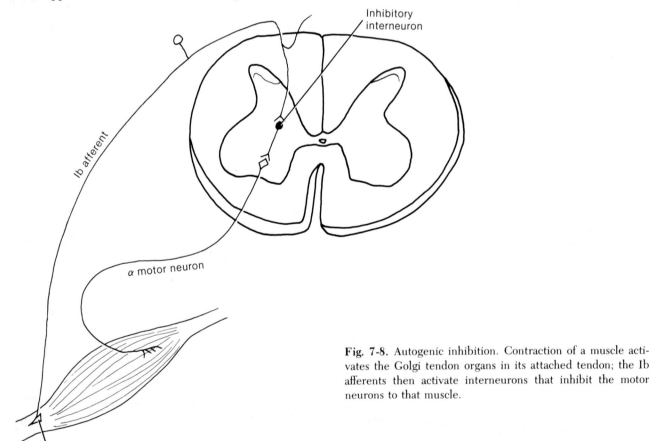

Fig. 7-8. Autogenic inhibition. Contraction of a muscle activates the Golgi tendon organs in its attached tendon; the Ib afferents then activate interneurons that inhibit the motor neurons to that muscle.

Flexor reflex

Whereas stretch reflexes and autogenic inhibition are initiated by muscle or tendon receptors and primarily involve the muscle stretched or tensed, the *flexor reflex* is initiated by cutaneous receptors and involves a whole limb. A familiar example is withdrawal from a painful stimulus: after accidentally touching something painfully hot, we automatically remove the offended hand from that vicinity by flexing the arm to which it is attached.

The flexor reflex pathways in the spinal cord are normally held in a somewhat inhibited state by descending influences from the brainstem, so that only noxious stimuli result in a strong reflex. If these descending influences are removed, either surgically in experimental animals or as a result of certain pathological conditions, reflex flexion can result from harmless tactile stimulation. This indicates that most or all cutaneous receptors feed into the pathway, but ordinarily only nociceptors have a powerful enough influence to cause a reflex withdrawal.

Since the flexor reflex involves an entire limb, its pathway must spread over several spinal segments to include the motor neurons innervating all the various flexor muscles of that limb. This spreading occurs in two ways. First, all primary afferent fibers bifurcate on entering the spinal cord, and their processes then extend one or more segments in both rostral and caudal directions. Second, the flexor pathway includes at least one interneuron, which itself may have processes extending over several segments (Fig. 7-9).

Although this reflex is usually called the flexor reflex, the term "withdrawal reflex" is also used and is perhaps more appropriate. The reflex is not an all-or-none phenomenon for a given limb but rather shows different

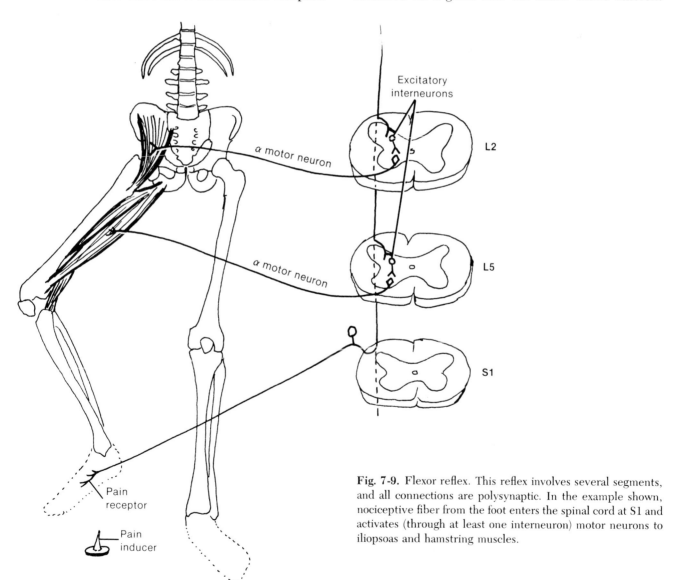

Fig. 7-9. Flexor reflex. This reflex involves several segments, and all connections are polysynaptic. In the example shown, nociceptive fiber from the foot enters the spinal cord at S1 and activates (through at least one interneuron) motor neurons to iliopsoas and hamstring muscles.

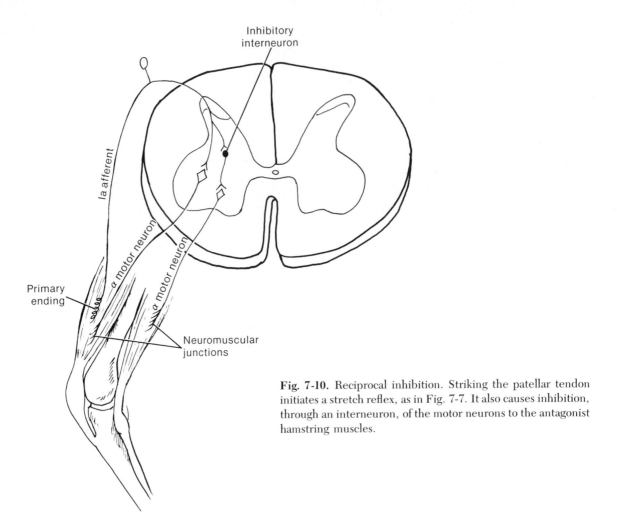

Inhibitory
interneuron

Ia afferent

α motor neuron

α motor neuron

Primary
ending

Neuromuscular
junctions

Fig. 7-10. Reciprocal inhibition. Striking the patellar tendon initiates a stretch reflex, as in Fig. 7-7. It also causes inhibition, through an interneuron, of the motor neurons to the antagonist hamstring muscles.

patterns depending on which portion of the limb is stimulated (the pattern being appropriate to withdraw the stimulated area). It would be imprudent to flex a lower extremity when a painful stimulus was applied to the anterior surface of its thigh, since this would drive the thigh into the stimulus. In such a situation, it would make much more sense to activate the extensors, which is in fact what happens. Modification of the reflex response so that it reflects the area being stimulated is called *local sign*.

Reciprocal and crossed effects

So far, we have given a simplified description of reflex circuits, including only the most direct and dominant motor effects. However, these reflexes also include weaker influences on other muscles of the same limb and even of contralateral limbs.

It would clearly be easier to shorten a stretched muscle if the motor neurons to its synergists were excited and those to its antagonists inhibited. This actually does occur and is a general principle in all reflexes: reflex activity in a given muscle produces similar activity in its ipsilateral synergists and the opposite activity in its ipsilateral antagonists (Fig. 7-10). Thus the standard tap on the patellar tendon causes not only excitation of quadriceps motor neurons but also inhibition (through an interneuron) of motor neurons to the hamstring muscles. If one extensor muscle of the thigh were selectively stretched, its motor neurons would be monosynaptically excited, as would those of all the other thigh extensors. After stimulation of a Golgi tendon organ the pattern is just the reverse. If tension is applied to the patellar tendon, the quadriceps is inhibited and the hamstring muscles are excited, both actions occurring through interneurons. Finally, the flexor reflex is accompanied by inhibition of the extensors of that limb.

The crossed effects in reflex actions are most easily understood with reference to the flexor reflex (Fig. 7-11). If the only effect of stepping on a tack with the right foot were withdrawal of the right leg, then the maladaptive behavior of falling over and possibly landing on the tack might follow. This is avoided by a simultaneous and opposite pattern of activity in the contralateral limb; as the right leg flexes and withdraws, the left leg extends

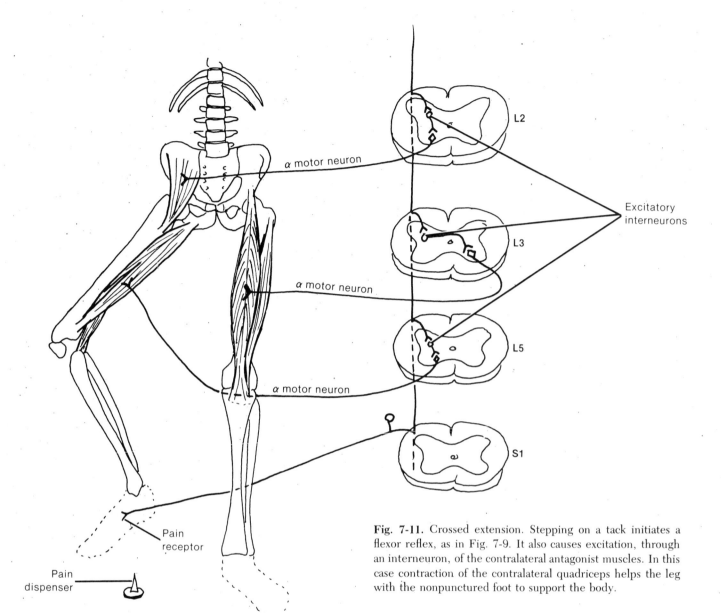

Fig. 7-11. Crossed extension. Stepping on a tack initiates a flexor reflex, as in Fig. 7-9. It also causes excitation, through an interneuron, of the contralateral antagonist muscles. In this case contraction of the contralateral quadriceps helps the leg with the nonpunctured foot to support the body.

and is thus better able to support the body. Similar observations have been made after stimulation of muscle spindles and Golgi tendon organs, although the effects on contralateral antagonists are not pronounced.

These crossed effects may be the basic building blocks for more complex subroutines, such as those for coordinated stepping movements referred to earlier.

SPINAL WHITE MATTER

The nerve fibers in the white matter of the spinal cord are of three general types:
1. Long ascending fibers projecting to the thalamus, the cerebellum, or various brainstem nuclei.
2. Long descending fibers projecting from the cerebral cortex or from various brainstem nuclei to the spinal gray matter.

3. Shorter *propriospinal* fibers interconnecting various spinal cord levels, such as the fibers responsible for the coordination of flexor reflexes.

Fibers having similar functions tend to travel together, forming the various tracts of the spinal cord. Propriospinal fibers mostly remain in a thin shell surrounding the gray matter called the *propriospinal tract* or *fasciculus proprius* (Latin, fasciculus = little bundle); descending tracts are found in the lateral and anterior funiculi; ascending tracts are found in the posterior, lateral, and anterior funiculi.

A great many ascending and descending tracts have been described, largely on the basis of their origins and terminations; the function of some is unknown. In this chapter we will describe the largest and best-known tracts descending from the cerebral cortex or ascending to the cerebellum or the thalamus. We will defer consideration of several other tracts until the structures where they arise or terminate are discussed.

Ascending pathways

There is a tendency to think of individual primary afferents as performing a single function (for example, either participating in a particular reflex arc or transmitting information to a single ascending tract). Single fibers are drawn that way in textbooks for convenience and clarity, but in fact each primary afferent probably participates in one or more reflex arcs and also in one or more ascending tracts. In a similar way, there is a tendency to think of particular sensory functions as uniquely associated with particular tracts (for example, pain with one tract and touch with another), so that damage to an ascending tract should result in total loss of some sensory function. This is not actually the case, and most kinds of sensory information reach the thalamus and the cerebellum by more than one route. It is not understood why this is so and what the consequences are in an intact nervous system, but one result is that the loss of a single tract can often be compensated for, to a surprising extent, by the remaining tracts.

The following section describes the principal pathways by which somatic sensory information reaches the thalamus and the cerebellum. Information that reaches the thalamus is relayed to the cerebral cortex and perceived consciously. Information that reaches the cerebellum is used in the regulation of motor patterns; we are not consciously aware of cerebellar activity.

Pathways to the thalamus and cortex. There are two traditionally important routes for somatic sensory information to reach the thalamus (the *posterior column– medial lemniscus* pathway and the *spinothalamic tract*), and one more recently discovered route (the *spinocervical tract*) that may also be of considerable importance. Two generalizations may be made about ascending somatosensory pathways of the spinal cord:

1. Most somatosensory information travels in more than one pathway.
2. Tracts in the posterior half of the cord ascend uncrossed (that is, ipsilateral to the dorsal roots whose information they carry), while those in the anterior half of the cord cross the midline as they form.

Posterior columns. The term "posterior column" refers to the entire contents of a posterior funiculus, exclusive of its share of the propriospinal tract (Fig. 7-12). The posterior columns consist mainly of ascending collaterals of large myelinated primary afferents carrying impulses from various kinds of mechanoreceptors. This has traditionally been considered the major pathway by which information from low-threshold cutaneous, joint, and muscle receptors reaches the cerebral cortex.

Almost all the fibers in a posterior column arise in ipsilateral dorsal root ganglia. Where the dorsal root enters the spinal cord, it segregates itself into *medial* and *lateral divisions*. The medial division contains large myelinated afferents, while the lateral division contains small, finely myelinated or unmyelinated afferents. Fibers of the medial division enter the posterior column. Most of them give off numbers of collaterals to the spinal gray matter and finally terminate at some spinal level, but some reach the caudal medulla and synapse there. Caudal to T6 each posterior column is an undivided bundle called the *fasciculus gracilis* (Latin, gracilis = slender). Rostral to T6, fibers may leave the fasciculus gracilis, but few, if any, are added. Afferents entering rostral to T6 accumulate in a second bundle lateral to the fasciculus gracilis called the *fasciculus cuneatus* (Latin, cuneus = wedge). A glial partition (the *posterior intermediate septum*) extends inward to partially separate the two.

At each successive spinal level, fibers entering the posterior columns add on laterally to those already present. A lamination results, with layers of fibers from sacral levels most medial and layers from cervical levels most lateral (Fig. 7-12). This sort of arrangement, in which particular portions of the body are represented in particular regions of a pathway or nucleus, is called *somatotopic* organization and is characteristic of most sensory and motor pathways.

Those posterior column fibers that reach the brainstem synapse in the *nucleus gracilis* or the *nucleus cuneatus* (the *posterior column nuclei*) in the caudal medulla. Second-order fibers arising in these nuclei cross the midline and form the *medial lemniscus* (Latin, lemniscus = ribbon), a flattened bundle of fibers that proceeds rostrally through the brainstem and terminates in the thalamus. Third-order fibers arising in the thalamus (specifically in the *ventral posterolateral nucleus* of the thalamus, or *VPL*) ascend through the internal capsule to synapse mainly in the cortex of the postcentral gyrus, the primary somatosensory cortex.

When the primary afferents of the posterior columns terminate in the posterior column nuclei, they maintain their somatotopic organization. Fibers from sacral levels terminate in the most medial portions of the nucleus gracilis, and fibers from cervical levels terminate in the most lateral portions of the nucleus cuneatus. A somatotopic arrangement is found throughout the rest of this pathway, so that information from sacral segments travels through a particular part of the medial lemniscus, projects to a particular portion of the VPL, and proceeds to a particular region of the postcentral gyrus. This does

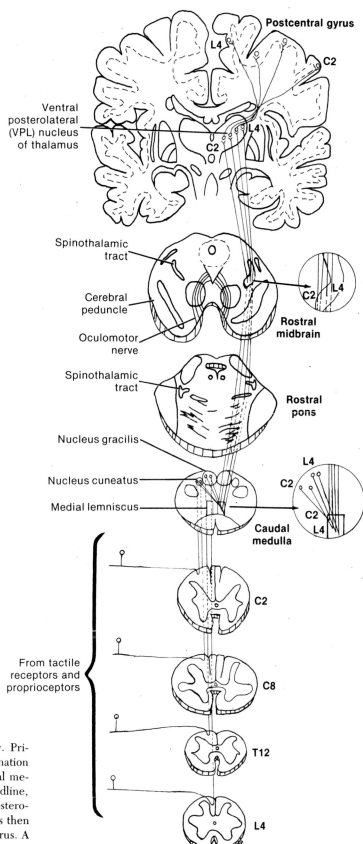

Fig. 7-12. Posterior column–medial lemniscus pathway. Primary afferents carrying tactile and proprioceptive information synapse in the posterior column nuclei of the ipsilateral medulla. The axons of second order cells then cross the midline, form the medial lemniscus, and ascend to the ventral posterolateral (VPL) nucleus of the thalamus. Third order fibers then project to the somatosensory cortex of the postcentral gyrus. A somatotopic arrangement of fibers is present at all levels.

not mean that the sacral-to-cervical sequence remains along a medial-to-lateral line throughout the pathway, but rather that sacral information remains segregated from cervical information at all points along the way to somatosensory cortex. You may find it easier to keep track of the somatotopic arrangement of the pathway at different levels if you envision it as an actual map of the body (a *homunculus*, Latin = little man), with sacral and lumbar levels corresponding to the legs, thoracic to the trunk, and cervical to the arms and neck. Viewed in this way, the homunculus is lying down with its feet toward the midline, up to the level of the posterior column nuclei. Its subsequent gyrations will be described in the next chapter.

As might be expected from the types of afferents contained in the posterior columns, this pathway carries information relevant to the conscious appreciation of cutaneous touch, pressure, and vibration and of joint position and movement. Since input from cutaneous receptors reaches the cortex by at least one, and probably two, other routes (to be described shortly), damage to the posterior columns causes impairment (but not abolition) of tactile sensibility. However, some types of tactile sensation are more affected than others. One of the most severely affected sensations is vibration perception; posterior column function is commonly tested clinically by touching a vibrating tuning fork to the skin. Other functions, such as *kinesthesia* (sense of body movement and position), are classically considered to be totally lost after posterior column destruction. The result is a distinctive type of *ataxia* (incoordination of muscular activity): the brain is unable to properly direct motor activity without sensory feedback as to the current position of parts of the body. This ataxia is particularly pronounced when the patient's eyes are closed.

Spinothalamic tract. Collaterals of some touch- and pressure-sensitive fibers in the posterior columns, as well as collaterals of mechanoreceptive, thermoreceptive, and nociceptive fibers of the lateral division of the dorsal root, enter the dorsal horn and synapse in or near the substantia gelatinosa. After one or more synapses, fibers that arise from cells of the nucleus proprius or intermediate gray matter (but not the substantia gelatinosa) cross the midline with a slight rostral inclination to form the *spinothalamic tract* (Fig. 7-13). This is one alternate pathway by which mechanoreceptive input reaches the thalamus and cerebral cortex and is the primary pathway for pain and temperature information. The tract occupies most of the ventral half of the lateral funiculus. New fibers join the spinothalamic tract at its ventromedial edge, so that the tract, like the posterior columns, is somatotopically organized. Fibers from the most caudal segments occupy its most dorsolateral portion, and those from more rostral segments occupy more ventromedial portions.

The spinothalamic tract has traditionally been subdivided into the lateral and ventral spinothalamic tracts, the former subserving pain and temperature sensation and the latter some aspects of tactile sensation. Recent studies, however, indicate that all these types of fibers are intermingled to a great extent, and there is a growing tendency to regard the whole complex as a single spinothalamic tract. On the other hand, the spinothalamic pathway can be subdivided on the basis of the destination and probable function of the fibers. One subset of spinothalamic fibers projects directly to the VPL of the thalamus in the same somatotopic fashion as the medial lemniscus. This has been called the *neospinothalamic tract*, and there is some evidence that it may have a special role in the appreciation of sharp, pricking, well-localized pain (the kind mediated by Aδ fibers). The second subset projects to a different part of the thalamus (the intralaminar nuclei) without a somatotopic arrangement. Many of the latter projections are indirect, following a polysynaptic course through the reticular formation of the brainstem (Chapter 8) and so are more properly called *spinoreticular* fibers. Those that do pass directly to the intralaminar nuclei have been called the *paleospinothalamic* tract. There is some evidence that these, together with the spinoreticular fibers, have a special role in the sensation of dull, aching, poorly localized pain of the sort mediated by C fibers. All these neospinothalamic, paleospinothalamic, and spinoreticular fibers are intermingled in the spinal cord, but the neospinothalamic component pursues a separate course in the brainstem, as discussed in the next chapter.

The role of the substantia gelatinosa in the transmission of pain information is incompletely understood at the present time. Anatomically it consists of large numbers of small cells among which finely myelinated and unmyelinated afferents terminate. Very few of these small cells give rise to long ascending axons; rather, the dendrites of more deeply situated tract cells and interneurons extend up into this region to receive input from pain and temperature afferents. The substantia gelatinosa is therefore strategically organized to regulate the access of pain and temperature information to the spinothalamic tract. The notion of the dependence of the perception of pain on the balance of activity in large and small afferents was referred to briefly in Chapter 6. Many workers think that the substantia gelatinosa is one site at which these activities are compared and the transmission of pain information is modulated.

Although the spinothalamic tract carries some tactile and pressure information, a great deal also travels in the posterior column system, so destruction of the spino-

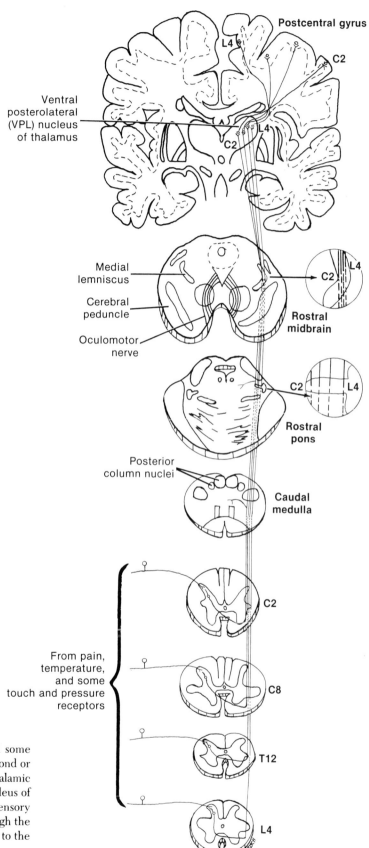

Fig. 7-13. Spinothalamic tract. Pain, temperature, and some touch and pressure afferents end in the dorsal horn. Second or higher order fibers cross the midline, form the spinothalamic tract, and ascend to the ventral posterolateral (VPL) nucleus of the thalamus. Thalamic cells then project to the somatosensory cortex of the postcentral gyrus. Along their course through the brainstem, spinothalamic fibers give off many collaterals to the reticular formation.

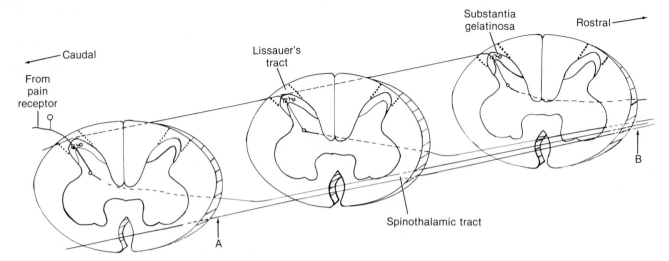

Fig. 7-14. Formation of the spinothalamic tract. Primary afferents ascend several segments in Lissauer's tract before all their branches terminate; fibers crossing to join the spinothalamic tract do so with a rostral inclination. As a result, a cordotomy incision at *A* would spare much of the pain information entering the most caudal segment shown, and an incision at *B* or higher would be necessary.

thalamic tract causes no detectable tactile deficit. There are, however, several types of sensation (in addition to pain and temperature) subserved more or less predominantly by the spinothalamic tract. These are itch (and probably tickle) sensations, pressure sensations from bladder and bowel, and sexual sensations. However, with the exception of itch (and possibly tickle), this information is carried bilaterally, so unilateral damage generally results in little dysfunction. This may be considered a particularly elegant example of the providence of nature.

The spinothalamic tract is, however, the principal pathway for somatic pain sensations, and its destruction produces a contralateral analgesia. An operation to destroy the tract (called a *cordotomy* or *chordotomy*) is sometimes performed on patients suffering from intractable pain. This operation consists of cutting the lateral funiculus from the dentate ligament to the line of ventral rootlets. The cut is usually made several segments rostral to the highest dermatomal level of pain, for two reasons (Fig. 7-14). First, collaterals of primary afferents may ascend one or more segments in the dorsolateral fasciculus before synapsing, so input from these would be spared if the cut were made at the highest dermatomal level of pain. Second, the axons that form the spinothalamic tract cross the midline with a rostral inclination, so a cut at any given level will spare fibers that arise contralaterally at that level, since they will join the tract rostral to the cut.

Cordotomy provides prompt contralateral analgesia, but surprisingly the analgesia is usually not permanent.

After a varying interval (generally several months), the patient's pain frequently returns. The reason is not known but may be the increasing efficacy of a few uncrossed fibers in the contralateral spinothalamic tract, of polysynaptic relays via the substantia gelatinosa and the dorsolateral fasciculus to the thalamus, or of both.

Spinocervical tract. In recent years a third route for the conduction of tactile (and, to a lesser extent, pain) information has been described in cats. Primary afferents, mostly related to hair receptors of various types, synapse on tract cells in the nucleus proprius. These *spinocervical tract* cells send their axons ipsilaterally through the most dorsal part of the lateral funiculus to terminate in the small *lateral cervical nucleus*, which is embedded in the lateral funiculus of the upper cervical cord. The axons of cells of the lateral cervical nucleus then cross the midline, join the medial lemniscus as it forms in the caudal medulla, and ascend to the VPL.

The size and importance of the spinocervical tract in humans is unknown, although it is known to be present in monkeys. It is mentioned here because evidence is slowly accumulating that it is a very important complement to the posterior column system. In monkeys, for example, combining a lesion of this small tract with one of the posterior column results in a much more severe and long-lasting tactile deficit than does damage to the posterior column alone.

Pathways to the cerebellum

Posterior spinocerebellar tract. Collaterals of posterior column fibers conveying tactile, pressure, and proprioceptive information (mainly the latter, from mus-

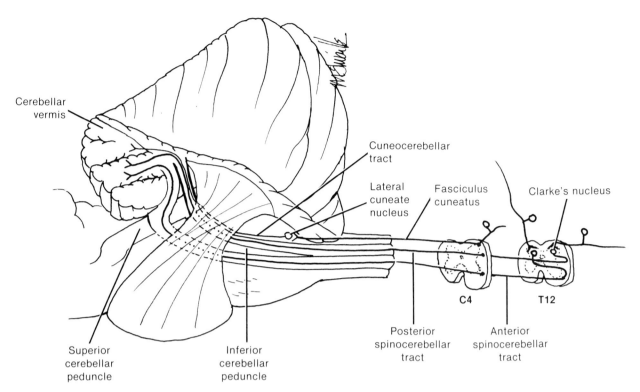

Fig. 7-15. Spinocerebellar and cuneocerebellar tracts. Mechanoreceptive afferents from the lower extremity synapse in Clarke's nucleus, whose cells give rise to the ipsilateral posterior spinocerebellar tract, which enters the inferior cerebellar peduncle and ends ipsilaterally in the vermis of the anterior lobe. Similar afferents also end on other cells of the spinal gray matter, whose axons form the contralateral anterior spinocerebellar tract; this tract ascends to the pons, loops over the superior cerebellar peduncle, and ends bilaterally in the vermis of the anterior lobe. Mechanoreceptive afferents from the upper extremity ascend to the medulla in the fasciculus cuneatus and end in the lateral cuneate nucleus (analogous to Clarke's nucleus); these cells give rise to the cuneocerebellar tract, which enters the inferior cerebellar peduncle and ends ipsilaterally in the vermis of the anterior lobe. The rostral spinocerebellar tract is not shown in this diagram. (Modified from Nieuwenhuys, R., et al.: The human central nervous system, New York, 1978, Springer-Verlag, Inc.)

cle spindles and Golgi tendon organs) synapse on neurons of Clarke's nucleus. These then send their axons into the lateral funiculus of the same side, forming the *posterior spinocerebellar tract* (Fig. 7-15). This tract, a curved band of fibers extending from the dorsal root entry zone to the dentate ligament, lies at the surface of the spinal cord. Fibers in the tract project ipsilaterally to the vermis of the cerebellum through the *inferior cerebellar peduncle*. Since Clarke's nucleus does not exist caudal to L2 or L3, neither does the posterior spinocerebellar tract. However, afferents from segments caudal to L2 or L3 ascend to that level in the fasciculus gracilis to synapse in Clarke's nucleus. This probably explains why Clarke's nucleus is so large at upper lumbar and lower thoracic levels (Fig. 7-5), since at these levels it has a large backlog of afferent input to process.

The posterior spinocerebellar tract is principally concerned with the ipsilateral leg. Most spinocerebellar-type afferents that enter in cervical and upper thoracic segments (for example, those representing the arm) do not project to Clarke's nucleus. Rather, they travel in the fasciculus cuneatus to a nucleus in the medulla analogous to Clarke's nucleus called the *lateral cuneate nucleus*, because it is located just lateral to the nucleus cuneatus (Fig. 8-6). Axons of these cells form the *cuneocerebellar tract*, which also projects ipsilaterally to the vermis of the cerebellum through the inferior cerebellar peduncle.

Anterior spinocerebellar tract. Collaterals of group I muscle afferents (mainly Golgi tendon organs) and of a wide variety of cutaneous afferents from the leg synapse on cells of the nucleus proprius and on other cells on the lateral surface of the ventral horn (called spinal border cells). These cells send their axons across the midline to form the *anterior spinocerebellar tract* (Fig. 7-15), which is anterior to and continuous with the posterior spinocerebellar tract. These fibers take a roundabout route to the cerebellum: they ascend as far as the rostral pons, then turn caudally and enter the cerebellum via the *superior cerebellar peduncle*. There they end bilaterally in the vermis of the anterior lobe.

A forelimb equivalent of the anterior spinocerebellar tract, called the *rostral spinocerebellar tract*, has been described in cats. It has not been studied in primates, so no one knows whether it exists in humans.

Clinically detectable deficits as a result of damage to the spinocerebellar tracts are rare, if they occur at all. In order to eliminate the information reaching the cerebellum from one leg via the spinal cord, the posterior spino-

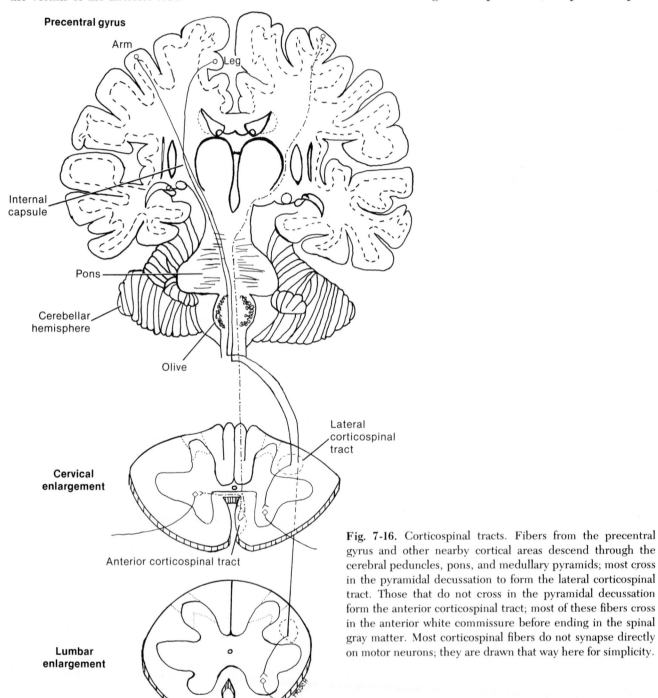

Fig. 7-16. Corticospinal tracts. Fibers from the precentral gyrus and other nearby cortical areas descend through the cerebral peduncles, pons, and medullary pyramids; most cross in the pyramidal decussation to form the lateral corticospinal tract. Those that do not cross in the pyramidal decussation form the anterior corticospinal tract; most of these fibers cross in the anterior white commissure before ending in the spinal gray matter. Most corticospinal fibers do not synapse directly on motor neurons; they are drawn that way here for simplicity.

cerebellar tract of one side and the anterior spinocerebellar tract of the other side would have to be destroyed. This would be unlikely unless the whole cord were damaged at that level, in which case the neurological deficits would be so great that cerebellar signs would be impossible to detect.

Descending pathways

The alpha and gamma motor neurons of the ventral horn are regulated in a variety of ways by supraspinal centers. Some of these centers are located in the brainstem and will be discussed in later chapters. The major descending outflow is from the cerebral cortex, particularly the precentral gyrus. This *corticospinal* system will be dealt with at length in Chapter 12, but a few basic concepts will be introduced here.

Lateral corticospinal tract. The *lateral corticospinal tract* (Fig. 7-16) is a large, crossed, descending tract that contains the approximately 85% of the fibers of the contralateral pyramid that cross in the pyramidal decussation. It is also known as the *pyramidal tract* and occupies the dorsal portion of the lateral funiculus deep to the posterior spinocerebellar tract. Its fibers originate in the cerebral cortex (principally in the precentral gyrus); descend through the cerebral peduncle, basis pontis, and medullary pyramid; decussate; and end in the ventral horn or intermediate gray matter. They terminate on the large motor neurons of the ventral horn or, more often, on smaller interneurons that in turn synapse on

these motor neurons. Lateral corticospinal fibers are arranged somatotopically, with those destined for more caudal cord levels located more laterally.

The difference between fibers of the pyramidal tract and the motor axons of the ventral root should be clearly understood. Alpha motor neurons (and the ventral root fibers these neurons give rise to) contact striated muscle directly and are called *lower motor neurons*. They are also sometimes called the "final common pathway" of the motor system, since, as noted earlier, they are the only means by which the nervous system can exercise control over body movements. Interruption of the lower motor neurons supplying a muscle causes flaccid paralysis and, eventually, atrophy of the muscle.

Fibers that originate in motor cortex and end on lower motor neurons (either directly or indirectly by way of an interneuron) are called *upper motor neurons*. The collection of upper motor neurons is more or less the same thing as the pyramidal system, although there are serious problems with this terminology, as will be discussed later. As the terms are used clinically, a lesion of the pyramidal system (an upper motor neuron lesion) has very different effects from those of a lower motor neuron lesion. Characteristically the muscles involved show hyperactive reflexes. Their resting tension is increased (that is, they are *hypertonic*). There is paralysis or weakness *(paresis)*, particularly of fine voluntary movements. This complex of symptoms is referred to as *spastic paralysis*. There are a number of pathological reflexes asso-

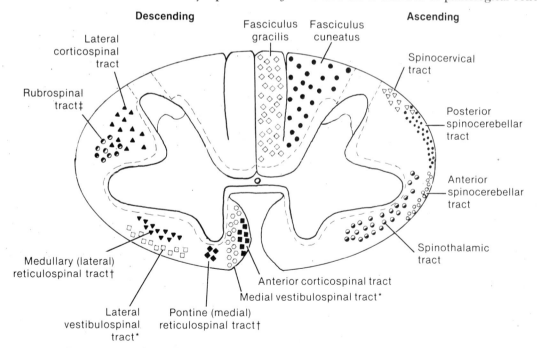

Fig. 7-17. Summary diagram of principal tracts present in lower cervical spinal cord. Not all of these tracts were mentioned in this chapter. *Discussed in Chapter 9. †Discussed in Chapter 8. ‡Discussed in Chapter 12.

ciated with upper motor neuron lesions. The best known is *Babinski's sign*—dorsiflexion of the big toe and fanning of the others in response to firmly stroking the sole of the foot. (Note that Babinski's sign is either present or not present; it is not "positive" or "negative.")

Anterior corticospinal tract. The 15% or so of the fibers in each pyramid that do not cross in the pyramidal decussation continue into the anterior funiculus (located adjacent to the anterior median fissure) as the *anterior corticospinal tract* (Figs. 7-16 and 7-17). These fibers also terminate on motor neurons or interneurons of the ventral horn or intermediate gray matter, mainly in cervical and thoracic segments. Many of them cross in the anterior white commissure before synapsing, but some do not. Strictly speaking, the term "pyramidal tract" refers to the combination of lateral and anterior corticospinal tracts.

VASCULAR SUPPLY OF THE SPINAL CORD

The arterial supply of the spinal cord is by way of the vertebral arteries and of branches, ultimately from the thoracic and abdominal aorta, called *radicular arteries.*

Each vertebral artery gives rise to a *posterior spinal artery*, which proceeds along the line of attachment of the dorsal roots, and to an *anterior spinal artery*. The two anterior spinal arteries fuse to form a single midline vessel that courses along the anterior median fissure of the spinal cord (Figs. 5-1 and 7-18). The posterior spinal arteries and the midline anterior spinal artery supply upper cervical levels with blood from the vertebral arteries. Below this, all three spinal arteries form a more or less continuous series of anastomoses with radicular arteries for the length of the cord. The spinal arteries are rather small; beginning with lower cervical segments, the spinal cord depends on these radicular arteries for its survival. One particular radicular artery, present at about L1 or L2 in most individuals, is called the *great radicular artery* (or *artery of Adamkiewicz*) and may provide the entire arterial supply for the caudal two thirds of the spinal cord.

The anterior spinal artery, which is usually a continuous vessel for the length of the spinal cord, gives rise to a series of central and circumferential branches that supply the anterior two thirds of the spinal cord, includ-

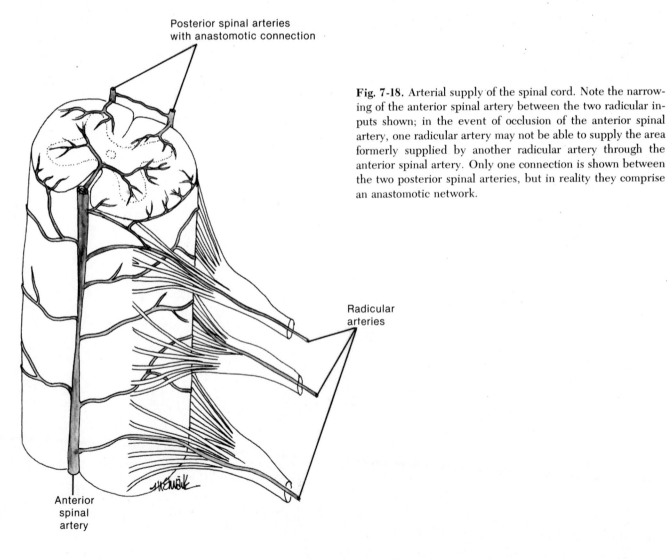

Posterior spinal arteries with anastomotic connection

Radicular arteries

Anterior spinal artery

Fig. 7-18. Arterial supply of the spinal cord. Note the narrowing of the anterior spinal artery between the two radicular inputs shown; in the event of occlusion of the anterior spinal artery, one radicular artery may not be able to supply the area formerly supplied by another radicular artery through the anterior spinal artery. Only one connection is shown between the two posterior spinal arteries, but in reality they comprise an anastomotic network.

ing the base of the dorsal horn and a variable portion of the lateral corticospinal tract (Fig. 7-18). The posterior spinal arteries, which are really more of a plexiform network of small arteries, supply the posterior columns, substantia gelatinosa, dorsal root entry zone, and a variable portion of the lateral corticospinal tract.

Venous drainage is by a series of six irregular, plexiform channels: one each along the anterior and posterior midlines and one along the line of attachment of the dorsal and ventral roots of each side. These are drained by *radicular veins*, which in turn empty into the *epidural venous plexus.*

SOME FUNCTIONAL ASPECTS OF THE SPINAL CORD

Spinal shock. If the spinal cord of a cat is transected at a midcervical level, you might expect, among other things, a spastic (upper motor neuron) paralysis of its whole body. This does happen eventually, but first there is a period, lasting for a few days, of more or less completely flaccid paralysis and areflexia. Deep tendon reflexes then begin to return and finally become hyperactive. The areflexic period is called *spinal shock.* The mechanism of spinal shock is incompletely understood, but the whole sequence of events is thought to be a consequence of interruption of fibers from the brainstem and cerebrum descending to spinal cord motor neurons. In addition to corticospinal tracts, there are a number of other descending influences, some facilitatory and some inhibitory. Spinal shock would thus be caused by sudden loss of descending facilitatory influences. After a period of adjustment, the effect of loss of descending inhibitory influences would predominate, and spastic paralysis would result.

Spinal shock occurs in humans as well, even in cases of contusion of the spinal cord, in which total or near-total recovery can be expected. It may last for weeks in cases of complete transection. A complicating factor in spinal shock is the complete loss of bladder function (and loss of a sensation of distention) that accompanies it. Early catheterization is called for to minimize bladder distention and consequent damage. With proper care, even in cases of complete cord transection a state of automatic or reflex emptying of the bladder develops.

Partial lesions of the spinal cord are (fortunately) much more common than complete transections. Complete transection of one side of the cord (hemisection), while rare, results in an instructional complex of symptoms called the *Brown-Séquard syndrome.* After a period of spinal shock (particularly prominent in those areas subserved by the damaged portion of the cord), a spastic paralysis develops below the lesion and ipsilateral to it because of interruption of the lateral corticospinal tract. Tactile, vibratory, and position senses are disturbed ipsilaterally below the lesion because of interruption of the

posterior column. There is loss of pain and temperature sensation *contralateral* to the lesion, beginning one or two segments caudal to the lesion, as a result of interruption of the lateral spinothalamic tract. This is one of many examples of crossed findings (that is, some symptoms referable to one side of the head or body and others to the other side).

Syringomyelia (Greek, syrinx = tube) is a disease of the central part of the spinal cord in which a tubelike enlargement of the central canal develops, typically at lower cervical or upper thoracic levels. As the syrinx enlarges, surrounding neural tissue is destroyed. The first damage is to fibers crossing through the limited available area around the central canal (Fig. 7-4). The next area damaged is usually the anterior horn. The result is a distinctive combination of loss of pain and temperature sensation bilaterally over the arms and shoulders (as a result of the damage to crossing fibers) and weakness and atrophy of the muscles of the hands (as a result of anterior horn damage). Of course, if the syrinx occurred at a different spinal level, the symptoms would be referred to a correspondingly different part of the body.

Posterior columns. The true function of the posterior columns is currently a matter of some controversy. Classical views of this pathway as the one principally involved in fine tactile discrimination and kinesthesia (sense of position and movement) were based mostly on clinical observations. However, selective lesions of the posterior columns are rare. For example, any process impinging on the posterior columns, such as a tumor, would probably also affect the adjacent posterior horns and dorsal roots as well as the spinocervical tract. *Tabes dorsalis* is a disease process traditionally regarded as typifying posterior column damage. Tabetic patients show all the symptoms one would expect if the classical view were correct: their two-point discrimination and vibratory sense are impaired; their sense of movement and position is impaired, and they have great difficulty walking unless they can watch their limbs; if they try to stand erect with eyes closed and feet together, they tend to sway and fall *(Romberg's sign).* Consistent with this, there is pronounced degeneration in the posterior columns. However, there is also degeneration of dorsal root fibers, particularly those of the medial division, so mechanoreceptive input to *all* spinal pathways is affected to some extent.

When the posterior columns of a monkey are selectively transected surgically, remarkably little chronic deficit results. There are slight losses in two-point discrimination and subtle deficits in tactile ability, but other sensations seem to be intact. If a lesion of the ipsilateral spinocervical tract is added, the tactile deficits are much more severe and prolonged, suggesting that this is an effective alternate route for tactile information.

It is hard to imagine that a system as large and well-organized as the posterior column system is largely redundant (and it is risky to apply animal findings to humans), but at this point the jury is still out.

ADDITIONAL READING

Applebaum, M.L., et al.: Organization and receptive fields of primate spinothalamic tract neurons, J. Neurophysiol. **38**:572, 1975.

Basbaum, A.I.: Conduction of the effects of noxious stimulation by short-fiber multisynaptic systems of the spinal cord in the rat, Exp. Neurol. **40**:699, 1973. *A series of experiments showing that rats can learn to avoid painful stimuli even after hemisection of both sides of the spinal cord, which should transect the long ascending fibers of both sides.*

Boivie, J.J.G., and Perl, E.R.: Neural substrates of somatic sensation. In Hunt, C.C., editor: Neurophysiology. MTP international review of science: physiology, series 1, vol. 3, Woburn, Mass., 1975, Butterworth Publishers, Inc. *An exhaustive review with a monstrous bibliography.*

Bryan, R.N., Coulter, J.D., and Willis, W.D.: Cells of origin of the spinocervical tract in the monkey, Exp. Neurol. **42**:574, 1974.

Calne, D.B., and Pallis, C.A.: Vibratory sense: a critical review, Brain **89**:723, 1966. *Interesting reading, with a review of old clinical observations.*

Coggeshall, R.E.: Law of separation of function of the spinal roots, Physiol. Rev. **60**:716, 1980.

Collins, W.F., Nulsen, F.E., and Randt, C.T.: Relation of peripheral nerve fiber size and sensation in man, Arch. Neurol. **3**:381, 1960. *Abolition after cordotomy of the painful consequences of controlled electrical stimulation of the sural nerve.*

Cook, A.W., and Browder, E.J.: Function of posterior columns in man, Arch. Neurol. **12**:72, 1965. *An influential paper describing the apparently minimal effects of sectioning parts of the posterior column as an experimental treatment for intractable pain.*

Creed, R.S., et al.: Reflex activity of the spinal cord, reprinted with annotations by D.P.C. Lloyd, New York, 1972, Oxford University Press.

Crock, H.V., and Yoshizawa, H.: The blood supply of the vertebral column and spinal cord in man, New York, 1977, Springer-Verlag, Inc.

Dennis, S.G., and Melzack, R.: Pain-signalling systems in the dorsal and ventral spinal cord, Pain **4**:97, 1977.

Gillilan, L.A.: The arterial blood supply of the human spinal cord, J. Comp. Neurol. **110**:75, 1958.

Glees, P., and Soler, J.: Fibre content of the posterior column and synaptic connections of nucleus gracilis, Z. Zellforsch. **36**:381, 1951. *Documents the fact that, at least in the cat, only about 25% of the fibers that enter the posterior columns actually reach the posterior column nuclei; the rest end within the spinal cord.*

Gordon, G., editor: Somatic and visceral sensory mechanisms, Br. Med. Bull. **33**:89, 1977.

Grillner, A.: Locomotion in the spinal cat. In Stein, R.B., et al., editors: Control of posture and locomotion: advances in behavioral biology, vol. 7. New York, 1973, Plenum Press. *Walking with the hindlimbs by cats whose spinal cords had been transected at low thoracic levels.*

Ha, H.: Cervicothalamic tract in the rhesus monkey, Exp. Neurol. **33**:205, 1971.

Hosobuchi, Y.: The majority of unmyelinated afferent axons in human ventral roots probably conduct pain, Pain **8**:167, 1980.

Keswani, N.H., and Hollinshead, W.H.: Localization of the phrenic nucleus in the spinal cord of man, Anat. Rec. **125**:683, 1956.

Kuhn, R.A.: Functional capacity of the isolated human spinal cord,

Brain **73**:1, 1950. *A careful study of the course of events after complete transection of the spinal cord, particularly spinal shock and its gradual fading.*

Liddell, E.G.T., and Sherrington, C.: Reflexes in response to stretch (myotatic reflexes), Proc. R. Soc. Lond., series B, **96**:212, 1924.

Melzack, R., and Wall, P.D.: Pain mechanisms: a new theory, Science **150**:971, 1965. *A seminal paper, in which the modulating effect of the substantia gelatinosa on pain transmission was proposed in a scheme called the "gate control theory" of pain. While apparently wrong in some of its details, the gate control theory has nevertheless been very influential on pain research since 1965.*

Miller, S., and van der Meché, F.G.A.: Coordinated stepping of all four limbs in the high spinal cat. Brain Res. **109**:395, 1976.

Morin, F.: A new spinal pathway for cutaneous impulses, Am. J. Physiol. **183**:245, 1955. *The original physiological description of the spinocervical tract.*

Norrsell, U.: Behavioral studies of the somatosensory system, Physiol. Rev. **60**:327, 1980.

Nyberg-Hansen, R.: Innervation and nervous control of the urinary bladder: anatomical aspects, Acta. Neurol. Scand. **42**(suppl. 20):7, 1966.

Oscarsson, O.: Functional organization of spinocerebellar paths. In Iggo, A., editor: Handbook of sensory physiology, vol. II.: Somatosensory system, New York, 1973, Springer-Verlag, Inc.

Perl, E.R.: Effects of muscle stretch on excitability of contralateral motoneurones, J. Physiol. **145**:193, 1959.

Rexed, B.: The cytoarchitectonic organization of the spinal cord in the cat, J. Comp. Neurol. **96**:415, 1952.

Shealy, C.N., Mortimer, J.T., and Hagfors, N.R.: Dorsal column electroanalgesia, J. Neurosurg. **32**:560, 1970. *Another example of treating pain by shifting the balance of activity toward large-fiber afferent systems, this time by stimulating the posterior columns.*

Siekert, R.G., and Dale, A.J.D.: Vascular disease of the spinal cord. In Goldensohn, E.S., and Appel, S.H., editors: Scientific approaches to clinical neurology, Philadelphia, 1977, Lea and Febiger.

Synder, R.: The organization of the dorsal root entry zone in cats and monkeys, J. Comp. Neurol. **174**:47, 1977.

Truex, R.C., et al.: The lateral cervical nucleus of cat, dog and man, J. Comp. Neurol. **139**:93, 1970.

Uddenberg, N.: Functional organization of long second-order afferents in the dorsal funiculus, Exp. Brain Res. **4**:377, 1968. *Physiological description of the minority of fibers in the posterior column that are not primary afferents.*

Vierck, C.J. Jr.: Alterations of spatio-tactile discrimination after lesions of primate spinal cord, Brain Res. **58**:69, 1973. *Some speculations on how primates compensate for loss of a posterior column, plus experiments to show the much greater deficits caused by damage to both a posterior column and the ipsilateral spinocervical tract.*

Vierck, C.J. Jr., and Luck, M.M.: Loss and recovery of reactivity to noxious stimuli in monkeys with primary spinothalamic cordotomies, followed by secondary and tertiary lesions of other cord sectors, Brain **102**:233, 1979.

Weaver, T.A., and Walker, A.E.: Topical arrangement within the spinothalamic tract of the monkey, Arch. Neurol. Psychiatr. **46**:877, 1941.

White, J.C., and Sweet, W.H.: Pain and the neurosurgeon: a forty year experience, Springfield, Ill., 1969, Charles C Thomas, Publisher.

Willis, W.D., and Coggeshall, R.E.: Sensory mechanisms of the spinal cord, New York, 1978, Plenum Press. *A well-written, thoroughly documented review of the literature through 1977.*

Willis, W.D., Kenshalo, D.R. Jr., and Leonard, R.B.: The cells of origin of the primate spinothalamic tract, J. Comp. Neurol. **188**:543, 1979.

BRAINSTEM

The spinal cord continues rostrally into the brainstem (Fig. 8-1), which performs spinal cord–like functions for the head. It contains the lower motor neurons for the muscles of the head and does the initial processing of general afferent information concerning the head. However, the brainstem does much more than this, and its activities may be divided (not very cleanly) into three general types: *conduit functions*, *cranial nerve functions*, and *integrative functions*.

The need for conduit functions is apparent, since the only way for ascending tracts to reach the thalamus or cerebellum (or for descending tracts to reach the spinal cord) is through the brainstem. Many of these tracts, however, are not straight-through affairs, and identifiable relay nuclei in the brainstem are frequently involved.

The cranial nerves contain not only the head's equivalent of spinal nerve fibers but also those involved in the special senses of olfaction, sight, hearing, equilibrium, and gustation (taste). The olfactory and optic nerves project directly to the telencephalon and diencephalon, respectively, but all the others project to the brainstem. Thus a wide assortment of sensory and motor nuclei related to cranial nerve function can be found at various brainstem levels.

A number of other functions are organized at the level of the brainstem, such as complex motor patterns, aspects of respiratory and cardiovascular activity, and even some regulation of the level of consciousness itself. Much of this is accomplished by the *reticular formation*, which forms the central core of the brainstem.

It is clear that these three general types of activity are far from mutually exclusive. For example, ascending pathways to the thalamus arise not only in the spinal cord, but also from cranial nerve nuclei. However, they do provide a useful framework on which to organize a treatment of the brainstem. It is difficult to learn about this portion of the nervous system all at once, so it will be presented in two parts. This chapter describes its

overall anatomy and presents a series of sections showing the locations of some prominent nuclei and of major ascending and descending tracts. The next chapter describes the central connections of cranial nerves III to XII.

GROSS ANATOMY
Medulla

The medulla is vaguely scoop shaped. The "handle" corresponds to the *caudal* or *closed* portion containing a central canal continuous with that of the spinal cord. The open portion of the scoop corresponds to the *rostral* or *open medulla*, in which the central canal expands as the fourth ventricle. The apex of the V-shaped caudal fourth ventricle, where it narrows into the central canal, is called the *obex* (Figs. 8-2 and 8-3).

The longitudinal grooves of the surface of the spinal cord continue into the medulla. They divide the surface of the caudal, and part of the rostral, medulla into a series of columns that completely encircle it (Fig. 8-2). The anterior median fissure is briefly interrupted by the pyramidal decussation at the junction between spinal cord and brainstem but then continues rostrally to the edge of the pons, separating the two pyramids (Figs. 8-2 and 8-3). Proceeding around in a posterior direction, the anterolateral sulcus marks the other side of the pyramid. The rootlets of the hypoglossal nerve (XII) emerge from it, mainly in the rostral medulla. The rootlets of the glossopharyngeal nerve (IX), vagus nerve (X), and the cranial part of the accessory nerve (XI) emerge from the same shallow groove as the spinal part of the accessory nerve (XI). In the rostral medulla, the column between the hypoglossal rootlets and the vagal and glossopharyngeal rootlets is enlarged to form an oval swelling called the *olive*. The posterolateral sulcus also continues into the medulla, and the area between it and the line of rootlets of IX to XI is referred to as the *tuberculum cinereum*. Beneath the tuberculum cinereum is the *spinal tract of the trigeminal nerve*, which, as explained

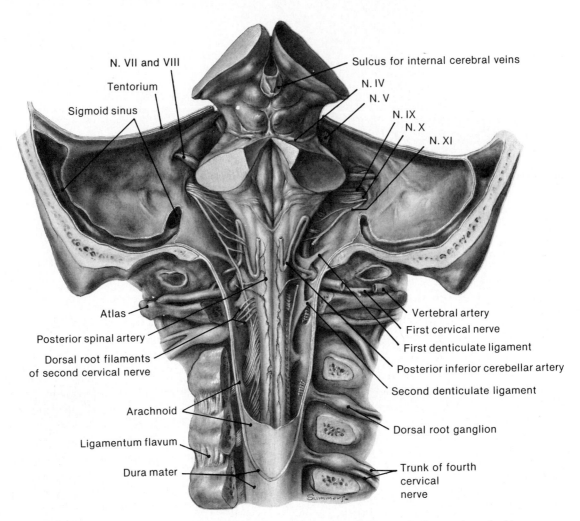

Fig. 8-1. Posterior aspect of the brainstem and upper spinal cord. The cerebellum and cerebral hemispheres have been removed. (From Mettler, F.A.: Neuroanatomy, ed. 2, St. Louis, 1948, The C.V. Mosby Co.)

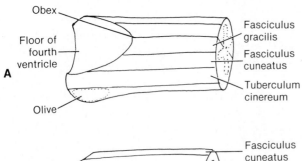

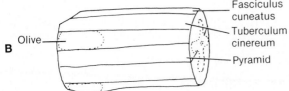

Fig. 8-2. Surface features of the medulla. **A,** Seen from above and to the left. **B,** Seen from below and to the left.

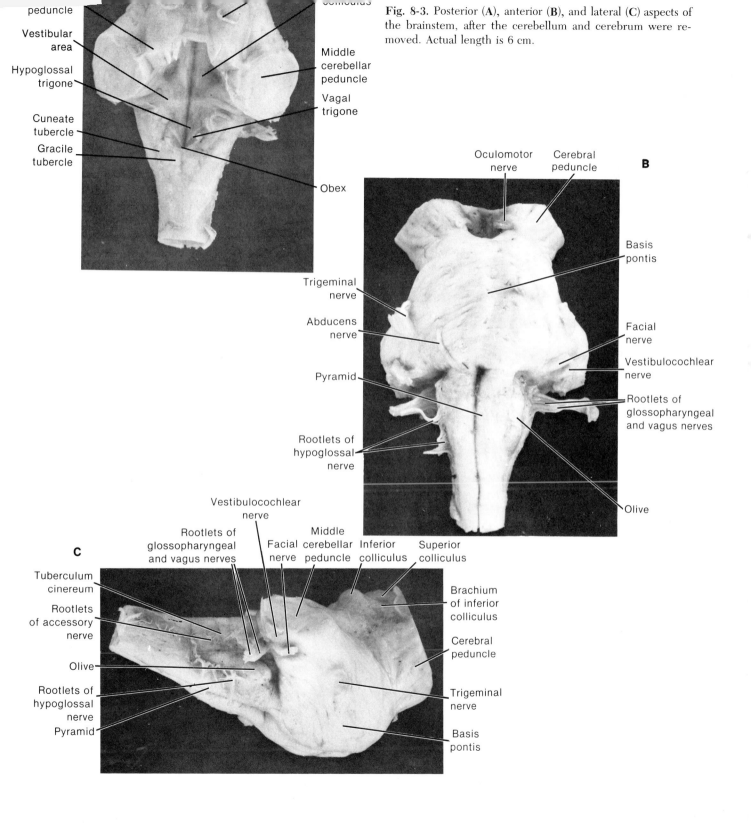

peduncle

Vestibular area

Hypoglossal trigone

Cuneate tubercle

Gracile tubercle

colliculus

Middle cerebellar peduncle

Vagal trigone

Obex

Fig. 8-3. Posterior (**A**), anterior (**B**), and lateral (**C**) aspects of the brainstem, after the cerebellum and cerebrum were removed. Actual length is 6 cm.

B

Oculomotor nerve

Cerebral peduncle

Basis pontis

Trigeminal nerve

Abducens nerve

Pyramid

Rootlets of hypoglossal nerve

Facial nerve

Vestibulocochlear nerve

Rootlets of glossopharyngeal and vagus nerves

Olive

C

Vestibulocochlear nerve

Rootlets of glossopharyngeal and vagus nerves

Facial nerve

Middle cerebellar peduncle

Inferior colliculus

Superior colliculus

Tuberculum cinereum

Rootlets of accessory nerve

Olive

Rootlets of hypoglossal nerve

Pyramid

Brachium of inferior colliculus

Cerebral peduncle

Trigeminal nerve

Basis pontis

in the next chapter, is the head's equivalent of Lissauer's tract. Finally, the posterior columns continue into the medulla. The fasciculus cuneatus, adjacent to the posterolateral sulcus, extends rostrally to a small swelling called the *cuneate tubercle*, which marks the site of the nucleus cuneatus. The fasciculus gracilis, adjacent to the midline, extends rostrally to a similar small swelling called the *gracile tubercle* (or *clava*), which marks the site of the nucleus gracilis.

If the cerebellum is removed (as it has been in Fig. 8-3), one can peer down on the floor of the fourth ventricle. Here, too, various grooves and elevations signify the presence of underlying nuclei. The sulcus limitans can sometimes be followed rostrally along the floor of the ventricle into the pons. As in the embryonic spinal cord, it is a line of separation between motor nuclei (now medial to it) and sensory nuclei (now lateral to it; see Fig. 1-10). The portion of the medulla and pons immediately beneath the floor of the ventricle, lateral to the sulcus limitans, is mostly occupied by vestibular nuclei and is referred to as the *vestibular area.* The area medial to the sulcus limitans overlies a series of motor nuclei, three of which make visible elevations. In the medulla, the hypoglossal nucleus and the dorsal motor nucleus of the vagus make small triangular swellings, appropriately called the *hypoglossal* and *vagal trigones*. Farther rostrally, in the

pons, is another elevation called the *facial colliculus.* This elevation is not caused by an underlying motor nucleus of the facial nerve but instead is the location of the abducens nucleus; fibers destined for the facial nerve loop over it at this location on their way out of the brainstem.

Pons

The pons is dominated by the massive, transversely oriented structure on its ventral surface from which it derives its name (Figs. 8-3 and 8-4). "Pons" is Latin for "bridge," and this portion of it (called the *ventral portion of the pons*, or *basis pontis*) looks like a bridge interconnecting the two cerebellar hemispheres. Actually, though, it does not interconnect them. Rather, many of the fibers descending in a cerebral peduncle synapse in scattered nuclei of the ipsilateral half of the basis pontis. These nuclei in turn project their fibers across the midline, after which they funnel into the middle cerebellar peduncle (*brachium pontis*) and enter the cerebellum.

The trigeminal nerve (V) enters the brainstem at the midpons, and three others enter (or leave) along the groove between the basis pontis and the medulla (Fig. 8-3). The abducens nerve (VI) is the smallest and most medially located of these three, exiting where the pyra-

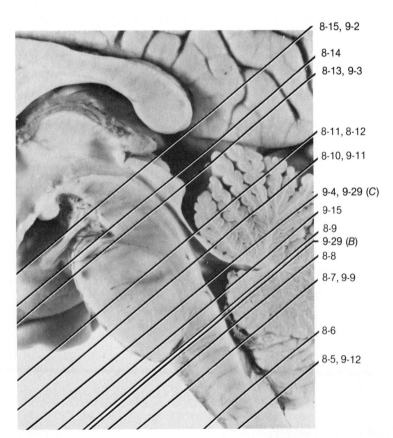

8-15, 9-2
8-14
8-13, 9-3

8-11, 8-12
8-10, 9-11

9-4, 9-29 (*C*)
9-15
8-9
9-29 (*B*)
8-8
8-7, 9-9

8-6

8-5, 9-12

Fig. 8-4. Planes of sections seen in Figs. 8-5 to 8-15.

is farther lateral and consists of two parts: a larger and more medial motor root and a smaller sensory root (sometimes referred to as the *nervus intermedius*). The vestibulocochlear nerve (VIII) is slightly lateral to the facial nerve and also has two parts: a vestibular division and a more lateral cochlear division.

The superior cerebellar peduncle *(brachium conjunctivum)* forms much of the roof of the fourth ventricle in the pons. It emerges from the cerebellum, moves toward the midline and the brainstem, and enters the latter near the junction between the pons and midbrain. At this same junction, the trochlear nerve (IV) emerges from the dorsal surface of the brainstem.

Midbrain

The midbrain is characterized by four bumps (the paired superior and inferior colliculi) on its posterior surface and by the large cerebral peduncles on its anterior surface. The oculomotor nerve (III) emerges from the interpeduncular fossa between the peduncles.

The broad low ridge extending rostrally from the inferior colliculus is the *brachium of the inferior colliculus* (usually shortened to *inferior brachium*). This is part of the ascending auditory pathway connecting the inferior colliculus and the thalamic relay nucleus for audition (the *medial geniculate nucleus*).

INTERNAL STRUCTURE

At any given brainstem level rostral to the obex, three general areas can be identified in cross section. These are (1) the area posterior to the ventricular space, (2) the area anterior to the ventricular space, and (3) large structures "appended" to the anterior surface of the brainstem. (In the caudal medulla, the central canal is surrounded by structures that will be anterior to the ventricular space at more rostral levels).

The only place where the portion posterior to the ventricular space contains a substantial amount of neural tissue is the midbrain. Here this region is called the *tectum* (Latin = roof) and consists of the superior and inferior colliculi. In the pons and rostral medulla, the fourth ventricle is covered posteriorly by the superior and inferior medullary vela (and, of course, the cerebellum).

The area anterior to the ventricular space is called the *tegmentum* (Latin = covering) as a general term. The tegmentum contains most of the structures to be described in this and the next chapter: the reticular formation, cranial nerve nuclei and tracts, ascending pathways from the spinal cord, and some descending pathways.

The structures appended to the anterior surface of the brainstem contain fibers descending from the cerebral cortex to the spinal cord, to certain cranial nerve nuclei, or to pontine nuclei, which in turn project to the cerebellum. These appended structures are the large fiber bundle of each cerebral peduncle, the basis pontis, and the pyramids of the medulla.

Although the brainstem is embryologically derived from a serial array of vesicles, in the adult it no longer possesses an organization quite so neat (Fig. 8-4). For example, the basis pontis usually extends rostrally to a point anterior to the tectum of the midbrain; the pineal gland and part of the thalamus extend caudally to a point posterior to the tectum of the midbrain. Since the most instructive way to study the brainstem is to consider a series of parallel sections through it (all perpendicular to its long axis), I have ignored minor inconveniences (for example, the intrusion of the basis pontis under the midbrain) and have used, for the purposes of the following discussion, reference transverse planes that subdivide the brainstem into six parts: caudal and rostral medulla, caudal and rostral pons, and caudal and rostral midbrain.

The following discussion points out major brainstem structures at these levels and locations of tracts that begin or end in the spinal cord. The next chapter deals with the cranial nerves and their tracts and nuclei.

Caudal medulla

The caudal (closed) medulla extends from the caudal edge of the pyramidal decussation (where it is continuous with the spinal cord) to the obex, which marks the caudal end of the fourth ventricle.

The caudal medulla (Figs. 8-5 and 8-6) looks somewhat like the spinal cord. Part of the anterior horn is still present caudally (Fig. 8-5), as are structures similar to Lissauer's tract and part of the posterior horn. The latter two are actually the *spinal tract* and *spinal nucleus of the trigeminal nerve*. These are the head's equivalent of Lissauer's tract and the substantia gelatinosa (that is, they deal with pain, temperature, and some tactile information).

The fasciculi gracilis and cuneatus continue into the caudal medulla but are gradually replaced by the posterior column nuclei (nucleus gracilis and nucleus cuneatus). The nucleus cuneatus begins and ends a bit rostral to the nucleus gracilis, so even in Fig. 8-6 part of the fasciculus cuneatus is still present. Postsynaptic fibers leave these two nuclei in a ventral direction and arch across the midline to form the contralateral medial lemniscus, a vertically oriented band of fibers (Fig. 8-6). These decussating fibers are part of the collection of *internal arcuate fibers* and are sometimes called the *sensory decussation*. Throughout the medulla, the medial lemniscus is organized so that fibers representing cervical segments are most posterior (that is, as though the homunculus were standing upright).

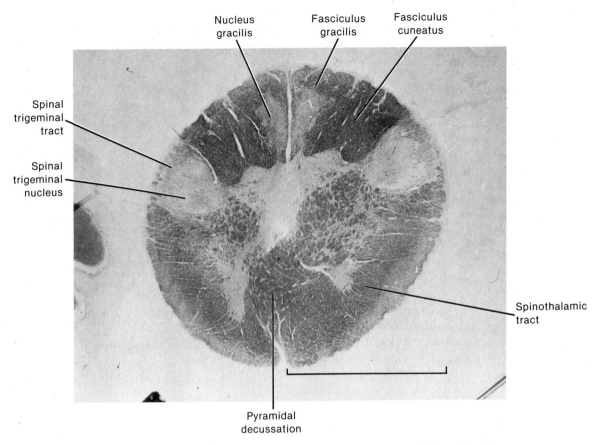

Nucleus gracilis

Fasciculus gracilis

Fasciculus cuneatus

Spinal trigeminal tract

Spinal trigeminal nucleus

Spinothalamic tract

Pyramidal decussation

Fig. 8-5. Caudal medulla, at the level of the pyramidal decussation. Scale mark = 5 mm.

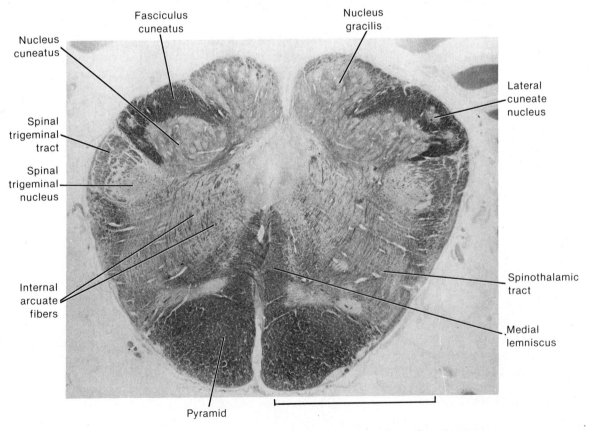

Fasciculus cuneatus

Nucleus gracilis

Nucleus cuneatus

Lateral cuneate nucleus

Spinal trigeminal tract

Spinal trigeminal nucleus

Internal arcuate fibers

Spinothalamic tract

Medial lemniscus

Pyramid

Fig. 8-6. Caudal medulla, just caudal to the obex. Scale mark = 5 mm.

Adjacent to the nucleus cuneatus and embedded in the fasciculus cuneatus is the *lateral* (or *accessory*) *cuneate nucleus* (Fig. 8-6). This is the forelimb equivalent of Clarke's nucleus, and the axons of these cells join the posterior spinocerebellar tract in the inferior cerebellar peduncle at a slightly more rostral level.

The spinothalamic tract is one of several that are not so compact or heavily myelinated as the medial lemniscus and therefore cannot be clearly distinguished in myelin-stained sections. However, this tract maintains more or less the same location (the ventrolateral portion of the tegmentum) during its passage through the brainstem, at least until it reaches the rostral midbrain.

The prominent pyramids and their decussation are located most anteriorly in the caudal medulla. Each pyramid consists of corticospinal fibers that originated in ipsilateral cerebral cortex and are (mostly) bound for the contralateral anterior horn.

Most of the area traversed by internal arcuate fibers in Fig. 8-6 is *reticular formation*. A casual observer, looking at this region in photographs like these, will not see much. This is, to a first approximation, what distinguishes the reticular formation from the rest of the brainstem; the posterior column nuclei, for example, *look* like nuclei, while the reticular formation just looks like the uniform neural tissue filling the gaps between identifiable structures throughout the brainstem tegmentum. In fact, though, the reticular formation is organized, but on a microscopic level, as discussed briefly later in this chapter.

Rostral medulla

The rostral (open) medulla, as defined here, extends from the obex to the rostral wall of the lateral recess, where the inferior cerebellar peduncle turns posteriorly to enter the cerebellum. The rostral medulla (Figs. 8-7 and 8-8) no longer looks much like the spinal cord, partly because the walls of the embryonic neural tube have been pushed outward to form the floor of the fourth ventricle (Fig. 1-10).

The caudal boundary (the obex) is approximately coincident with the caudal edge of the *inferior olivary nucleus*, a prominent structure that is responsible for the surface swelling called the olive (Fig. 8-3). The inferior cerebellar peduncle is located dorsolaterally at these levels and grows progressively larger as it continues

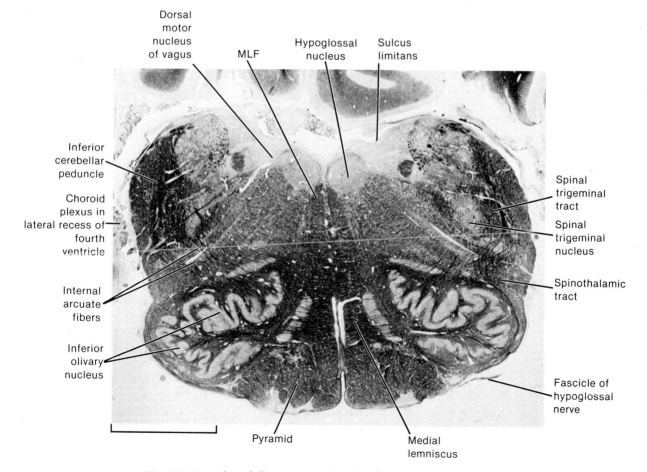

Fig. 8-7. Rostral medulla, just rostral to the obex. Scale mark = 4 mm.

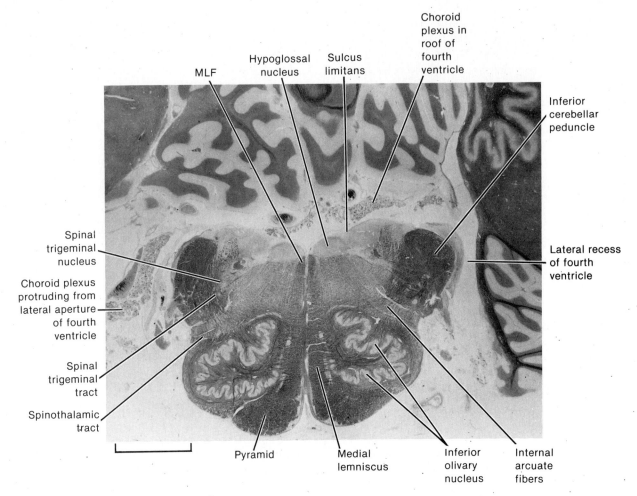

MLF   Hypoglossal nucleus   Sulcus limitans   Choroid plexus in roof of fourth ventricle

Inferior cerebellar peduncle

Spinal trigeminal nucleus

Choroid plexus protruding from lateral aperture of fourth ventricle

Spinal trigeminal tract

Spinothalamic tract

Lateral recess of fourth ventricle

Pyramid   Medial lemniscus   Inferior olivary nucleus   Internal arcuate fibers

Fig. 8-8. Rostral medulla, near the pontomedullary junction. Scale mark = 5 mm.

rostrally (compare Figs. 8-7 and 8-8). Fibers can be seen leaving the medially facing mouth (or *hilus*) of the inferior olivary nucleus, arching across the midline, and joining the contralateral inferior cerebellar peduncle. These too are internal arcuate fibers. More and more are added at progressively more rostral levels of the medulla, increasing the size of the peduncle.

Medial to the inferior olivary nucleus is the medial lemniscus, which still has the shape of a flattened band with a dorsal-ventral axis. Anterior to the medial lemniscus is the pyramid. Fascicles of the hypoglossal (XII) nerve (Figs. 8-3 and 8-7) emerge lateral to the pyramid in the groove between it and the inferior olivary nucleus. Posterior to the medial lemniscus, near the floor of the fourth ventricle, is a small but distinctive bundle of fibers that can be followed all the way to the midbrain. This is the *medial longitudinal fasciculus (MLF)*, which is involved in vestibular functions and eye movements.

The spinothalamic tract remains in the ventrolateral portion of the tegmentum, just above the inferior olivary nucleus, as does the anterior spinocerebellar tract. The

posterior spinocerebellar tract moves posteriorly and joins the inferior cerebellar peduncle.

Caudal pons

The caudal pons, as defined here, extends from the rostral wall of the lateral recess of the fourth ventricle to the point of attachment of the trigeminal nerve. In the caudal pons the inferior olivary nucleus ends, and the inferior cerebellar peduncle bends posteriorly and enters the cerebellum (Fig. 8-9). The MLF is in the same relative position as it was previously, adjacent to the midline and the floor of the fourth ventricle.

As the inferior olivary nucleus ends, the medial lemniscus assumes a more oval shape, as though it had previously been held upright against the midline. Now the homunculus is allowed to slump down slowly into a horizontal position, with its feet directed laterally (Fig. 8-10).

The pyramidal tract becomes dispersed in the basis pontis, which contains bundles of longitudinally oriented fibers, bundles of transversely oriented fibers, and *pon-*

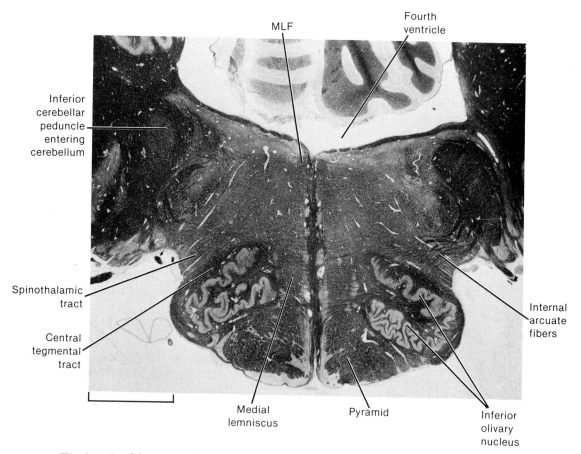

MLF

Fourth
ventricle

Inferior
cerebellar
peduncle
entering
cerebellum

Spinothalamic
tract

Central
tegmental
tract

Internal
arcuate
fibers

Medial
lemniscus

Pyramid

Inferior
olivary
nucleus

Fig. 8-9. Caudal pons, in the transition region from medulla to pons. Scale mark = 5 mm.

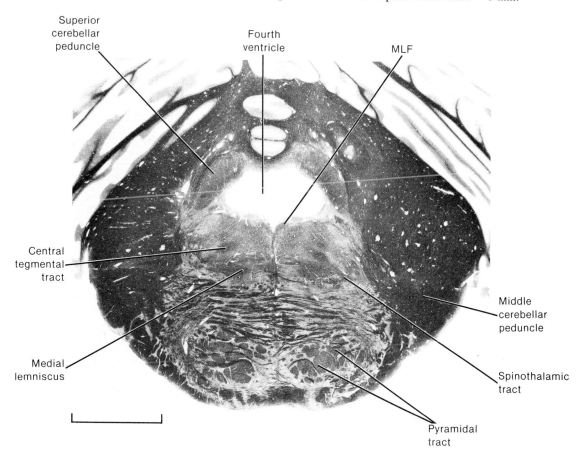

Superior
cerebellar
peduncle

Fourth
ventricle

MLF

Central
tegmental
tract

Middle
cerebellar
peduncle

Medial
lemniscus

Spinothalamic
tract

Pyramidal
tract

Fig. 8-10. Midpons, near the level of entry of the trigeminal nerve. Scale mark = 8 mm.

tine nuclei scattered among these bundles (Fig. 8-10). Some of the longitudinally oriented fibers are those of the pyramidal tract. Most of the others are *corticopontine fibers*, originating in many areas of the cerebral cortex and terminating in ipsilateral pontine nuclei. Fibers arising in the pontine nuclei cross the midline and form the massive middle cerebellar peduncle (brachium pontis).

The spinothalamic tract and the anterior spinocerebellar tract remain in the ventrolateral portion of the tegmentum. Spinoreticular fibers related to the spinothalamic system terminate medial to the direct spinothalamic fibers in the reticular formation throughout the brainstem, as do collaterals of direct spinothalamic fibers.*

---

*All direct spinothalamic fibers in humans (that is, those that project directly to the thalamus from the spinal cord) follow the classic spinothalamic pathway through the brainstem. That is, both neospinothalamic and paleospinothalamic fibers, in the strict sense of the term, travel together. However, the spinoreticular fibers leave the spinothalamic tract and travel somewhat more medially, particularly in the pons and midbrain. Some authors include the polysynaptic spinoreticulothalamic pathway in the term "paleospinothalamic," so the reader may encounter descriptions of a medial paleospinothalamic tract, as opposed to a more laterally situated neospinothalamic tract.

Rostral pons

The rostral pons extends from the attachment point of the trigeminal nerve (V) to the beginning of the cerebral aqueduct, which is about at the point of emergence of the trochlear nerve (IV). The MLF is visible throughout the rostral pons, as is the basis pontis (Fig. 8-11). The fourth ventricle narrows as the cerebral aqueduct is approached, and the superior cerebellar peduncle (brachium conjunctivum) becomes apparent in the wall of the ventricle. This is the major outflow from the cerebellum, projecting to the thalamus and to other structures.

The medial lemniscus gradually takes on a more flattened profile, now with a medial-lateral axis, and assumes a transverse orientation at the junction between the basis pontis and the pontine tegmentum. As in the caudal pons, the homunculus is arranged so that its feet are most lateral. As the medial lemniscus moves laterally, it approaches the spinothalamic tract; from here through the midbrain, the two are adjacent.

The anterior spinocerebellar tract moves posteriorly onto the surface of the superior cerebellar peduncle (Fig. 8-12). From here it turns caudally and enters the cerebellum, traveling "backwards" along the peduncle.

Near the floor of the fourth ventricle is a collection of

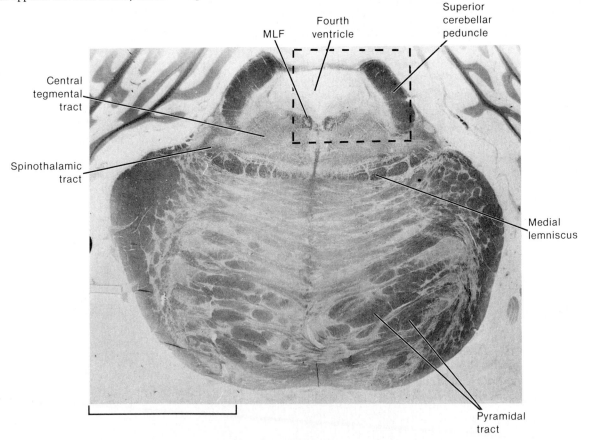

Fig. 8-11. Rostral pons, slightly rostral to Fig. 8-10. Scale mark = 1 cm.

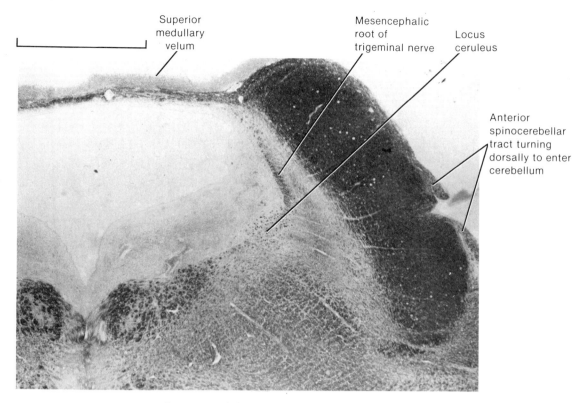

Fig. 8-12. Enlargement of the outlined area of Fig. 8-11. Scale mark = 2 mm.

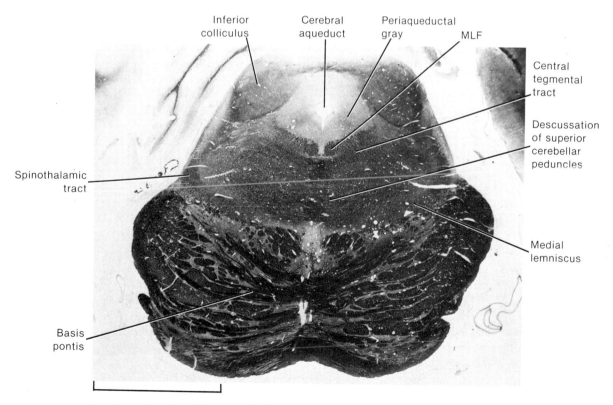

Fig. 8-13. Caudal midbrain, at the level of the inferior colliculus. Scale mark = 1 cm.

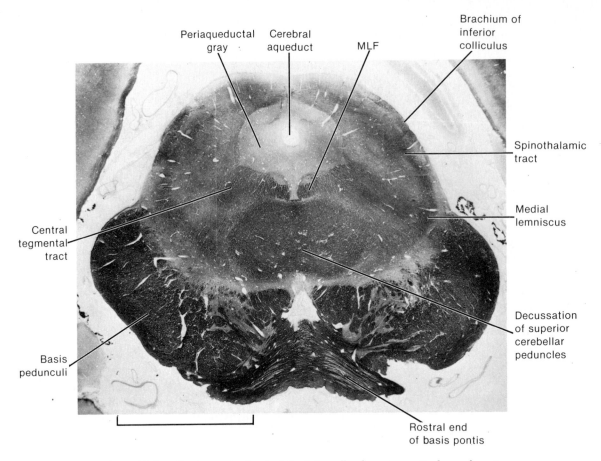

Fig. 8-14. Mid-midbrain, at the level of the intercollicular groove. Scale mark = 1 cm.

pigmented cells that contain neuromelanin and appear blue-black in unstained brain tissue (Fig. 8-12). This is the *locus ceruleus* (Latin = blue spot), a long thin nucleus that has been the subject of much research and interest in recent years. Cells of the locus ceruleus contain the neurotransmitter norepinephrine and innervate virtually the entire CNS, from spinal cord to cerebral cortex. In fact, there is some evidence that individual cells have branched axons that innervate the spinal cord, the diencephalon, and the cerebral cortex. (It had previously been thought that no fibers arising caudal to the diencephalon reached the cortex.) The function of the locus ceruleus is not yet known, but it has been surmised from its widespread connections that it has some sort of an overall biasing effect and might be important in regulating states of consciousness or arousal.

Caudal midbrain

The caudal midbrain is essentially the part that contains the inferior colliculi. It extends from the point of emergence of the trochlear nerve to the *intercollicular groove*. The fourth ventricle has narrowed into the cerebral aqueduct (Fig. 8-13), the superior cerebellar peduncles sink deeper into the midbrain tegmentum and begin

to decussate, and the MLF continues on its usual course. The basis pontis protrudes rostrally under the caudal midbrain tegmentum. The inferior colliculus is (literally) a prominent nuclear mass. Ventromedial to it, encircling the aqueduct, is a particularly pale-staining region of gray matter called, appropriately enough, the *periaqueductal gray*.

The medial lemniscus is still a flattened band of fibers, now curving a bit laterally, and the spinothalamic tract is lateral to it at the surface of the brainstem. At slightly more rostral levels (Fig. 8-14), the spinothalamic fibers are arranged in a band just beneath the brachium of the inferior colliculus. Damage here would be expected to abolish pain and temperature sensations over the entire contralateral body. This was done for a time in a surgical procedure called *mesencephalic tractotomy*, in the hope of relieving intractable pain. However, because of unexpected and undesirable side effects (discussed later), the operation is no longer performed.

Rostral midbrain

The rostral midbrain contains the superior colliculi. It extends from the intercollicular groove to the *posterior commissure*. Fig. 8-15 shows a section through the

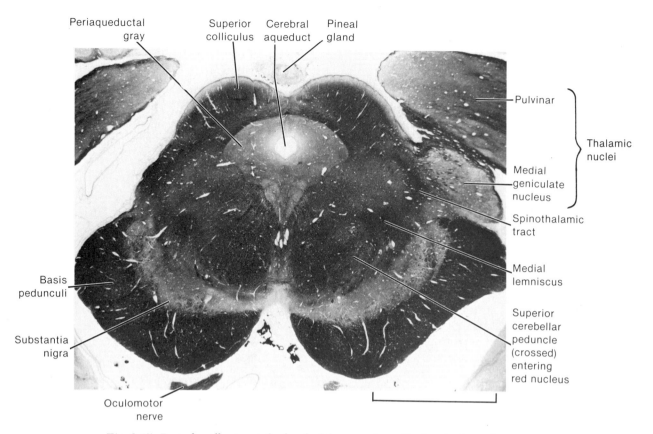

Periaqueductal gray Superior colliculus Cerebral aqueduct Pineal gland

Pulvinar

Thalamic nuclei

Medial geniculate nucleus

Spinothalamic tract

Medial lemniscus

Superior cerebellar peduncle (crossed) entering red nucleus

Basis pedunculi

Substantia nigra

Oculomotor nerve

Fig. 8-15. Rostral midbrain, at the level of the superior colliculus. Scale mark = 1 cm.

rostral portion of the rostral midbrain. At this level the MLF is ending, decussation of the superior cerebellar peduncles is complete, and in their place the large *red nucleus* becomes visible on each side. Some fibers from the contralateral superior cerebellar peduncle end here, but most continue on to the thalamus. Anterior to the red nucleus is the *substantia nigra* (pale in myelin-stained preparations but dark in unstained or cell-stained preparations), and ventral to the substantia nigra is the cerebral peduncle. Strictly speaking, the term "cerebral peduncle" refers to all of the midbrain anterior to the superior colliculus, and the term "basis pedunculi" (or "crus cerebri") refers to the massive fiber bundle in the anterior part of the peduncle. However, in common usage, "basis pedunculi" and "cerebral peduncle" are becoming more or less interchangeable, both referring to the fiber bundle. This bundle consists principally of descending corticopontine and corticospinal fibers. The oculomotor nerve (III) emerges into the space between the cerebral peduncles (the interpeduncular fossa). Several parts of the diencephalon (the pineal gland and some thalamic nuclei) hang back over and alongside the rostral midbrain.

At rostral midbrain levels, the medial lemniscus and the spinothalamic tract form a continuous curved band of fibers. Many fibers traveling with the more medial, spinoreticular fibers terminate in the periaqueductal gray and in certain portions of the superior colliculus. The latter fibers are sometimes considered separately as a spinotectal tract.

RETICULAR FORMATION
Nature

The reticular formation is an apparently (but not actually) diffusely organized area that forms the central core of the brainstem (Fig. 8-16). It has been likened to a hot dog surrounded by a bun of discrete tracts and nuclei.* The reason it appears to be diffusely organized is twofold:

1. Its pattern of connectivity is characterized by a great deal of convergence and divergence, so that a single cell may respond to several different sensory modalities or to stimuli applied practically anywhere on the body.
2. Although it is involved in several quite separate functions, the areas involved in these functions overlap considerably, almost as though several nuclei had been scrambled together and dispersed

---

*Earnest, Michael: Personal communication, 1974.

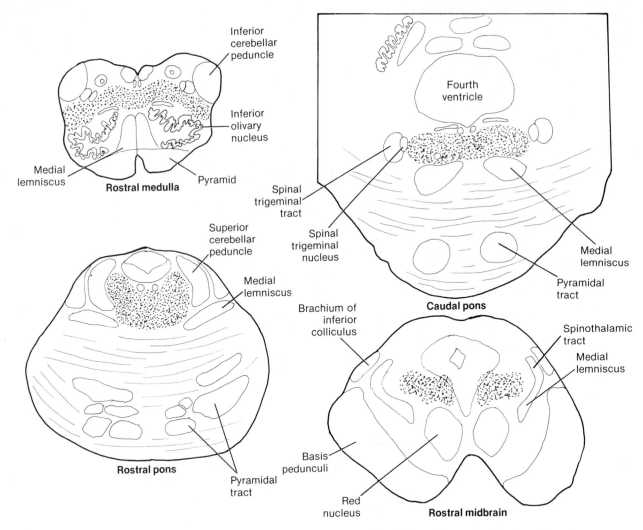

Fig. 8-16. Approximate extent of the reticular formation at four different brainstem levels, indicated by stippling.

along the brainstem, while their constituent cells retained their original connections.

Histologically the reticular formation can be divided into a lateral third and a medial two thirds; this division is particularly clear-cut in the pons and rostral medulla. The medial zone in the rostral medulla contains some very large cells and is often referred to as the *gigantocellular reticular nucleus*. The medial zone in the pons is customarily subdivided into rostral and caudal portions called, respectively, the *oral pontine* and the *caudal pontine reticular nucleus*. The lateral zone consists of small cells with short axons that receive most of the afferent input and project to the medial zone. The medial zone contains, in addition to small cells, a complement of larger cells with long axons that carry the output of the reticular formation. These axons often bifurcate and then give rise to enormous numbers of collaterals, and a single cell may send processes to both the spinal cord

and the diencephalon (but generally not to the cortex*) while sending collaterals to many structures along the way (Fig. 8-17). Reticular cells also have large fields of dendrites that tend to spread out in a plane perpendicular to the long axis of the brainstem, receiving numerous synapses from ascending sensory pathways, descending cortical axons, and many other sources. A look at the processes of a single reticular cell in a single plane (Fig. 8-17) should demonstrate why the reticular formation has been a tremendously difficult area of the brain to study, even though some progress has been made.

Functions and connections

The reticular formation is involved in four general types of function: motor control, sensory con-

---

*Groups of monoamine-containing cells, like these of the locus ceruleus, are an exception. Certain of these cell groups are considered to be part of the reticular formation.

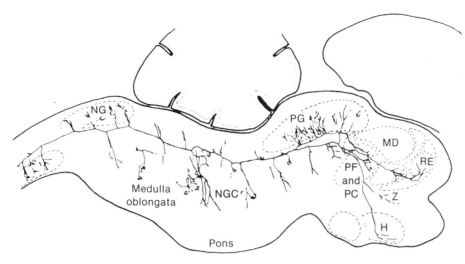

Fig. 8-17. Drawing of a Golgi-stained parasagittal section from the brain of a young rat. The single stained cell in the pontine reticular formation has an axon that bifurcates and ends in wide areas of the CNS. If one cell has projections this extensive, imagine the complexity of the reticular formation as a whole. *H*, Hypothalamus; *MD, PC, PF,* and *RE*, thalamic nuclei (dorsomedial, paracentral, parafascicular, and reuniens); *NG*, nucleus gracilis; *NGC*, part of the pontine reticular formation (gigantocellular nucleus); *PG*, periaqueductal gray; *Z*, zona incerta (part of the diencephalon). (From Scheibel, M.E., and Scheibel, A.B.: Structural substrates for integrative patterns in the brain stem reticular core. In Jasper, H.H., et al., editors: Reticular formation of the brain, Boston, 1958, Little, Brown and Co.)

trol, visceral control, and control of consciousness.

Motor control. Motor control has several different aspects.

1. Certain reticular regions are closely related to the cerebellum and its motor control functions. A fairly discrete collection of cells in the medullary reticular formation called the *lateral reticular nucleus* can often be resolved in conventionally prepared brainstem sections adjacent to the spinothalamic tract. It extends rostrally to midolivary levels and caudally into the caudal medulla, receiving direct spinoreticular fibers and collaterals of spinothalamic fibers and projecting to the cerebellum. It also receives input from the red nucleus, so it is more than a straightforward somatosensory relay to the cerebellum. Collections of reticular neurons near the medullary midline, collectively called the *paramedian reticular nucleus*, also project to the cerebellum. Afferents to the paramedian nucleus arise in the cerebellum and in the other locations, including the cerebral cortex.

2. There are two *reticulospinal tracts* arising from the medial two thirds of the pontine and the rostral medullary reticular formation. Those from the pons descend with the ipsilateral MLF and travel through the ventral funiculus in the spinal cord (Fig. 8-18). Those from the medulla descend bilaterally in the ventral part of the lateral funiculus.

The reticulospinal tracts are a major alternate route

(to the pyramidal tract) by which spinal motor neurons are controlled. These reticular neurons receive projections from many areas, including the basal ganglia, red nucleus, and substantia nigra. Input from widespread areas of the cerebral cortex, particularly the somatosensory and motor cortex, seems to be especially important. Most of these descending fibers travel to their reticular terminations in the *central tegmental tract* (Figs. 8-9 to 8-15). This is a complex tract containing afferents to, and efferents from, the reticular formation and descending projections from the red nucleus to the inferior olivary nucleus.

3. The reticulospinal tracts also carry descending motor commands generated within the reticular formation itself. Just as the spinal cord contains the basic neural machinery for simple (and some not-so-simple) reflexes, so the reticular formation contains the neural machinery for considerably more complex patterns of movement. A cat whose brainstem has been surgically separated from its diencephalon can, after a recovery period, walk and run spontaneously, properly right itself if tipped over, and assume a variety of complex postures. There have been cases of human infants born without cerebral hemispheres who were, nevertheless, capable of apparently normal yawning, stretching, suckling, and orienting behavior. It is assumed that their reticular formations formed the basis for these activities.

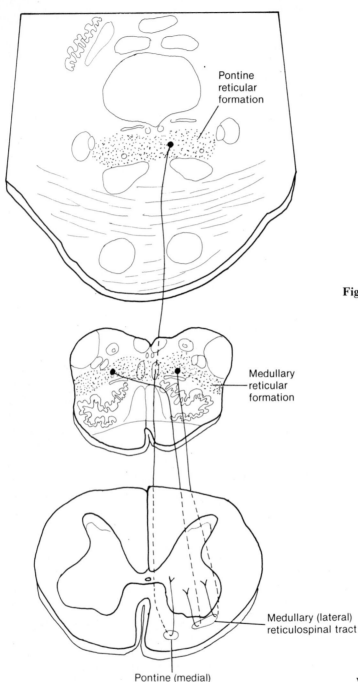

Pontine
reticular
formation

Medullary
reticular
formation

Medullary (lateral)
reticulospinal tract

Pontine (medial)
reticulospinal tract

Fig. 8-18. Medullary and pontine reticulospinal tracts.

Sensory control. Reticular neurons exert some control over activity in spinal reflex arcs and also over the access of sensory information to ascending pathways. Tonic inhibition of flexor reflexes originates in the reticular formation, with the result that only noxious stimuli can normally evoke such a reflex. In addition, stimulation of certain regions of the medullary reticular formation causes inhibition of some sensory interneurons and tract cells in the spinal cord. This seems to be important in the regulation of pain perception, as discussed a little later in this chapter.

Visceral control. Numerous visceral afferents synapse in the reticular formation, which programs appropriate responses to environmental changes and projects to the autonomic nuclei of the brainstem and spinal cord. Centers controlling inspiration, expiration, and the normal rhythm of breathing have been identified physiologically in the medulla and pons. Other centers controlling heart rate and blood pressure have been identified in the medullary reticular formation.

The hypothalamus also gives rise to numerous fibers concerned with autonomic regulation. Many of those involved in sympathetic control traverse the brainstem near the spinothalamic tract and reach mainly the ipsilateral (but to some extent the contralateral) intermediolateral cell column of the spinal cord. The numbers and types of synapses in the pathway are poorly understood, but at least some of the fibers reach the spinal cord directly from the hypothalamus. Interruption of the descending sympathetic pathway causes ipsilateral *Horner's syndrome*, which refers to a combination of miosis (small pupil), ptosis (drooping eyelid), and enophthalmos (recession of the eyeball; this is more apparent than real). Horner's syndrome may be accompanied by flushing and lack of sweating in ipsilateral skin of the face and part of the body.

Control of consciousness. Ascending projections from the reticular formation terminate in the thalamus, subthalamus, hypothalamus, and basal ganglia. The functions of most of these are poorly understood, but those to the thalamus seem to be particularly important. They terminate (as do the paleospinothalamic fibers) in the intralaminar nuclei, which in turn project to widespread areas of the cortex. Activity in this pathway is essential for the maintenance of a normal state of consciousness, and bilateral damage to these fibers as they traverse or originate in the midbrain reticular formation results in prolonged coma. This is an astounding notion: a normal, intact cerebrum is incapable of functioning in a conscious manner by itself; sustaining input from the brainstem reticular formation is required. The portion of the reticular formation that provides this input is known as the *ascending reticular activating system* (ARAS). It is important to understand that the ARAS is defined by physiological criteria; it is not synonymous with the anatomically defined reticular formation but rather is a portion of it. Modulation of the ARAS has a basic role in the sleep-wakefulness cycle, as discussed later in this book.

VASCULAR SUPPLY

The brainstem depends chiefly on the vertebral-basilar system for its blood supply. The caudal medulla has a supply much like that of the spinal cord. Anterior and lateral portions are supplied by the anterior spinal artery and/or small branches of the vertebral artery. Posterior portions are supplied by the posterior spinal artery and/or small branches of the posterior inferior cerebellar artery (PICA). The rostral medulla receives a varying supply. Anterior and medial structures, such as the pyramid and the medial lemniscus, depend on some combination of vertebral branches and the anterior spinal artery. Lateral and posterior structures, such as the spinothalamic tract and the inferior cerebellar peduncle, depend on the PICA and, to a lesser extent, on the posterior spinal artery.

Most of the pons is supplied by unnamed *paramedian* and *circumferential* branches of the basilar artery. The anterior inferior cerebellar artery (AICA) and the superior cerebellar artery contribute branches to the middle and superior cerebellar peduncles and to lateral portions of the pontine tegmentum.

The supply of the midbrain is chiefly from the posterior cerebral artery, with some contribution from the superior cerebellar artery caudally. In addition, the anterior choroidal artery and the posterior communicating artery may send branches to the cerebral peduncle.

SOME FUNCTIONAL ASPECTS OF THE BRAINSTEM
Pain pathways

As noted in Chapter 7, cordotomy is sometimes used for the surgical relief of intractable pain. When the pain involves an entire side of the body, the spinothalamic tract is occasionally sectioned in the medulla (an operation known as a *medullary tractotomy*). This is a rather more serious operation than a cordotomy, partly because of the difficulty of obtaining surgical access to the medulla and partly because of the risk to vital structures located in the medulla. Therefore attempts have been made in the past to cut the spinothalamic tract in other, less risky sites in the brainstem. Mesencephalic tractotomy, where the tract is near the surface of the brainstem (Fig. 8-14), seems feasible on anatomical grounds and has been attempted in several instances. However, while medullary tractotomies abolish contralateral pain over the whole body (much as a high cervical cordotomy would), a mesencephalic tractotomy often had a less favorable outcome. In a large percentage of the latter cases, the patients developed a new form of pain shortly after the operation. A pinprick, or sometimes just a light touch, on the contralateral body would cause an excruciating, deep, burning pain that was frequently felt to be worse than the original problem. The operation therefore is no longer performed. What was the cause of this unfortunate outcome? Medullary tractotomy, like cordotomy, interrupts both spinothalamic and spinoreticular fibers, but mesencephalic tractotomy interrupts only the spinothalamic fibers, since the spinoreticular fibers have by this time moved medially and terminated in the reticular formation. Apparently activity in this spinoreticulothalamic pathway, in the absence of direct spinothalamic activity, somehow causes the *dysesthesia*.

Endorphins and enkephalins

Opium and its derivatives, especially morphine, have long been used for pain control. The mechanism of their action has been a topic of great interest; if this mechanism could be understood, it might then be possible to design new pain-killing drugs that would not cause tolerance and addiction to develop. In recent years, pharmacological and anatomical-physiological studies have converged to produce extremely exciting data about this mechanism.

Electrical stimulation (through implanted electrodes) of the periaqueductal gray of the midbrain of rats causes an analgesia so profound that major surgery can then be performed without the aid of an anesthetic. This electrically induced analgesia is blocked by drugs that antagonize the action of morphine. Similar stimulation of the periaqueductal gray of humans can abolish intractable pain, an effect also blocked by opiate antagonists. This seems to imply that morphine mimics a pain-killing substance that is produced by the brain and released by stimulation of the periaqueductal gray. Two closely related pentapeptides called *enkephalins* (Greek = in the head), having powerful opiate properties, have now been isolated from mammalian brains and are found in high concentration in the periaqueductal gray.

One way in which midbrain stimulation (or morphine administration) depresses pain transmission is via a pathway that travels through the posterior part of the lateral funiculus, terminates in the ipsilateral posterior horn, and inhibits the interneurons and the tract cells of the spinothalamic tract. At least part of this descending pathway involves a relay in the reticular formation. Groups of cells along the midline of the brainstem (not including the paramedian nucleus) are collectively called the *raphe nuclei*. The raphe nuclei of the rostral medulla are known to project to the spinal cord through the dorsal part of the lateral funiculus and appear to be the part of the reticular formation involved in the descending pain-control pathway.

The study of endogenous substances with opiate activity (collectively called *endorphins*) is in its infancy, but it is already known that they are part of much more than a midbrain pain-control system. The two enkephalins, other endorphins, and the receptor molecules to which they bind are widespread in the brain and are also found in other parts of the body. They are concentrated not only in the periaqueductal gray but also (among other places) in the caudate nucleus, the locus ceruleus, the substantia gelatinosa, much of the limbic system, and the small intestine. How they relate to emotions and to intestinal motility is mainly a matter of speculation at present.

ADDITIONAL READING

Amaral, D.G., and Sinnamon, H.M.: The locus coeruleus: neurobiology of a central noradrenergic nucleus, Prog. Neurobiol. **9**:147, 1977. *A recent, extensive review.*

Basbaum, A.I., Clanton, C.H., and Fields, H.L.: Opiate and stimulus-produced analgesia: functional anatomy of a medullospinal pathway, Proc. Nat. Acad. Sci. USA **73**:4685, 1976. *An exciting paper with anatomical and physiological evidence that reticulospinal fibers from the raphe nuclei, stimulated from the periaqueductal gray matter, can inhibit the spinal pain-transmission pathways.*

Basbaum, A.I., and Fields, H.L.: Endogenous pain control mechanisms: review and hypothesis, Ann. Neurol. **4**:451, 1978.

Beecher, H.R.: Pain in men wounded in battle, Ann. Surg. **123**:96, 1946. *A fascinating paper showing that wounds we would expect to be terribly painful may not be, depending in part on the circumstances surrounding the incurrence of the injury.*

Bonica, J.J.: Pain, Res. Publ. Ass. Res. Nerv. Ment. Dis., vol. 58, 1980.

Cohen, M.I.: Neurogenesis of respiratory rhythm in the mammal, Physiol. Rev. **59**:1105, 1979.

Drake, C.G., and McKenzie, K.G.: Mesencephalic tractotomy for pain, J. Neurosurg. **10**:457, 1953.

Engberg, I., Lundberg, A., and Ryall, R.W.: Reticulospinal inhibition of transmission in reflex pathways, J. Physiol. **194**:201, 1968.

Hobson, J.A., and Brazier, M.A.B., editors: The reticular formation revisited: specifying function for a nonspecific system, International Brain Res. Organization monograph series, vol. 6, New York, 1980, Raven Press.

Hosobuchi, Y., Adams, J.E., and Linchitz, R.: Pain relief by electrical stimulation of the central gray matter in humans and its reversal by naloxone, Science **197**:183, 1977. *Evidence that the analgesia caused by stimulation of the periaqueductal gray has properties in common with morphine analgesia.*

Hughes, J.: Isolation of an endogenous compound from the brain with pharmacological properties similar to morphine, Brain Res. **88**:295, 1975.

Klee, W.A.: Endogenous opiate peptides. In Gainer, H., editor: Peptides in neurobiology, New York, 1977, Plenum Press.

Kneisley, L.W., Biber, M.P., and La Vail, J.H.: A study of the origin of brain stem projections to monkey spinal cord using the retrograde transport method, Exp. Neurol. **60**:116, 1978.

Kuhar, M.J., Pert, C.B., and Snyder, S.H.: Regional distribution of opiate receptor binding in monkey and human brain, Nature **245**:447, 1973.

Loewy, A.D., Araujo, J.C., and Kerr, F.W.L.: Pupillodilator pathways in the brain stem of the cat: anatomical and electrophysiological identification of a central autonomic pathway, Brain Res. **60**:65, 1973.

Mayer, D.J., Price, D.D., and Rafii, A.: Antagonism of acupuncture analgesia in man by the narcotic antagonist naloxone, Brain Res. **121**:368, 1977. *A provocative paper providing initial evidence that acupuncture works by somehow causing the release of enkephalins.*

Mehler, W.R.: Some neurological species differences—a posteriori, Ann. N.Y. Acad. Sci. **167**:424, 1969. *Tracing ascending tracts through the brainstem in a phylogenetic series of mammals from opossums to people.*

Moore, R.Y., and Kromer, L.F.: The organization of central catecholamine neuron systems. In Haber, B., and Aprison, M.H., editors: *Neuropharmacology and behavior*, New York, 1978, Plenum Press.

Nyberg-Hansen, R.: Sites and modes of termination of reticulo-spinal fibers in the cat: an experimental study with silver impregnation methods, J. Comp. Neurol. **124**:71, 1965.

Nygren, L.-G., and Olson, L.: A new major projection from locus coeruleus: the main source of noradrenergic nerve terminals in the ventral and dorsal columns of the spinal cord, Brain Res. **132**:85, 1977.

Olszewski, J., and Baxter, D.: Cytoarchitecture of the human brainstem, Philadelphia, 1954, J.B. Lippincott Co.

Pompeiano, O.: Reticular formation. In Iggo, A., editor: Handbook of sensory physiology, vol. II: Somatosensory system, New York, 1973, Springer-Verlag, Inc. *An extensive review with a long bibliography.*

Reynolds, D.V.: Surgery in the rat during electrical analgesia induced by focal brain stimulation, Science **164**:444, 1969.

Riley, H.A.: An atlas of the basal ganglia, brain stem and spinal cord, New York, 1960, Hafner.

Saper, C.B., et al.: Direct hypothalamo-autonomic connections, Brain Res. **117**:305, 1976.

Willis, W.D., Haber, L.H., and Martin, R.F.: Inhibition of spinothalamic tract cells and interneurons by brain stem stimulation in the monkey, J. Neurophysiol. **40**:968, 1977.

CHAPTER 9

CRANIAL NERVES

The caudal medulla looks somewhat similar to the spinal cord, but this similarity seems to disappear at more rostral levels of the brainstem. One of the complicating factors is the arrangement of the tracts and nuclei associated with cranial nerves III to XII. These tracts and nuclei appear discouragingly intricate on first inspection, but there is a commonly used way of systematizing the cranial nerves so that their central connections make sense. This is in terms of the *functional components* contained within each nerve.

Spinal nerves contain sensory and motor fibers. Some of each kind are related to visceral structures and some to somatic structures. A given spinal nerve fiber can therefore be placed in one of the following four categories, each of which is prefixed by the word "general":

1. *General somatic afferent (GSA)* fibers are related to receptors for pain, temperature, and mechanical stimuli in somatic structures such as skin, muscles, and joints.

2. *General visceral afferent (GVA)* fibers are related to receptors in visceral structures such as the walls of the digestive tract.

3. *General visceral efferent (GVE)* fibers are preganglionic autonomic fibers.

4. *General somatic efferent (GSE)* fibers innervate skeletal muscle (that is, they are alpha and gamma motor neurons).

The cell bodies on which spinal afferents synapse and the cell bodies of spinal efferent fibers are located by and large in portions of the spinal gray matter predictable from its embryological development (Fig. 9-1, *A*). The sulcus limitans separates the alar plate (which will develop into the dorsal horn) from the basal plate (which will develop into the ventral horn). Within both the alar and the basal plate, cells concerned with visceral function tend to be located nearer the sulcus limitans. This is shown most clearly in the adult by the location of the cell bodies of GVE fibers in the intermediolateral cell column. Thus for each of the four spinal functional com-

ponents there is a corresponding column of cells in the spinal gray matter. The GSA and GSE columns extend the length of the cord; the GVA and GVE columns are found at spinal levels T1 to L2 or L3 and S2 to S4.

All four of the spinal functional components are found in various cranial nerves, where they subserve the same functions for the head. Three additional components are also found among the cranial nerves; these new components are prefixed by the word "special":

1. *Special somatic afferent (SSA)* fibers are related to the special senses of sight, hearing, and equilibrium.

2. *Special visceral afferent (SVA)* fibers are related to the special senses of smell and taste.

3. *Special visceral efferent (SVE)* fibers innervate the branchiomeric muscles. Structures that develop into the gill arches (or branchial arches) in fish develop instead into various structures in and near the head and neck in humans. Branchiomeric muscles (notably the muscles of the larynx, pharynx, and face) are associated with these branchial arch structures. Functionally and histologically, branchiomeric muscles are identical to ordinary skeletal muscle. However, since they tend to be concentrated around the mouth at the junction between visceral and somatic areas, the motor fibers that innervate them are conventionally called SVE fibers. The classification is sometimes confusing (particularly since the sensory fibers to these muscles are called GSA fibers), but it is a tradition of long standing.

There are no special somatic efferent fibers, so GSE fibers are often referred to simply as *somatic efferent (SE)* fibers.

As in the case of the spinal cord, the locations of the cell bodies where cranial nerve afferents terminate or cranial nerve efferents originate can be predicted (to some extent) from the embryology of the brainstem. The walls of the neural tube spread apart in the medulla and

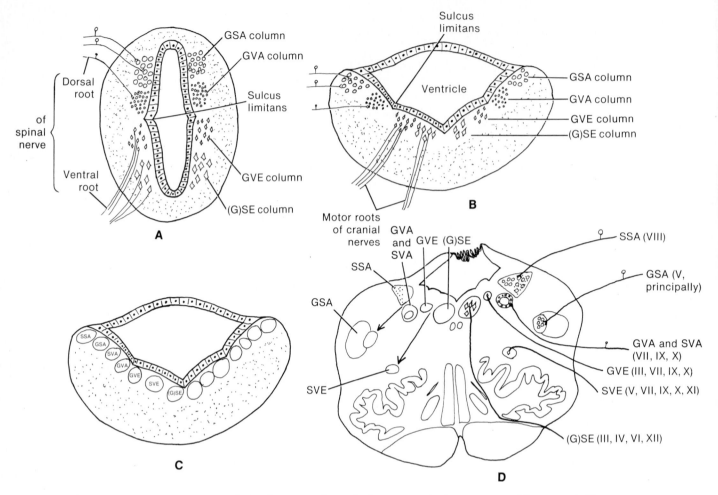

Fig. 9-1. Arrangement of cranial nerve nuclei in the brainstem. A, Arrangement of the general afferent and efferent cell columns in the embryonic spinal cord. B, Movement of these columns to the floor of the fourth ventricle in the embryonic rhombencephalon. C, Further subdivision of these cell columns, showing the "ideal" locations of the cranial nerve nuclei, corresponding to the seven functional components. D, Drawing of an actual section through the rostral medulla of an adult brain. On the left the nuclei corresponding to the seven functional components are indicated. On the right the cranial nerves containing each of these components are indicated; cranial nerves I and II are not included, nor are some minor components such as the few GSA fibers in cranial nerve VII. Not all the nerves listed actually emerge at this brainstem level; they are included here for summary purposes.

pons to form the floor of the fourth ventricle (Fig. 1-10). The sulcus limitans runs longitudinally along the floor of the adult ventricle, still separating sensory alar plate derivatives (now lateral) from motor basal plate derivatives (now medial) (Fig. 9-1, B). As in the case of the spinal cord, cells concerned with visceral function tend to be located nearer the sulcus limitans.

Ideally the cell columns subserving the special components of the cranial nerves would be located adjacent to those for the corresponding general components, as indicated in Fig. 9-1, C. The actual arrangement in the adult brainstem is not quite so simple as in this idealized diagram, for two principal reasons. First, the cell columns of the brainstem are not continuous like those of

the spinal cord; rather, they are interrupted and form a series of nuclei, so that all components may not be present in a given transverse plane. Second, in a few instances, portions of a cell column migrate away from their expected locations. For example, most SVE neurons are located in the ventrolateral part of the tegmentum rather than in the floor of the ventricle adjacent to other efferent neurons. The actual locations of cranial nerve nuclei in the rostral medulla are shown in Fig. 9-1, D; also indicated are the types of functional components in each of the cranial nerves of the brainstem. Please understand, however, that this is meant to be a convenient summary, and not all cranial nerves project to or originate from the rostral medulla.

TABLE 4

Contents of the cranial nerves

Nerve	Functional component	Origin or termination within CNS	Peripheral sensory or motor ending
I	SVA	Olfactory bulb	Olfactory epithelium
II	SSA	Lateral geniculate nucleus, principally	Ganglion cells of retina
III	(G) SE	Oculomotor nucleus	Superior, inferior, and medial recti; inferior oblique; levator palpebrae superioris
	GVE	Edinger-Westphal nucleus (part of oculomotor nucleus)	Sphincter pupillae, ciliary muscle*
IV	(G) SE	Trochlear nucleus	Superior oblique
V	GSA	Spinal and main sensory nuclei	Skin and deep tissues of head; dura mater
		Mesencephalic nucleus	Muscle spindles and other mechanoreceptors
	SVE	Trigeminal motor nucleus	Muscles of mastication, tensor tympani, and a few others
VI	(G) SE	Abducens nucleus	Lateral rectus
VII	GSA	Spinal trigeminal nucleus	Outer ear
	SVA	Solitary nucleus	Taste buds of anterior two thirds of tongue
	GVA	Solitary nucleus	Small portion of nasopharynx
	GVE	Superior salivatory nucleus	Submandibular, sublingual salivary glands; lacrimal gland*
	SVE	Facial motor nucleus	Muscles of facial expression; stapedius
VIII	SSA	Cochlear and vestibular nuclei	Organ of Corti; cristae of semicircular canals; maculae of utricle and saccule
IX	GSA	Spinal trigeminal nucleus	Outer ear
	SVA	Solitary nucleus	Taste buds of posterior third of tongue
	GVA	Solitary and spinal trigeminal nuclei	Carotid body and sinus; mucous membranes of nasal and oral pharynx
	GVE	Inferior salivatory nucleus	Parotid gland*
	SVE	Nucleus ambiguus	Pharynx (stylopharyngeus)
X	GSA	Spinal trigeminal nucleus	Outer ear
	SVA	Solitary nucleus	Taste buds of epiglottis
	GVA	Solitary and spinal trigeminal nuclei	Thoracic and abdominal viscera; mucous membranes of larynx and laryngeal pharynx
	GVE	Dorsal motor nucleus	Thoracic and abdominal viscera*
	SVE	Nucleus ambiguus	Larynx and pharynx
Cranial XI	SVE	Nucleus ambiguus	Larynx and pharynx
Spinal XI	SVE	Accessory nucleus, cervical cord	Sternocleidomastoid; trapezius
XII	(G) SE	Hypoglossal nucleus	Muscles of tongue

*Final destination after synapse in a parasympathetic ganglion.

It can be seen from Fig. 9-1, *D*, that no cranial nerve contains all seven functional components. If the components of all the nerves are tabulated (as in Table 4), it becomes apparent that there are three types of cranial nerve. Some nerves (III, IV, VI, and XII) contain GSE fibers and little or nothing else, so they may be referred to as *somatic efferent nerves*. Others (I, II, and VIII) contain special sensory fibers (SSA or SVA) and nothing else. The remaining nerves (V, VII, IX, X, and XI) are somewhat more complex and tend to contain several components; all innervate branchial arch musculature (that is, they contain SVE fibers), so they are called *branchiomeric nerves*.

Presenting the cranial nerves requires dealing with a considerable amount of material; the remainder of this chapter is divided into three more or less distinct sections discussing the somatic efferent nerves, the branchiomeric nerves, and a particular special sensory nerve, the eighth nerve. Since cranial nerves I and II are not attached to the brainstem but rather are directly related to the forebrain, they are considered separately in later chapters.

SOMATIC EFFERENT NERVES (III, IV, VI, and XII)

The somatic efferent nerves are the simplest of the cranial nerves, since each contains only one functional component (GSE fibers), except for cranial nerve III, which has a small but important complement of GVE fibers.* The nuclei of origin of all these nerves are located adjacent to the midline near the aqueduct or the floor of the fourth ventricle, as would be expected from their embryological origins.

Oculomotor nerve (III)

Cranial nerve III supplies the levator palpebrae superioris and all the internal and external muscles of the ipsilateral eye except the lateral rectus, superior oblique, and dilator pupillae. The fibers originate in the wedge-shaped *oculomotor nucleus*, which is located at the ventral edge of the periaqueductal gray in the rostral midbrain (Fig. 9-2). They then proceed ventrally and arch through the midbrain tegmentum in several separate bundles that join to form the nerve just as they emerge into the interpeduncular fossa.

The oculomotor nucleus actually consists of a series of longitudinal cell columns, or subnuclei. The column supplying the levator palpebrae superioris is located in

*The course of proprioceptive fibers (for example, from muscle spindles) from extraocular muscles and muscles of the tongue has long been a matter of contention. The hypoglossal nerve almost certainly contains lingual proprioceptive fibers for part or all of its course. Those from the extraocular muscles probably travel in cranial nerves III, IV, and VI within the orbit, then join the trigeminal nerve for the rest of their course to the brainstem. Since the function of these afferents is largely unknown, and since so much uncertainty surrounds their anatomy, they are usually just ignored.

the midline and innervates this muscle on both sides. The column supplying the superior rectus projects to the contralateral eye. The columns supplying the medial rectus, inferior oblique, and inferior rectus all project to the ipsilateral eye. Finally, a column of preganglionic parasympathetic (GVE) neurons, which straddles the midline and is known by the tenacious eponym of *Edinger-Westphal nucleus*, projects to the ipsilateral ciliary ganglion. The ciliary ganglion in turn innervates the sphincter pupillae and the ciliary muscle.

The partly crossed/partly uncrossed nature of the oculomotor nerve is a curious fact but one of very limited clinical significance. This is because the oculomotor nuclei of the two sides are so close to one another that a central lesion in this vicinity is likely to damage both nuclei. On the other hand, once a given oculomotor nerve emerges from the brainstem, it supplies only ipsilateral muscles, so a third nerve lesion affects only one eye. Therefore the dissociated finding of paralysis of the superior rectus on one side and of other extraocular muscles on the opposite side is rarely (if ever) encountered.

Damage to one oculomotor nerve causes a series of deficits. The eye ipsilateral to the lesion is deviated laterally, since the medial rectus is now paralyzed and the lateral rectus is unopposed. This is called *lateral strabismus*, indicating that the eyes are misaligned because one of them is deviated away from the midline. As

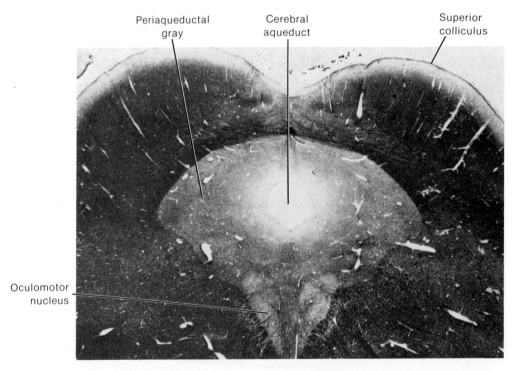

Fig. 9-2. Section through the rostral midbrain showing the oculomotor nucleus. This figure is an enlargement of part of a section similar to that shown in Fig. 8-15.

a result, the patient complains of *diplopia* (double vision) and is unable to move the affected eye vertically or medially. The ipsilateral levator palpebrae superioris is paralyzed, so *ptosis* occurs. In addition, the sphincter pupillae and ciliary muscle are nonfunctional. The pupil on the affected side is dilated *(mydriasis)* as a result of the now unopposed dilator pupillae and does not constrict in response to light*; the lens cannot be focused on near objects.

Along the course of the oculomotor nerve from brainstem to orbit, the GVE fibers from the Edinger-Westphal nucleus travel in a superficial location and are therefore especially susceptible to external pressures. A dilated pupil, unresponsive to light, may therefore be the first clinically detectable sign of something pressing on the third nerve.

Since ptosis and pupils of unequal size accompany Horner's syndrome, one might think this could be confused with third nerve damage. However, in Horner's syndrome the ptosis is on the same side as a nonfunctional dilator pupillae, hence on the same side as the *smaller* pupil. On the other hand, the ptosis following third nerve damage is on the same side as a nonfunctional sphincter pupillae, hence on the same side as the *larger* pupil. In addition, the ptosis following third nerve

damage is more pronounced and is usually accompanied, of course, by defective eye movements and lateral strabismus.

Trochlear nerve (IV)

Cranial nerve IV supplies the superior oblique muscle. Its cell bodies of origin are located in the contralateral *trochlear nucleus*. This is a small nucleus (since it has only one small muscle to supply) located at the level of the inferior colliculus, where it indents the MLF (Fig. 9-3). Fibers leaving the nucleus turn caudally in the periaqueductal gray, then arch dorsally to decussate and leave the brainstem at the pons-midbrain junction. The trochlear nerve is thus unique in two respects: it is the only cranial nerve attached to the dorsal aspect of the brainstem and the only one to originate entirely from a contralateral nucleus.

Damage to the trochlear nerve results in much less drastic and noticeable deficits than does damage to either the oculomotor or the abducens nerve. The superior oblique muscle moves the eye downward and laterally, so attempted movement in these directions (typically in reading or in descending stairs) may cause diplopia.

Abducens nerve (VI)

Cranial nerve VI supplies the lateral rectus muscle. The fibers originate from the ipsilateral *abducens nu-*

---

*Both pupils normally constrict when light is shone into either eye. This is the *pupillary light reflex*, which is discussed further in Chapter 11.

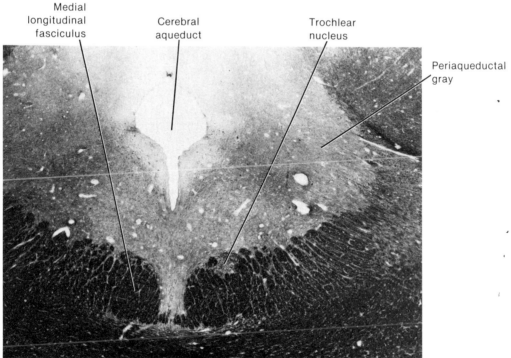

Fig. 9-3. Section through the caudal midbrain showing the trochlear nucleus. This figure is an enlargement of part of a section similar to that shown in Fig. 8-13.

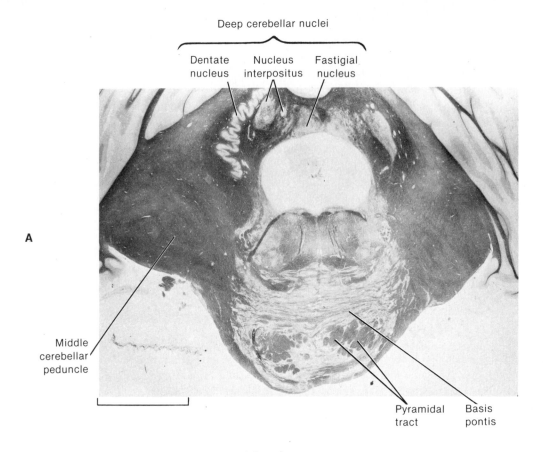

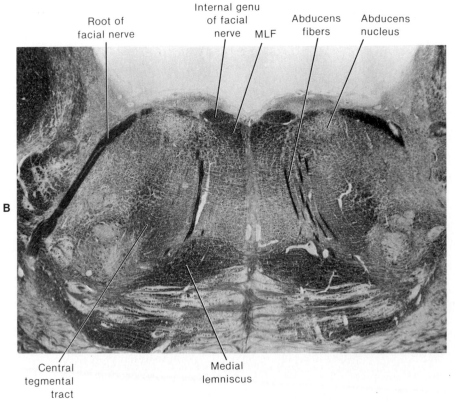

Fig. 9-4. Section through the caudal pons showing the abducens nucleus and fibers of the facial nerve cut at different points along their course. **A,** Scale mark = 1 cm. **B,** Enlargement of a portion of **A.**

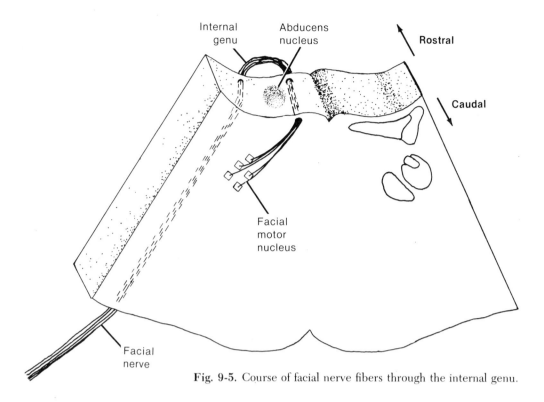

Fig. 9-5. Course of facial nerve fibers through the internal genu.

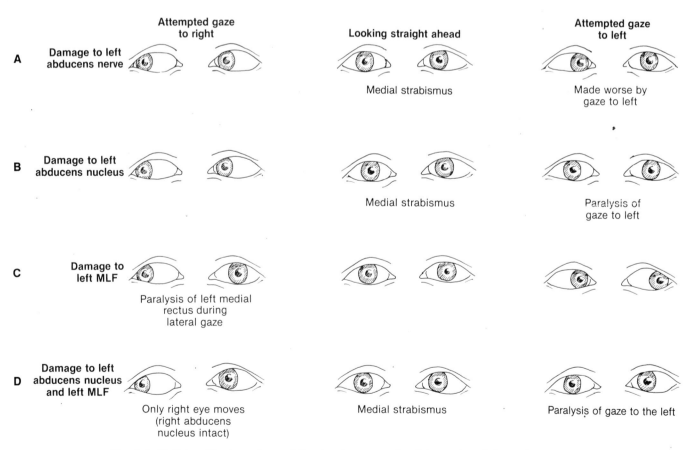

	Attempted gaze to right	Looking straight ahead	Attempted gaze to left
A Damage to left abducens nerve		Medial strabismus	Made worse by gaze to left
B Damage to left abducens nucleus		Medial strabismus	Paralysis of gaze to left
C Damage to left MLF	Paralysis of left medial rectus during lateral gaze		
D Damage to left abducens nucleus and left MLF	Only right eye moves (right abducens nucleus intact)	Medial strabismus	Paralysis of gaze to the left

Fig. 9-6. Deficits of horizontal gaze following damage to the abducens/parabducens/MLF system as indicated in Fig. 9-7. **A**, Abducens palsy. **B**, Lateral gaze paralysis. **C**, Internuclear ophthalmoplegia. **D**, A "one-and-a-half" (combination of **B** and **C**).

cleus, which is located in the caudal pons beneath the floor of the fourth ventricle (Fig. 9-4). Medial to this nucleus are two bundles of fibers. The more medial of the two is the MLF. Between the MLF and the abducens nucleus are motor fibers of the facial nerve, which take a most unusual course in leaving the brainstem. They originate in the facial nucleus (Fig. 9-15), which is slightly caudal to the abducens nucleus. They project dorsomedially, wrap around the abducens nucleus, and turn back ventrally to exit from the brainstem (Fig. 9-5). The place where these fibers wrap around the abducens nucleus is called the *internal genu of the facial nerve.* The abducens nucleus, together with the internal genu, is responsible for the facial colliculus in the floor of the fourth ventricle (Fig. 8-3).

Lateral gaze. Damage to the abducens nerve causes a *medial strabismus* (that is, the affected eye deviates medially) as a result of the action of the now-unopposed medial rectus muscle. The individual may be able to move the affected eye to the midline (but not past it) by relaxing its medial rectus muscle (Fig. 9-6). Damage to the abducens nucleus causes the same deficit but with a significant addition. In this case, not only can the individual not move the ipsilateral eye laterally, but he is also unable to move the contralateral eye medially when he tries to look toward the side of the lesion (Fig. 9-6, *B*). This is called *lateral gaze paralysis.* Such clinical findings led to the postulate that there is a second nucleus, overlapping the abducens nucleus, that controls the medial movement of the contralateral eye. This postulated nucleus is called the *parabducens nucleus.* It has recently been demonstrated that there are interneurons in the abducens nucleus whose axons project through the MLF to the motor neurons that control the contralateral medial rectus muscle (Fig. 9-7). The conclusion is that the motor neurons of the abducens nucleus and

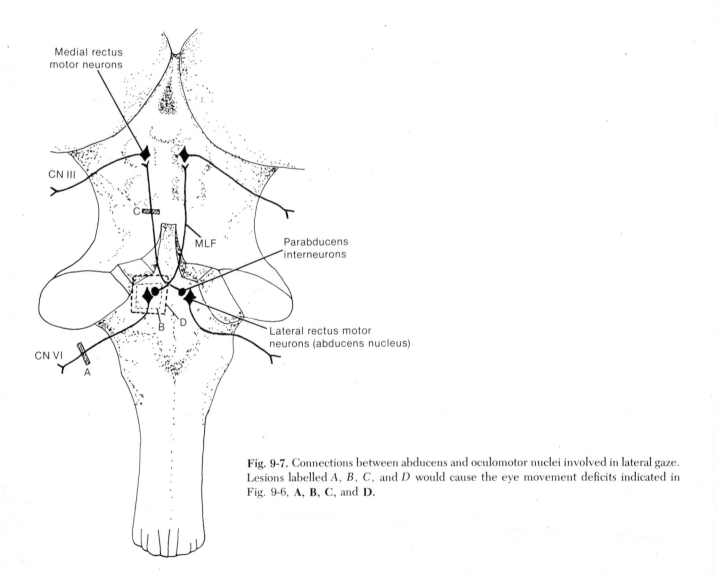

Fig. 9-7. Connections between abducens and oculomotor nuclei involved in lateral gaze. Lesions labelled *A, B, C,* and *D* would cause the eye movement deficits indicated in Fig. 9-6, **A, B, C,** and **D.**

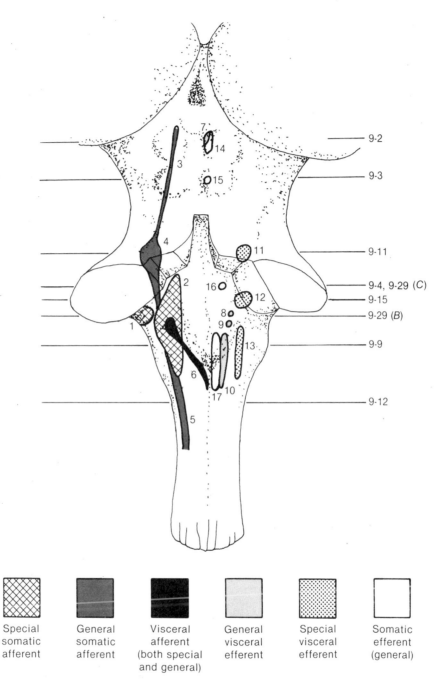

Fig. 9-8. Locations of cranial nerve nuclei within the brainstem. Sensory nuclei are shown on the left and motor nuclei on the right. Different hatchings and stipplings indicate the functional components that originate or terminate in particular nuclei. Horizontal lines indicate the planes of section of various photographs in this chapter. *1*, Cochlear nuclei; *2*, vestibular nuclei; *3*, mesencephalic nucleus of trigeminal; *4*, main sensory nucleus of trigeminal; *5*, spinal trigeminal nucleus (shown here as ending abruptly, whereas actually it blends gradually with the posterior horn of upper cervical segments); *6*, solitary nucleus; *7*, Edinger-Westphal nucleus (part of oculomotor nuclear complex); *8*, superior salivatory nucleus; *9*, inferior salivatory nucleus; *10*, dorsal motor nucleus of vagus; *11*, trigeminal motor nucleus; *12*, facial motor nucleus; *13*, nucleus ambiguus; *14*, oculomotor nucleus; *15*, trochlear nucleus; *16*, abducens nucleus; *17*, hypoglossal nucleus.

the interneurons of the parabducens nucleus are mixed up together in the same place. Nevertheless the two nuclei are still spoken of as separate entities.

The function of the MLF may be understood by considering that both eyes normally work together. For example, when we look to one side, one lateral rectus muscle contracts, and the contralateral medial rectus muscle also contracts. The pathway that interconnects the abducens, trochlear, and oculomotor nuclei to make these sorts of movements possible is the MLF. Vertical movements and the higher centers that direct coordinated eye movements are discussed in a later chapter, but for purely horizontal movements the crucial interconnecting fibers are those that arise from the interneurons in the parabducens nucleus (Fig. 9-7). These cells send their axons across the midline at the level of the abducens/parabducens nucleus to the contralateral MLF. These axons then ascend to the oculomotor nucleus, where they make excitatory synapses on medial rectus motor neurons. Simultaneous firing of abducens motor neurons and parabducens interneurons results in coordinated lateral gaze.

Damage to one MLF removes this excitatory influence from medial rectus motor neurons, so the eye ipsilateral to the lesion fails to move medially past the midline during attempted horizontal gaze (Figs. 9-6 and 9-7). Since both abducens nuclei are intact, full lateral movements of both eyes are still possible. This condition has the ponderous name of *internuclear ophthalmoplegia*.

Another eye movement disorder, clinically called a *one-and-a-half*, is rarely seen but is nevertheless instructive. It is caused by damage in the vicinity of the abducens nucleus and is characterized by the patient's inability to move either eye toward the side of the lesion in lateral gaze and inability to move the eye on the side of the lesion in gaze toward the opposite side (Fig. 9-6, *D*). Thus of the two directions of horizontal gaze (right and left), the patient has only half of one intact. This is presumed to be caused by destruction of one abducens/parabducens nucleus plus destruction of fibers from the contralateral parabducens nucleus as they join the MLF on the side of the lesion (Fig. 9-7).

Hypoglossal nerve (XII)

Cranial nerve XII supplies the intrinsic muscles of the tongue. The fibers originate in the ipsilateral *hypoglossal nucleus,* which extends from the caudal medulla to the rostral part of the rostral medulla (Figs. 9-8 and 9-9). This nucleus is situated adjacent to the midline just beneath the floor of the fourth ventricle and forms an elevation there called the hypoglossal trigone or triangle (Fig. 8-3). Hypoglossal axons proceed ventrally and emerge as a series of rootlets in the groove between the pyramid and the olive (Figs. 8-3 and 8-7).

Damage to the hypoglossal nerve causes weakness of

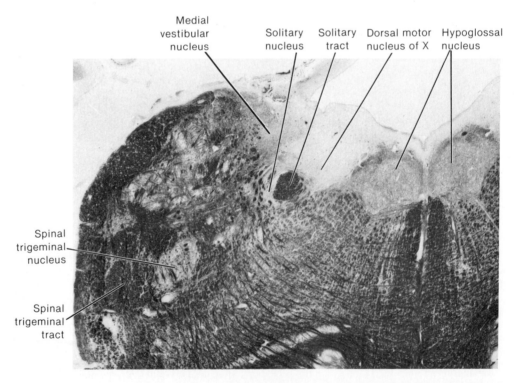

Fig. 9-9. Section through the rostral medulla showing the hypoglossal nucleus and other cranial nerve nuclei. This figure is an enlargement of part of a section similar to that shown in Fig. 8-7.

one side of the tongue and, since this would be a lower motor neuron lesion, atrophy of that side of the tongue as well. This weakness is most easily demonstrated by asking the patient to protrude his or her tongue; the tongue will deviate *toward* the side of the lesion (that is, toward the weak side). Bilateral hypoglossal lesions may cause difficulties in both speaking and eating.

BRANCHIOMERIC NERVES (V, VII, IX, X, AND XI)

The branchiomeric nerves all innervate striated muscle of branchial arch origin (that is, they all contain SVE fibers). With the possible exception of cranial nerve XI, they all contain other components as well. In spite of this, each has one function with which it tends to be associated: the trigeminal nerve (V) is the major general sensory nerve for the head; the facial nerve (VII) is the motor nerve for facial expression; the glossopharyngeal nerve (IX) is the most important conveyor of taste and pharyngeal sensations; the vagus nerve (X) carries the parasympathetic outflow to the thoracic and abdominal viscera; and the accessory nerve (XI) is the motor nerve for the sternocleidomastoid and trapezius muscles.

Trigeminal nerve (V)

With respect to somatic sensory innervation, cranial nerve V and its connections are to the head what the dorsal roots and spinal cord are to the body. That is, the trigeminal system is ultimately responsible for the transmission of tactile, proprioceptive, and pain and temperature information from the head to the cerebral cortex, cerebellum, and reticular formation. The primary afferent fibers are distributed peripherally in the three divisions of the trigeminal nerve (the *ophthalmic* [V$_1$],

maxillary [V$_2$] and *mandibular* [V$_3$] divisions), in the pattern shown in Fig. 9-10.

Trigeminal motor nucleus. There is also one motor nucleus, a special visceral efferent (SVE) nucleus, associated with the trigeminal nerve. This nucleus is called the *trigeminal motor nucleus*. It innervates the muscles of the first branchial arch, which consist mainly of the muscles of mastication. They also include the tensor tympani (discussed later) and several other small muscles. The nucleus is located in the midpons at the level of attachment of the trigeminal nerve to the brainstem (Fig. 9-11). Fibers arising in the trigeminal motor nucleus emerge as a separate motor root and are then distributed peripherally with the mandibular division.

Sensory nuclei. There are three sensory nuclei associated with trigeminal afferents, and they form a long, almost continuous column of cells that extends from the rostral midbrain to the upper cervical spinal cord (Fig. 9-13). The *main sensory nucleus* (Fig. 9-11) forms an enlargement in this column in the midpons and is lateral and slightly dorsal to the trigeminal motor nucleus. The *spinal nucleus* extends caudally from this level, and the very slender *mesencephalic nucleus* extends rostrally.

Entering trigeminal afferent (GSA) fibers, whose cell bodies are in the *trigeminal (gasserian or semilunar) ganglion*, do one of three things: (1) Most fibers bifurcate and send a very short ascending branch to the main sensory nucleus and a longer descending branch into the *spinal trigeminal tract*, which is just lateral to the spinal trigeminal nucleus. The remaining fibers do not bifurcate and either (2) terminate directly in the main sensory nucleus or (3) turn caudally and enter the spinal tract (Fig. 9-13).

Spinal trigeminal nucleus. The primary afferent colla-

Fig. 9-10. Peripheral distribution of the ophthalmic, maxillary, and mandibular branches of the trigeminal nerve.

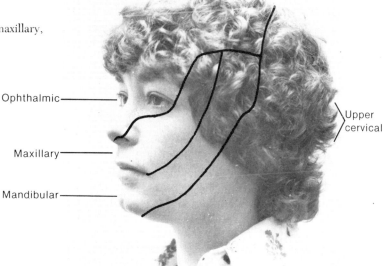

Ophthalmic

Maxillary

Mandibular

Upper cervical

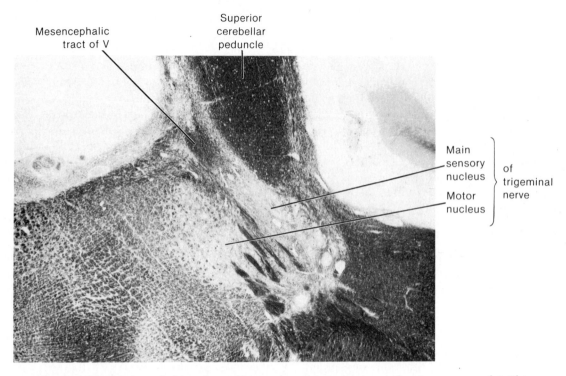

Fig. 9-11. Section through the midpons showing the trigeminal motor and main sensory nuclei. This figure is an enlargement of part of a section similar to that shown in Fig. 8-10.

terals of the spinal trigeminal tract are somatotopically arranged, with mandibular division fibers most dorsal, ophthalmic division fibers most ventral, and maxillary division fibers in between. They terminate in the medially adjacent spinal trigeminal nucleus. Both nucleus and tract extend caudally to about the third cervical segment of the spinal cord, the nucleus gradually blending with the dorsal horn and the tract gradually blending with Lissauer's tract. This may seem like a peculiar arrangement, unless it is remembered that the cutaneous areas innervated by the trigeminal nerve are adjacent to those innervated by upper cervical dorsal roots (Fig. 9-10).

The spinal trigeminal nucleus has been subdivided into three regions on the basis of its histology. The most caudal part, extending from the spinal cord to the obex, is the *nucleus caudalis.* The most rostral part, extending from the main sensory nucleus to about the pontomedullary junction, is the *nucleus oralis.* Between these two is the *nucleus interpolaris* in the rostral medulla. There are differences among these nuclei in terms of the types of afferents that terminate at each level and the types of secondary connections made from each level. The functional correlates of these differences are poorly understood for the nucleus oralis and nucleus interpolaris, but the nucleus caudalis is known to be particularly important for the processing of pain and temperature information from the head. This fits nicely with its

appearance (Fig. 9-12): the nucleus caudalis looks much like the dorsal horn of the spinal cord, with a cap of cells resembling the substantia gelatinosa.

The nucleus caudalis gives rise to a crossed ascending pain pathway analogous to the spinothalamic tract. It is called the *ventral trigeminal* (or *ventral trigeminothalamic*) *tract* and is located in or near the medial lemniscus throughout its course to the thalamus (Fig. 9-14). These trigeminothalamic fibers terminate in the *ventral posteromedial (VPM) nucleus* of the thalamus, adjacent to the VPL.* Trigeminal pain information also reaches the thalamus indirectly (via relays in the reticular formation) in a manner thought to be similar to spinoreticulothalamic projections. It is often assumed that this similarity holds in a functional sense as well (that is, that the ventral trigeminal tract is responsible for sharp, well-localized pain, while indirect trigeminal projections through the reticular formation are responsible for dull, aching pain). However, clinical evidence for such a functional similarity seems to be relatively scanty.

It was thought at one time that the spinal trigeminal nucleus and tract could be subdivided longitudinally according to the peripheral distribution of the fibers ending at a given level, with ophthalmic division fibers terminating most caudally and mandibular division fi-

---

*VPL and VPM are sometimes referred to together as the *ventrobasal complex.*

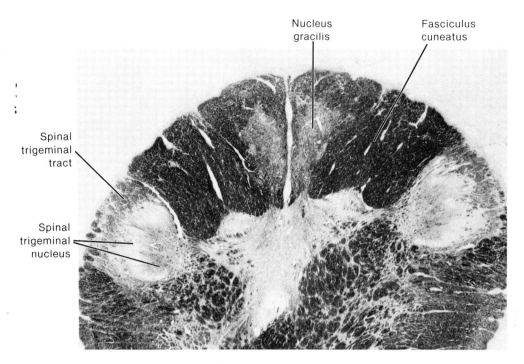

Nucleus gracilis

Fasciculus cuneatus

Spinal trigeminal tract

Spinal trigeminal nucleus

Fig. 9-12. Section through the caudal medulla where the spinal trigeminal tract and nucleus have an appearance much like that of Lissauer's tract and the dorsal horn in the spinal cord. At levels rostral to the obex (for example, Fig. 9-9), the spinal trigeminal tract and nucleus do not have this appearance.

bers terminating most rostrally. This seems to be incorrect, and the longitudinal division is now made according to types of afferents and secondary connections. Thus pain fibers from all three divisions reach the most caudal levels of the tract and nucleus.

The spinal nucleus has other connections in addition to the direct and indirect pain pathways just described. Some fibers project to the cerebellum (through the inferior cerebellar peduncle), and some fibers carrying tactile information travel in the ventral trigeminal tract. These are presumably similar to spinocerebellar fibers and to the tactile component of the spinothalamic tract, respectively. There are also reflex connections within the brainstem involving the reticular formation and other cranial nerve nuclei. One of these, the *corneal reflex*, is of considerable clinical importance and is discussed in conjunction with the facial nerve. The relative contributions of the three portions of the spinal nucleus to these various functions are not well understood.

Main sensory nucleus. The main sensory nucleus of the trigeminal nerve (Fig. 9-11), located near the motor nucleus, is generally considered to be analogous to the posterior column nuclei. Thus it is primarily concerned with discriminative tactile and proprioceptive sensations. It receives large-diameter, heavily myelinated tactile afferents and gives rise to two ascending pathways.

One is a collection of fibers that crosses the midline, joins the ventral trigeminal tract, and terminates in the VPM (Figs. 9-13 and 9-14). The other is a completely ipsilateral projection from the dorsomedial portion of the main sensory nucleus (an area that does not project through the ventral trigeminal tract). This is called the *dorsal trigeminal (dorsal trigeminothalamic) tract;* it travels through the dorsomedial part of the brainstem tegmentum and ends in its own separate portion of the VPM. Its significance is unknown, but since it arises from the part of the main sensory nucleus that is particularly concerned with the mouth, it may be of some significance in the processing of taste information (discussed later).

Since tactile information from the head is processed in the main sensory nucleus as well as in the spinal trigeminal nucleus, lesions in the medulla affecting the spinal tract and nucleus leave the sense of touch relatively intact and cause a more or less selective impairment of pain sensation.

Mesencephalic trigeminal nucleus. Afferents from muscle spindles in the muscles of mastication and some from mechanoreceptors of the gums, teeth, and hard palate have their cell bodies not in the trigeminal ganglion but rather within the CNS. They are located in a slender column of cells called the *mesencephalic trigeminal nucleus* (Fig. 9-13), which is quite unusual, since all

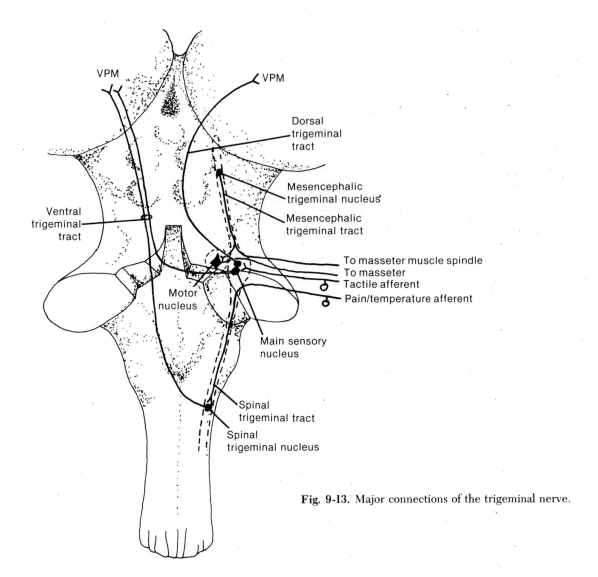

Fig. 9-13. Major connections of the trigeminal nerve.

other primary somatic sensory fibers have their cell bodies located in peripheral ganglia. The name of the nucleus refers to the fact that it extends rostrally all the way to the posterior commissure, although it is very small at midbrain levels. The cells of the mesencephalic nucleus are pseudounipolar (in every way analogous to dorsal root ganglion cells), and their myelinated processes collect in a bundle, called the *mesencephalic trigeminal tract* or *root*, adjacent to the nucleus (Figs. 8-12 and 9-11). The peripheral processes of these fibers travel in the trigeminal motor root and are distributed through the mandibular division to the structures mentioned previously. Some of the central processes end in the motor and main sensory nuclei, while others enter the cerebellum through the superior cerebellar peduncle.

The function of the mesencephalic trigeminal nucleus is rather obscure. It is often assumed that it is important for the coordination of chewing movements, since its afferents carry relevant proprioceptive information. However, fairly discrete lesions of the mesencephalic nucleus in monkeys produce no gross abnormalities of chewing movements. Since this is a small but extended nucleus, it is unlikely to be selectively affected in disease processes, so no clinical observations on humans are available.

The one function definitely established for the mesencephalic trigeminal nucleus is its participation in the *jaw jerk reflex*. Stretching the masseter, typically by a downward tap on the chin, causes it to contract (bilaterally) in a reflex fashion. This is a monosynaptic reflex basically similar to the knee jerk reflex: the afferent limb is a mesencephalic trigeminal neuron whose peripheral process innervates a masseter muscle spindle and whose central process synapses on a trigeminal motor neuron; the efferent limb is the axon of the trigeminal motor neuron, which travels back to the masseter.

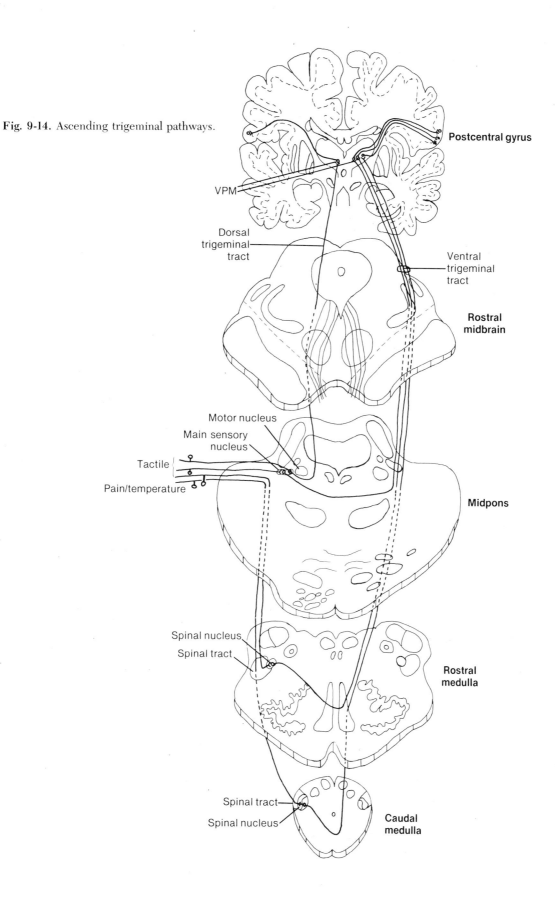

Fig. 9-14. Ascending trigeminal pathways.

Postcentral gyrus

VPM

Dorsal
trigeminal
tract

Ventral
trigeminal
tract

Rostral
midbrain

Motor nucleus

Main sensory
nucleus

Tactile

Pain/temperature

Midpons

Spinal nucleus

Spinal tract

Rostral
medulla

Spinal tract

Spinal nucleus

Caudal
medulla

Facial nerve (VII)

Cranial nerve VII, like IX and X, contains fibers belonging to several different functional components; certain aspects of all three nerves will be described together in this section.

General afferents. All three nerves contain general somatic afferent (GSA) fibers from the skin of the outer ear and its immediate vicinity. The exact distribution and the division of these fibers among the three nerves varies somewhat from one individual to another. These GSA fibers of nerves VII, IX, and X all enter the spinal trigeminal tract and thereafter behave exactly like trigeminal afferents. They are the most dorsomedial fibers in the spinal tract and occupy a position adjacent to those from the mandibular division of nerve V.

Nerves VII, IX, and X also contain general visceral afferent (GVA) fibers. In the case of the facial nerve this is a very small collection of afferents that innervate parts of the nasal cavity and soft palate; these fibers are seldom of clinical importance and are frequently omitted from accounts of the cranial nerves.

The GVA fibers from all three nerves enter a discrete bundle called the *solitary tract* (Fig. 9-9). This bundle received its name as a result of its somewhat unusual appearance, since it is a collection of afferents surrounded by the nucleus of termination of these afferents (the *solitary nucleus*) and looks rather isolated in cross sections. Both tract and nucleus extend through most of the medulla, dealing with facial afferents at rostral levels, vagal afferents at caudal levels, and glossopharyngeal afferents in between. The solitary nucleus in turn projects to the reticular formation, to brainstem visceral motor nuclei, and to the intermediolateral cell column of the spinal cord.

Taste. Although we tend to associate the sense of taste with the tongue, taste buds are in fact widely distributed not only over the tongue but also over the palate and pharynx. The pharyngeal and palatal taste buds are probably more important for normal gustatory experience than is generally realized. Special visceral afferent (SVA) fibers that innervate taste buds travel in the facial, glossopharyngeal, and vagus nerves. Those in the facial nerve are from the palate and the anterior two thirds of the tongue, those in the glossopharyngeal nerve are from the pharynx and the posterior third of the tongue, and the few in the vagus nerve are from the epiglottis.

The solitary nucleus is the principal visceral afferent nucleus of the brainstem and receives (via the solitary tract) gustatory afferents as well as the GVA fibers mentioned earlier. However, the SVA fibers end in the rostral third of the solitary nucleus, as opposed to the GVA fibers, which end at all levels. For this reason, the rostral portion of the solitary nucleus is sometimes referred to as the *gustatory nucleus*.

Second order taste fibers are usually said to cross the midline, join the contralateral medial lemniscus, and terminate in the thalamus. This pathway has long been accepted on the basis of old and possibly faulty anatomical studies and is at odds with physiological findings that indicate that gustatory information from one side of the tongue somehow reaches the thalamus bilaterally. More recent studies on rats and cats indicate that in fact secondary taste fibers arising in the solitary nucleus project ipsilaterally through the dorsomedial portion of the brainstem tegmentum to a small nucleus in the midpons dorsal to the main sensory nucleus of nerve V. This small nucleus, so far simply called the *pontine taste area*, then projects bilaterally through the dorsomedial tegmentum to the VPM in the thalamus. There is, in addition, a direct ipsilateral projection from the gustatory nucleus to the VPM via the central tegmental tract. The importance of this direct projection in primates (relative to the pathway through the pontine taste area) is not yet known. It is interesting to note that the pontine taste area is adjacent to the portion of the main sensory nucleus that deals with intraoral structures and gives rise to the dorsal trigeminal tract. This tract also projects through the same dorsomedial part of the tegmentum to the VPM. This may indicate that intraoral sensations of several different modalities are processed in an interrelated fashion that is not yet understood.

Efferents. A small collection of general visceral efferent (GVE) fibers, innervating the submandibular and sublingual salivary glands and the lacrimal gland, travel in the facial nerve. These fibers originate from a scattered group of cells called the *superior salivatory nucleus*, located in the reticular formation near the internal genu of the facial nerve.

Most of the fibers of the facial nerve are SVE fibers that innervate muscles derived from the second branchial arch. These are the muscles of facial expression and the stapedius, a small muscle in the middle ear. The large nucleus of origin of all these fibers, the *facial motor nucleus*, is located in the ventrolateral tegmentum of the caudal pons (Fig. 9-15). The peculiar course of these fibers, through the internal genu of the facial nerve, was described earlier.

The facial motor nucleus is involved in a reflex of considerable clinical importance, the *corneal blink reflex*. If either cornea is touched by a foreign object (in testing situations, typically a wisp of cotton), both eyes automatically blink. Sensory innervation of the cornea is by way of the ophthalmic division of the trigeminal nerve, so this is the afferent limb of the reflex. The afferents enter the spinal trigeminal tract and synapse on interneurons in the spinal trigeminal nucleus, mostly rostral to the obex. These interneurons then project bilaterally to motor neurons of the facial motor nucleus, forming the efferent limb. Thus by touching each of an individ-

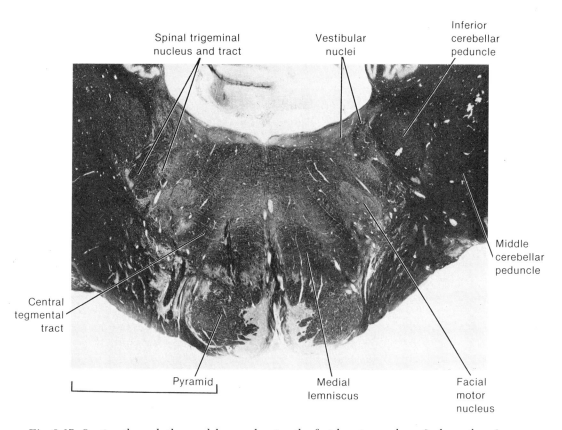

Spinal trigeminal nucleus and tract

Vestibular nuclei

Inferior cerebellar peduncle

Middle cerebellar peduncle

Central tegmental tract

Pyramid

Medial lemniscus

Facial motor nucleus

Fig. 9-15. Section through the caudal pons showing the facial motor nucleus. Scale mark = 1 cm.

ual's corneas in turn and observing the resulting blinks, it is possible to test, in a crude fashion, the integrity of both trigeminal nerves, both facial nerves, and some of their central connections.

Glossopharyngeal nerve (IX)

The glossopharyngeal nerve contains a number of general visceral afferent (GVA) fibers, among them afferents from the carotid body, carotid sinus, medial surface of the eardrum, posterior third of the tongue, and the walls of the pharynx. Most of these enter the solitary tract and synapse in the solitary nucleus. However, clinical evidence (described shortly) indicates that the fibers conveying information about pain from the pharynx and posterior part of the tongue (or at least collaterals of these fibers) enter the spinal trigeminal tract and terminate in the spinal nucleus. The same may be true of those fibers subserving tactile and temperature sensations. This fits with common experience: even though the pharynx is technically a visceral structure, it "feels" like a somatic structure in the way in which we can localize and discriminate stimuli applied there. Thus it is not surprising that the afferents involved should enter the trigeminal system.

A small group of general visceral efferent (GVE) fibers supplying the parotid gland also travel with the glossopharyngeal nerve. These arise from scattered cells in the reticular formation of the rostral medulla, collectively called the *inferior salivatory nucleus*.

Finally, a number of special visceral efferent (SVE) fibers, partially responsible for the innervation of muscles of the pharynx, travel in cranial nerve IX. Specifically, they innervate the stylopharyngeus. Most or all of the remaining pharyngeal musculature is innervated by the vagus nerve. All these SVE fibers arise in the *nucleus ambiguus*, which is aptly named since it is embedded in the medullary reticular formation and is sufficiently noncompact that it is difficult to distinguish in myelin-stained sections. It is located in the ventrolateral medullary tegmentum just dorsal to, and roughly coextensive with, the inferior olivary nucleus.

The GSA (skin of outer ear) and SVA (taste buds) fibers of cranial nerve IX have connections similar to those of the facial nerve and were described in conjunction with that nerve.

Vagus nerve (X)

Cranial nerve X has components and connections similar to, and partially overlapping, those of the glossopharyngeal nerve. GSA and SVA components were described in the section on the facial nerve. The vagus also contains a large collection of GVA fibers innervating the thoracic and abdominal viscera, including pressure receptors and chemoreceptors of the aortic arch. Vagal GVA fibers innervating the larynx, esophagus, and lower pharynx, like similar fibers from the glossopharyngeal nerve, are thought to enter the spinal trigeminal tract and terminate in the spinal trigeminal nucleus. The remaining vagal GVA fibers enter the solitary tract and terminate in caudal portions of the solitary nucleus.

A major collection of GVE fibers travels in the vagus nerve to thoracic and abdominal viscera generally. These arise in the *dorsal motor nucleus of the vagus*, which is the principal parasympathetic nucleus of the brain. It is located in the floor of the fourth ventricle just dorsolateral to the hypoglossal nucleus (Fig. 9-9), underlying the vagal trigone (Fig. 8-3).

Vagal SVE fibers arise in the nucleus ambiguus and supply striated muscles of the larynx and pharynx (which are of branchial arch origin). The stylopharyngeus is innervated by glossopharyngeal fibers, and most or all of the remaining pharyngeal muscles are innervated by vagal fibers. Laryngeal muscles are supplied mainly by SVE fibers of the cranial part of the accessory nerve, but since all these fibers arise in the nucleus ambiguus, and since those of cranial nerve XI join the vagus near the brainstem, laryngeal muscles generally behave as though they were innervated by the vagus.

A clinically useful (though unpleasant for the patient) reflex is the *gag reflex*. Touching the wall of the pharynx on one side in a normal individual elicits the unpleasant bilateral response. The afferent limb is via the glossopharyngeal nerve, while the efferent limb is mainly via the vagus. The central connections are not at all clear and may involve the spinal trigeminal tract and nucleus, the solitary tract and nucleus, or both, in addition to the nucleus ambiguus. Nevertheless, the gag reflex, like the blink reflex, can be used to test two cranial nerves (in this case IX and X) and some of their central connections.

Accessory nerve (XI)

Cranial nerve XI is considered by most to be purely a motor nerve and to have two portions. The *cranial root* consists of SVE fibers that arise from caudal portions of the nucleus ambiguus and innervate muscles of the larynx. These fibers are distributed with the vagus, as noted above. The *spinal root* consists of fibers that originate from lateral portions of the ventral horn of the upper five or six cervical segments, exit just dorsal to the dentate ligament, and innervate the sternocleidomastoid and part of the trapezius. The spinal root, like the cranial root, is usually considered to be SVE fibers. In addition, some workers think that some GVE fibers arising in the dorsal motor nucleus of the vagus leave the brainstem in the cranial root.

Some functional aspects of the branchiomeric nerves

Trigeminal neuralgia. *Trigeminal neuralgia* (also called *tic douloureux*) is characterized by brief (usually less than a minute) attacks of excruciating pain in the distribution of one, or sometimes more than one, division of the trigeminal nerve. Between attacks, no significant sensory abnormalities can be found. There is frequently a "trigger zone" in the involved area, where tactile stimulation may precipitate an attack. The mechanism is unknown and could be peripheral (for example, in the trigeminal ganglion) or central (for example, in the spinal trigeminal nucleus). Most cases can now be treated pharmacologically, but a number of surgical treatments are available if absolutely necessary. These include sectioning the involved nerve root and destroying or mechanically disturbing the trigeminal ganglion. The destructive procedures have a serious disadvantage in that the patient loses all tactile sensibility, in addition to pain, in the area. A more complex operation (but one that avoids this problem) is to section the trigeminal spinal tract slightly caudal to the obex. Tactile sensibility remains intact, and the corneal blink reflex is usually preserved. The fact that this operation abolishes pain sensations over one entire half of the face is a major piece of evidence that the caudal part of the trigeminal spinal nucleus deals with pain and that afferents from all three divisions of the trigeminal extend at least into the caudal medulla.

Glossopharyngeal neuralgia. *Glossopharyngeal neuralgia* is rare, but particularly distressing. The pain attacks usually begin in the posterior tongue or walls of the pharynx and radiate to the vicinity of the ear. One reason this condition is so distressing is that the trigger zone is often on the tongue or pharyngeal wall, and attacks may be set off by simply swallowing or talking. Pharmacological relief is usually available, but if it is not, the dorsomedial portion of the spinal trigeminal tract may be sectioned in the caudal medulla. The fact that this surgical procedure is effective provides evidence that the involved pain fibers (technically GVA fibers) travel in the spinal trigeminal tract.

Spinal trigeminal tract. In view of the somatotopic organization of the spinal trigeminal tract, partial lesions in the trigeminal system might be expected to result in sensory deficits related basically to the peripheral distribution of the nerve (for example, a selective loss in the distribution of the ophthalmic division). In fact, the losses resulting from central lesions tend to be in more or less circular zones centered around the mouth (usually referred to as an "onion-skin" distribution). This probably has to do with the pattern of termination of afferents in the spinal trigeminal nucleus. For example, there is some evidence that for each trigeminal division, afferents from areas close to the mouth terminate in the nucleus caudalis near the obex, and those from areas farther from the mouth terminate at progressively more caudal levels.

Facial paralysis. Pyramidal system upper motor neurons originating in the cortex of the frontal lobe supply motor nuclei of the cranial nerves, much as corticospinal fibers supply alpha motor neurons of the spinal cord. These upper motor neurons are called *corticobulbar fibers* (*bulbar* is a loosely used term referring to just the medulla in some applications and to the medulla, pons, and midbrain in others).

There are a number of peculiarities about the organization of the corticobulbar fiber system that will be discussed in some detail in a later chapter; the pattern of innervation of the facial motor nucleus is a good example. Corticobulbar fibers from one frontal lobe contact three groups of facial motor neurons: those for both the ipsilateral and the contralateral upper face and those for the contralateral lower face. The consequence of this pattern is that a lesion of the corticobulbar fibers on one side produces weakness of only the lower facial muscles of the opposite side, since the upper face is bilaterally innervated. This can be useful in distinguishing facial weakness resulting from a supranuclear lesion from that resulting from a nuclear or root lesion, since the latter would cause paralysis of the entire ipsilateral half of the face.

Other brainstem syndromes. The Brown-Séquard syndrome (Chapter 7), which follows hemisection of the spinal cord, demonstrates the possibility of crossed or *alternating* syndromes, in which some symptoms are referred to one side of the body and others to the other side. In the brainstem, most descending pathways are contralateral to the side on which they will terminate, and most ascending pathways are contralateral to the

side on which they arose. However, all the exiting cranial nerves are *ipsilateral* to the side that they will innervate; in addition, most of the cranial nerve nuclei deal with ipsilateral structures. As a result, alternating syndromes, in which long tract symptoms are referred to one side and cranial nerve symptoms to the other side, are the hallmark of brainstem lesions. For example, consider the effects of a lesion involving the medial portion of one side of the rostral medulla (Fig. 9-16), which could be caused by occlusion of a branch of one vertebral artery. The symptoms involved in the resulting *medial medullary syndrome* include contralateral spastic paralysis (damage to the pyramid), contralateral tactile and kinesthetic deficits (damage to the medial lemniscus), and ipsilateral paralysis with eventual atrophy of the tongue muscles (damage to the exiting hypoglossal nerve). This syndrome is also referred to as *alternating hypoglossal hemiplegia*.

More lateral damage at the same brainstem level (which could be caused by occlusion of branches of one vertebral or posterior inferior cerebellar artery) results in the *lateral medullary* (or *Wallenberg's*) *syndrome* (Fig. 9-16). The damaged structures may include the spinothalamic tract, the spinal trigeminal tract, the nucleus ambiguus, and descending sympathetic fibers. Symptoms of such damage would be loss of pain and temperature sensations over the contralateral body (with relative sparing of tactile sensation), loss of pain and temperature sensations over the ipsilateral face, hoarseness and difficulty in swallowing (as a result of paralysis of the ipsilateral larynx and pharynx), and ipsilateral Horner's syndrome. If the inferior cerebellar peduncle and adjacent vestibular nuclei are included in the lesion, vertigo and ipsilateral cerebellar deficits such as ataxia may also result.

A final example involves a lesion of the cerebral pe-

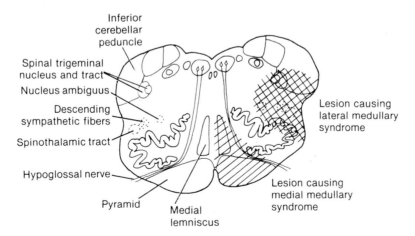

Fig. 9-16. Lesions that would cause a lateral medullary (Wallenberg's) syndrome or a medial medullary syndrome. The structures whose damage leads to prominent symptoms are indicated on the left.

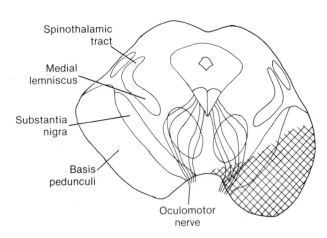

Fig. 9-17. A lesion that would cause Weber's syndrome.

duncle on one side of the rostral midbrain (Fig. 9-17) as might result from occlusion of branches of one posterior cerebral artery. This would damage descending corticospinal fibers, causing contralateral spastic paralysis; it would also damage one oculomotor nerve, causing ipsilateral ptosis, pupillary dilation, and lateral strabismus. This symptom complex is called *Weber's syndrome*.

VESTIBULOCOCHLEAR NERVE (VIII)

The eighth cranial nerve carries two special somatic afferent (SSA) components, one in a *vestibular division* and one in a *cochlear division*. Both divisions innervate specialized sensory end organs containing ciliated mechanoreceptors (called *hair cells*), but the end organs are such that the two divisions carry very different types of information. The vestibular division signals positions and movements of the head in space, whereas the cochlear division carries auditory information.

The structures innervated by the eighth nerve are embedded in the temporal bone (Fig. 9-18), where the

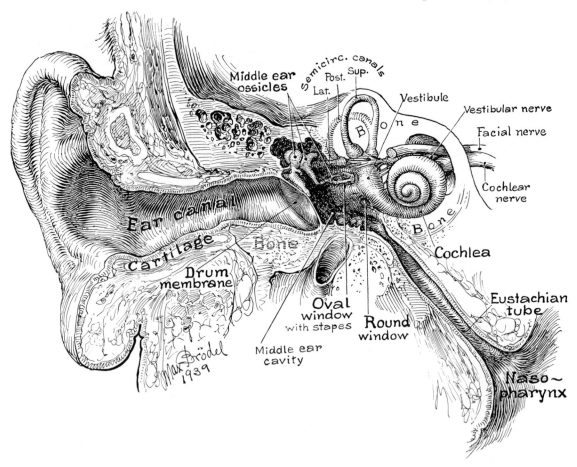

Fig. 9-18. The outer, middle, and inner ears, showing the bony labyrinth embedded in the temporal bone. The lateral and superior semicircular canals in this drawing are called horizontal and anterior, respectively, in this chapter. (From Brödel, M.: Three unpublished drawings of the anatomy of the human ear, Philadelphia, 1946, W.B. Saunders Co.)

receptor cells form parts of the walls of a convoluted, membranous tube that is suspended within a bony tube (Fig. 9-19). The walls of the bony tube are formed by a particularly dense portion of the temporal bone; since the tube consists of so many twists and turns, it is called the *bony labyrinth*. The membranous tube suspended within it, which follows most of its contours, is called the *membranous labyrinth*. The bony labyrinth is filled with *perilymph*, which is similar in composition to cerebrospinal fluid (and therefore to extracellular fluid generally; that is, low potassium concentration and high sodium concentration); the subarachnoid space around the brain is actually continuous with the perilymphatic space of the bony labyrinth through a tiny canal in the temporal bone. The membranous labyrinth, in contrast, is filled with *endolymph*, which is similar in ionic composition to intracellular fluids (that is, high potassium concentration and low sodium concentration). As might be expected from its different composition, the membranous labyrinth is a closed system and does not communicate with perilymphatic spaces. The resulting ionic concentration gradients across the walls of the membranous labyrinth are assumed to be important for the proper functioning of the receptors contained within these walls, but the mechanism is incompletely understood.

The type of stimulus to which a particular hair cell responds is determined by its relationship to various accessory structures, as well as by the way in which its portion of the membranous labyrinth is suspended within the bony labyrinth.

Vestibular division

Peripheral apparatus. The vestibular portion of the bony labyrinth consists of a central area called the *vestibule* and three *semicircular canals* that are attached to the vestibule (Fig. 9-18). Within each semicircular canal is a *semicircular duct*, which is the corresponding part of the membranous labyrinth. Within the vestibule are two dilations of the membranous labyrinth, the *utricle* and the *saccule*. The semicircular canal system is often referred to as the *kinetic labyrinth* (responding to head movement), while the utricle and saccule are referred to as the *static labyrinth* (responding to head position, but to linear acceleration as well).

Each semicircular duct communicates at both ends with the utricle. At one end of each duct is a dilation called an *ampulla*. Each ampulla contains a *crista*, which is a transversely oriented ridge of tissue (Fig. 9-20). The surface of each crista consists of supporting cells and sensory hair cells. Each hair cell bears a tuft of specialized microvilli called *stereocilia*. At one edge of the tuft of stereocilia is a single cilium called the *kinocilium*. Pushing the collection of cilia toward the kinocilium causes

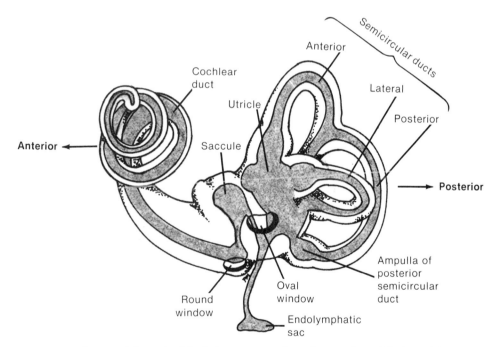

Fig. 9-19. Membranous labyrinth of the left ear as seen through an outline of the bony labyrinth. The endolymphatic sac is located beneath the dura on the surface of the temporal bone. It contains no receptor cells but rather is thought to be the principal site of absorption of endolymph. (Modified from Warwick, R., and Williams, P.L.W., editors: Gray's anatomy, Br. ed. 35, Philadelphia, 1973, W.B. Saunders Co.)

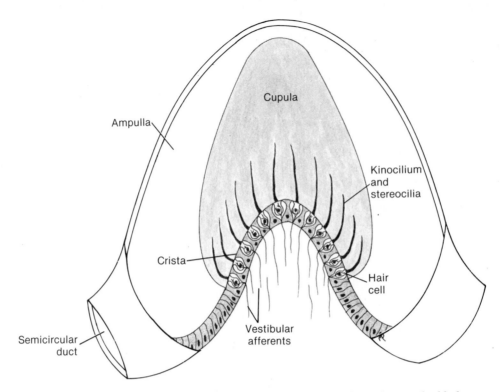

Fig. 9-20. Interior of an ampulla, showing the way in which the cupula, with its embedded sensory hairs, impedes the movement of endolymph through the semicircular duct.

the hair cell to depolarize, while pushing in the opposite direction causes the hair cell to hyperpolarize. The entire crista is covered by a flap of gelatinous material called the *cupula*, in which the "hairs" of the hair cells are embedded. A deflection of the cupula will distort these hairs and excite or inhibit the hair cells, depending on the direction in which the hairs are pushed. The hair cells in turn synapse on the dendrites of vestibular afferents, and excitation or inhibition of the hair cells causes an increase or decrease in the resting firing rate of these afferents. Each hair cell of a given crista is aligned with its kinocilium facing in the same direction, so deflection of the cupula in one direction will cause all the afferents that innervate that crista to increase their firing rate, and deflection in the opposite direction will cause them to decrease their firing rate.

The most straightforward way to deflect a cupula is to rotate its semicircular duct about an axis perpendicular to it (like a wheel on an axle). As such a rotation begins, the endolymph lags behind because of inertia; this motion of duct and endolymph relative to one another deflects the cupula and stimulates the hair cells. However, as the rotation continues, the endolymph "catches up" because of factors such as friction and the elasticity of the cupula, and the stimulation ceases. At the end of the rotation, the endolymph continues to move for a short period of time (again because of inertia), and the cupula

is deflected in the opposite direction. Thus each semicircular canal responds best to *changes* in speed of rotation in a particular plane. Since the three semicircular canals are arranged in orthogonal planes, and since most head movements have a rotational component, movements in any direction can be sensed. The fact that the semicircular canals cannot sense maintained rotation is not a great disadvantage since (except at amusement parks) we usually do not experience maintained rotations.

The relative orientations of the three semicircular canals should be noted in Figs. 9-19 and 9-21. One canal is roughly *horizontal* (actually, it is tilted backward about 30°), while the other two (the *anterior* and *posterior* canals) are roughly vertical. However, the anterior and posterior canals are also arranged at an angle of about 45° to the sagittal plane. The anterior canal of one side is therefore parallel to the posterior canal of the other side, so movements that stimulate one will stimulate the other. Thus the horizontal canals of the two sides form a functional pair, whereas the anterior canal of one side forms a functional pair with the posterior canal of the other side.

There are no cristae in the utricle and saccule, but each has in its wall a patch of supporting cells and hair cells called a *macula*. The utricular macula, lying at the bottom of the utricle, is roughly horizontal when one

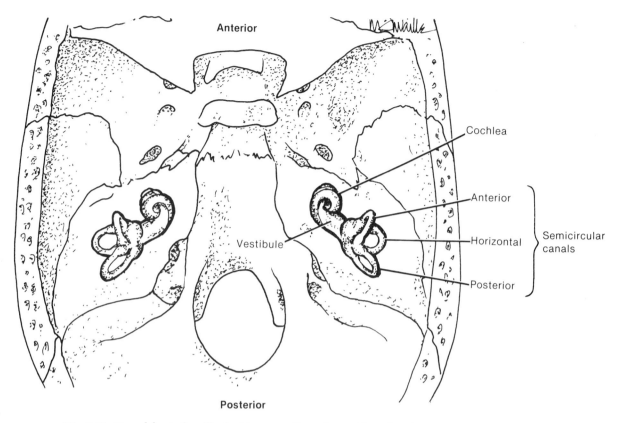

Fig. 9-21. Bony labyrinths of both sides, seen from above. Note that the anterior semicircular canal of one side is in a plane roughly parallel to that of the posterior semicircular canal of the other side.

(or one's head) is in an upright posture. The saccular macula is on the medial wall of the saccule and is roughly vertical. The sensory hairs of the macular receptors are also embedded in a gelatinous membrane similar in composition to the cupula. However, in the case of the macula, the gelatinous substance also contains minute crystals of calcium carbonate called *otoconia* or *otoliths* * and so is called an *otolithic membrane* (Fig. 9-22). The otoconia make the otolithic membrane denser than the endolymph so the membrane flops around and stays flopped when the position of the head is changed. This stimulates the hair cells, which then signal the new position of the head. In this case, the macula is responding to the force of gravity, but it responds equally well to other accelerating forces, such as those experienced in elevators and automobiles.

As might be expected from the orientation of its macula, the utricle is most sensitive to tilts beginning from a head-upright position. The saccule, in contrast, is more

_____

*Technically speaking, the very small crystals in the human otolithic membrane are otoconia (Greek = ear dust), while the somewhat larger concretions of some other vertebrates are otoliths (Greek = ear stones). However, the two terms are often used interchangeably.

sensitive to tilts beginning from a head-sideways position. The hair cells of a given macula are arranged with their kinocilia facing in several different directions, so any tilt will stimulate some cells more than others. The result is that every different head position causes a unique pattern of activity in the branches of the eighth nerve that innervate the utricle and saccule.

Central connections. Vestibular primary afferents have their cell bodies in the *vestibular* (or *Scarpa's*) *ganglion* in the internal auditory meatus. Their peripheral processes end about the hair cells just described. Their central processes enter the brainstem at the pontomedullary junction. Some proceed directly to the cerebellum, passing through the *juxtarestiform body*, which is located on the medial aspect of the inferior cerebellar peduncle. They end in the *flocculus, nodulus,* and nearby areas, as discussed in more detail in Chapter 14. Most primary vestibular afferents, however, end in the *vestibular nuclear complex* of the rostral medulla and caudal pons (Fig. 9-23).

Four vestibular nuclei have been distinguished on the basis of their histology and connections: the *inferior* (also called the *spinal* or *descending*), *medial, lateral* (or

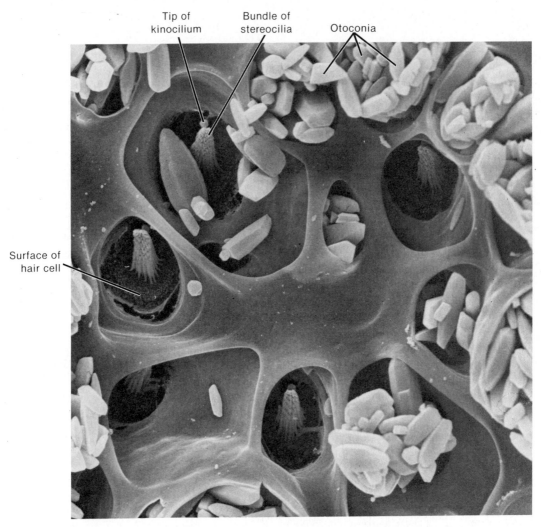

Fig. 9-22. Scanning electron micrograph of the otolithic membrane of the saccule of a bullfrog. Bundles of sensory hairs, each bundle consisting of a single kinocilium and numerous stereocilia, can be seen projecting from individual hair cells into small holes in the otolithic membrane. (Courtesy of R. Jacobs, D.P. Corey, and A.J. Hudspeth, California Institute of Technology. From Biophys. J. **26:** 499, 1979. Reproduced with the permission of Rockefeller University Press.)

Deiters'), and *superior vestibular nuclei* (Fig. 9-23). Each particular semicircular canal and otolithic organ has its own pattern of termination in the vestibular nuclei, and each vestibular nucleus has its own pattern of secondary connections. For the sake of simplicity, these patterns, for the most part, will be ignored and the vestibular nuclear complex treated as a uniform entity.

The connections of the vestibular nuclei are varied and widespread but not surprising in view of their function. We use the vestibular system principally to regulate posture and to coordinate eye and head movements; the anatomical substrates of these functions are connections with the spinal cord and with the motor nuclei of the extraocular muscles. The cerebellum is also involved in both these functions, and correspondingly there are substantial interconnections between it and the vestibular nuclei. We also have a conscious awareness of movement through space; there is a corresponding vestibular projection through the thalamus to cerebral cortex. Finally, there are connections between the vestibular nuclei and the reticular formation (including visceral centers of the reticular formation, as anyone who has been seasick can attest).

Inputs to the vestibular nuclei (in addition to primary vestibular afferents) include projections from the cerebellum (by way of the juxtarestiform body), the spinal cord, and the contralateral vestibular nuclei (Fig. 9-23). The cerebellar projections arise directly from the floc-

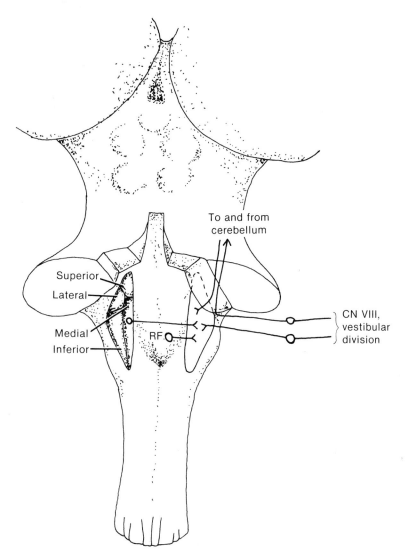

Fig. 9-23. Termination of right vestibular nerve and principal inputs to right vestibular nuclei. Not all commissural connections between vestibular nuclei arise in the medial vestibular nuclei; the diagram is drawn that way for reasons of simplicity. *RF*, Input from reticular formation.

culonodular lobe and indirectly from other cerebellar areas as well, as discussed further in Chapter 14. Input from the spinal cord makes reasonable sense, since it would be difficult to adjust posture properly in response to a movement or a tilt without knowledge of the current orientation of the body. A small amount of this information travels with the dorsal spinocerebellar tract as direct spinovestibular fibers, but most of it reaches the vestibular nuclei indirectly via relays in the cerebellum or reticular formation. Finally, the left and right vestibular apparatus normally function together as a coordinated pair, and the vestibular nuclear complexes of the two sides are extensively interconnected.

Secondary fibers arising in the vestibular complex

project to (1) the same cerebellar areas as do primary vestibular afferents (again, via the juxtarestiform body), (2) the spinal cord, in the lateral and medial vestibulospinal tracts, (3) the thalamus, (4) the motor nuclei of the extraocular muscles, and (5) the vestibular apparatus (Fig. 9-24). (This is in addition to the previously mentioned projections to the reticular formation and the contralateral vestibular nuclei.)

The *lateral vestibulospinal tract* arises in the lateral vestibular nucleus and projects to all levels of the ipsilateral spinal cord, where it is located in the ventral part of the lateral funiculus. This is the principal route by which the vestibular system brings about postural changes to compensate for tilts and movements of the

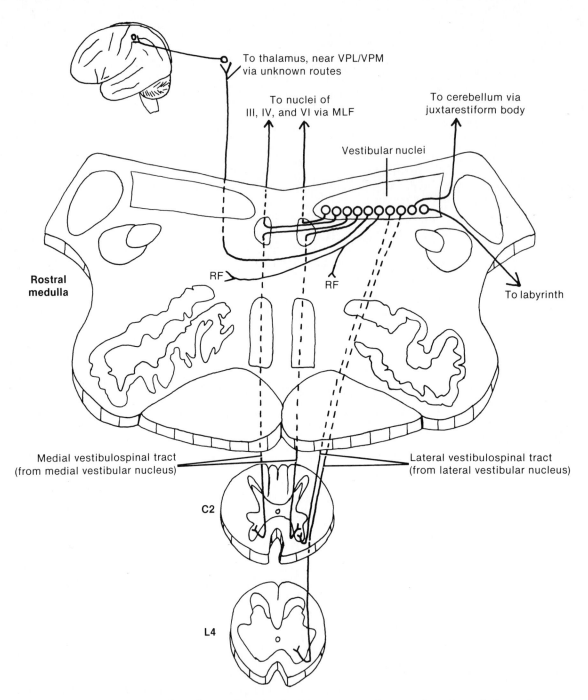

To thalamus, near VPL/VPM
via unknown routes

To nuclei of
III, IV, and VI via MLF

To cerebellum via
juxtarestiform body

Vestibular nuclei

Rostral
medulla

RF

RF

To labyrinth

Medial vestibulospinal tract
(from medial vestibular nucleus)

Lateral vestibulospinal tract
(from lateral vestibular nucleus)

C2

L4

Fig. 9-24. Some outputs from the vestibular nuclei. Projections to the contralateral vestibular nuclei are not shown but are extensive. *RF*, Reticular formation.

body. If as a child (or an adult) you ever spun yourself around until you felt dizzy and then proceeded to stagger, you have experienced the effects of exaggerated activity in your lateral vestibulospinal tract.

The *medial vestibulospinal tract* arises mainly in the medial vestibular nucleus and projects bilaterally to the cervical spinal cord. It is responsible for postural changes of the neck muscles.

Vestibular projections to the thalamus, and from there to the cerebral cortex, have been a matter of some controversy. The thalamic relay seems to be in a small nucleus in the inferior part of the thalamus near the VPL and VPM. The path taken by secondary vestibular fibers to reach the thalamus is unknown, but it probably does not include the MLF. There may be an intermediate synapse in the midbrain, but this too is uncertain. The primary vestibular cortical area is located in the parietal lobe at the junction between the intraparietal and postcentral sulci; this is adjacent to the portion of the postcentral gyrus where the head is represented. This makes some sense, as the somatosensory cortex of the postcentral gyrus is concerned with conscious appreciation of body position. It was thought for some time that the primary vestibular cortex was located in the superior temporal gyrus adjacent to the primary auditory cortex, but for a variety of reasons it now appears that this is incorrect.

Many secondary vestibular fibers project directly through the MLF to the motor neurons of the oculomotor, trochlear, and abducens nuclei. This forms much of the basis of the *vestibulo-ocular reflex,* by means of which a person's gaze can stay fixed on an object even though the head is moving or being moved. One might think that this is a form of visual tracking, but the reflex works even in the dark in normal individuals and works relatively poorly in individuals with bilateral vestibular damage; thus it seem clear that the vestibular division of cranial nerve VIII forms a major part of the afferent limb.

Some fibers arising in the vestibular nuclei project back through the eighth nerve and end on the hair cells of the vestibular apparatus. These efferents are another example of the widespread phenomenon of feedback from a higher level to a lower level of a sensory system. The role of such efferents, in general, is poorly understood, and the vestibular system is no exception. One common suggestion is that the efferents could suppress self-generated activity in the sensory system. For example, the horizontal semicircular canals receive the same stimulation if you rotate your head as they do if someone begins to rotate the chair in which you are sitting. However, the reflex postural adjustments to the two rotations are quite different. If the efferent system suppressed the hair cell response to self-generated rotation, then the reflex postural adjustments would also be suppressed. There is some experimental evidence that this may be the case, but there is also evidence that this is not the sole role of the efferents.

It should be noted that the vestibular system is not the only means available for detecting the position and motion of the head in space. The visual system also plays a major role, and humans can compensate reasonably well for total loss of vestibular function, as long as visual cues are available. Most of us have experienced illusion of movement when we were stationary and a nearby large object (such as a train on the next track) moved. It should also be noted that the vestibular apparatus can give no information about the position of the *body,* so additional information is required for such tasks as reaching with a hand for a seen object. Much of the additional information is provided by mechanoreceptors in the neck that detect the orientation of the head relative to the body. If the first three cervical dorsal roots of a monkey are anesthetized bilaterally, a remarkably severe disorientation results, involving not only eye-hand coordination but also such basic activities as walking and climbing.

Cochlear division

Peripheral apparatus. The auditory system faces a basic mechanical problem, since the sound vibrations that it must detect are propagated in air, whereas the auditory receptor cells (like other elements of the nervous system) live in a fluid-filled environment. Nearly all (99.9%) of the sound energy incident on an air-water interface is reflected, since water is harder to move than air. Therefore if the auditory receptor organ (the *organ of Corti*) and its fluid surroundings were mechanically coupled to the outside world by a simple membrane, it could utilize no more than 0.1% of the sound energy available to it. One major task of the air-filled *outer* and *middle ears* (Fig. 9-18) is, therefore, to transfer sound as efficiently as possible to the fluid-filled *inner ear.*

The outer ear is basically a complicated funnel consisting of the *auricle* (or *pinna*) and the *external auditory meatus;* it conducts sound to the *tympanic membrane.* Sound-induced vibrations are transferred along a chain of three small bones or ossicles that traverse the middle ear cavity (a cavity in the temporal bone). The handle of the *malleus* is attached to the medial surface of the tympanic membrane, so movements of this membrane are transferred directly to the malleus. The malleus in turn is attached to the *incus,* which is attached to the *stapes*—so sound-induced vibrations eventually reach the oval-shaped footplate of the stapes. The footplate of the stapes occupies a hole in the temporal bone called the *oval window* (or *fenestra vestibuli*); on the other side of the oval window is the perilymph-filled vestibule of the bony labyrinth. The vestibule leads directly to the cochlea, which contains the organ of Corti. Thus vibration of the tympanic membrane ultimately results in vibration of the fluids of the inner ear.

The chain of middle ear ossicles acts as a lever system with a small mechanical advantage, so a given force at the tympanic membrane results in a slightly greater force at the footplate of the stapes. More importantly, the area of the tympanic membrane is about 15 times that of the footplate of the stapes. The net result of the mechanical advantage and the size difference is that stapedial vibrations have a much greater force *per unit area* of the footplate; this force is sufficient to move the perilymph, and nearly all the sound energy incident on the tympanic membrane is successfully transferred to the inner ear. The effectiveness of this system is quite

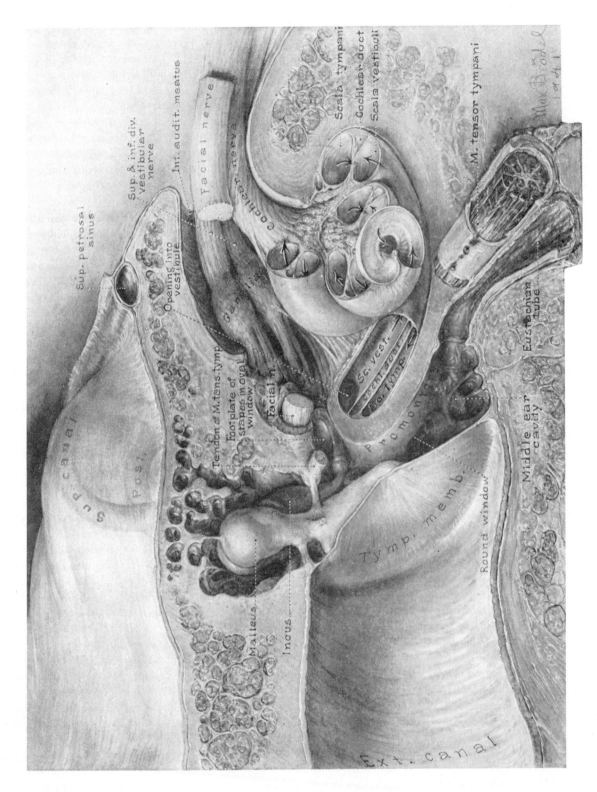

Fig. 9-25. Drawing of a dissection of the right cochlea showing the continuous perilymphatic path from the vestibule into the scala vestibuli and from there into the scala tympani, finally ending at the round window membrane. (From Brödel, M.: Three unpublished drawings of the anatomy of the human ear, Philadelphia, 1946, W.B. Saunders Co.)

extraordinary. At threshold at 3000 Hz (the frequency to which we are most sensitive) the tympanic membrane moves a distance somewhat less than the diameter of a single hydrogen atom.

Two tiny muscles are attached to the middle ear bones. One, the *tensor tympani*, is attached to the handle of the malleus; when it contracts, it increases the tension on the tympanic membrane and decreases the transmission of vibrations through the ossicular chain. The other muscle, the *stapedius*, is attached to the neck of the stapes; it too decreases the transmission of vibrations when it contracts. The tensor tympani receives motor innervation from the trigeminal nerve and the stapedius from the facial nerve; both muscles are involved in certain auditory reflexes to be described shortly.

The auditory part of the inner ear, like the vestibular part, consists of a portion of the endolymph-filled membranous labyrinth suspended within a portion of the perilymph-filled bony labyrinth.

The bony part is the cochlea (Latin = snail), which coils through 2½ turns from its relatively broad base to its apex. The cochlea lies on its side in the temporal bone, with its base facing medially and posteriorly (Figs. 9-18 and 9-21), but for the sake of simplicity it is usually discussed as though it sat upright on its base. The bony core of the cochlea is the *modiolus*, from which the *osseous spiral lamina* projects like the threads of a screw. A winding cavity within the modiolus houses the *spiral ganglion*, which contains the cell bodies of the primary auditory afferent fibers. The central processes of these cells collect at the base of the cochlea to form the cochlear division of the eighth nerve, while the peripheral processes pass in bundles through a series of canals in the osseous spiral lamina to innervate the auditory receptors.

The *cochlear duct* (the auditory portion of the membranous labyrinth) is firmly anchored to the bony labyrinth in such a way that the duct is triangular in cross section (Fig. 9-25). One corner of the triangle is attached to the edge of the osseous spiral lamina, and the other two corners are attached to the outer wall of the bony cochlea. The result is that the cochlear duct and osseous spiral lamina act as a partition separating two perilymphatic spaces from each other (except at the apex of the cochlea, where perilymph can pass from one space to the other through a small opening called the *helicotrema*). The perilymphatic space above the cochlear duct is called the *scala vestibuli*, because it is directly continuous with the perilymph of the vestibule. The space below the cochlear duct is called the *scala tympani*, because it ends blindly at the *secondary tympanic membrane* (or *round window membrane*). Vibrations reaching the stapedial footplate are transferred to the perilymph. Although perilymph is incompressible, the round win-

dow membrane is elastic, allowing these vibrations to enter the labyrinth. When the stapedial footplate moves inward, the round window membrane bulges out; when the footplate moves outward, the membrane is drawn inward. In the process, small quantities of perilymph oscillate within the cochlea. Most of this vibratory energy passes directly from the scala vestibuli to the scala tympani, deforming the cochlear duct. The cochlear duct contains the auditory receptors, and this deformation stimulates some of them.

The space enclosed by the cochlear duct is filled with endolymph and is called the *scala media*. As noted above, the scala media is triangular in cross section, and each of the three walls of the cochlear duct has a different structure. The thin *vestibular* (or *Reissner's*) *membrane* borders the scala vestibuli and probably serves mainly as a barrier between the endolymph and perilymph, playing no great role in the mechanical properties of the cochlea. The *stria vascularis* forms the second wall, adhering to the outer wall of the bony cochlea; it is a specialized area, rich in capillaries, that produces most of the endolymph in the membranous labyrinth. The *basilar membrane* completes the cochlear duct, separating the scala media from the scala tympani. Passing from the base to the apex of the cochlea, the osseous spiral lamina becomes narrower and the basilar membrane becomes broader. Because of this change in its width and progressive changes in its mechanical properties, the basilar membrane is vibrated most efficiently by sounds of progressively lower frequencies as one moves from the base to the apex of the cochlea. Since the organ of Corti (which contains the auditory receptor cells) rests on the basilar membrane, different receptor cells will respond best to sounds of different frequencies. This is the beginning of a *tonotopic organization* within the auditory system, quite analogous to the somatotopic organization of the somatosensory system; in this case particular frequencies are mapped in an orderly fashion onto particular areas of relay nuclei and auditory cortex.

The organ of Corti (Figs. 9-26 and 9-27) is a long strip of hair cells and supporting cells that rests on the basilar membrane. The hair cells are arranged in two groups: a single row of *inner hair cells* near the osseous spiral lamina and a band of *outer hair cells* 3 to 5 cells wide. The two groups are separated by a space called the *tunnel of Corti*, through which the peripheral processes of auditory afferents must pass on their way to the outer hair cells. The sensory hairs (all stereocilia, which are modified microvilli) of the outer hair cells are inserted into the gelatinous *tectorial membrane* so that vibration of the basilar membrane causes bending of the hairs and excitation of the hair cells. Anatomical evidence indicates that the stereocilia of the inner hair cells may not

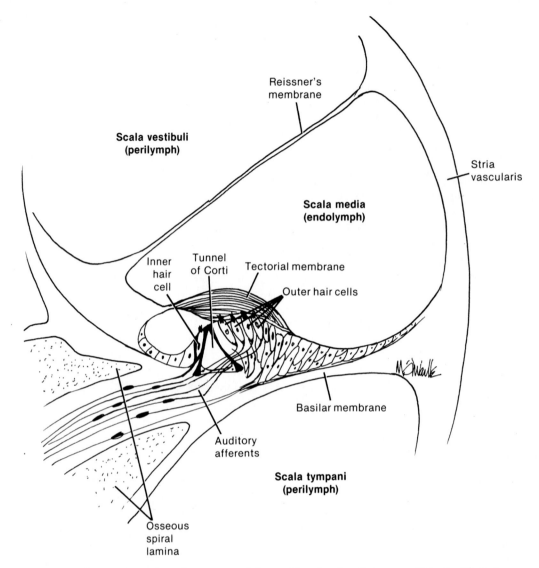

Fig. 9-26. Cross section through one turn of the cochlea showing the organ of Corti with its inner and outer hair cells.

Fig. 9-27. Micrographs of the organ of Corti. In both cases, the orientation is reversed left-to-right from that in Fig. 9-26 (that is, in the photographs, the modiolus would have been on the right). **A,** Light micrograph of the organ of Corti of a guinea pig; three outer hair cells can be seen, but only the top of an inner hair cell is present in this section. **B,** Scanning electron micrograph of the organ of Corti of a guinea pig. The tectorial membrane has been removed, and the stereocilia of the three rows of outer hair cells can be seen protruding into the scala media; normally these stereocilia would be embedded in the tectorial membrane. No inner hair cells are present in this view, but their stereocilia can also be seen protruding into the scala media. (**A** courtesy of Dr. David Asher, University of Colorado Medical Center; **B** with permission from Bredberg, G. In Evans, E.F., and Wilson, J.P., editors: Psychophysics and physiology of hearing, New York, 1977. Copyright by Academic Press, Inc. [London] Ltd.)

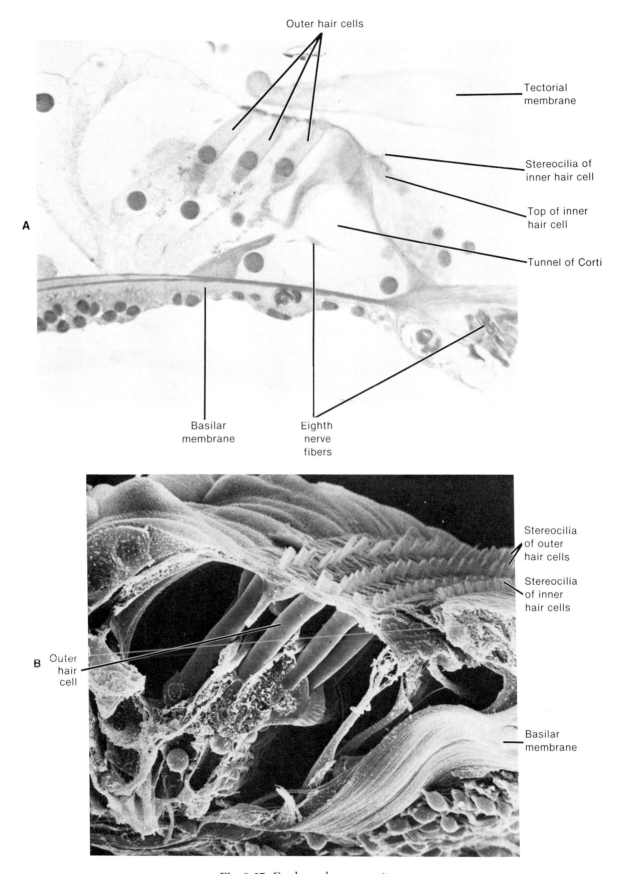

Outer hair cells

Tectorial membrane

Stereocilia of inner hair cell

Top of inner hair cell

Tunnel of Corti

A

Basilar membrane

Eighth nerve fibers

Stereocilia of outer hair cells

Stereocilia of inner hair cells

B   Outer hair cell

Basilar membrane

Fig. 9-27. For legend see opposite page.

be attached to the tectorial membrane and that these hair cells may be stimulated directly by movement of endolymph within the cochlear duct.

The roles of inner and outer hair cells in the hearing process seem to differ. There are about 20,000 outer hair cells and 3,500 inner hair cells per inner ear, but approximately 90% of auditory afferents end on inner hair cells. On the other hand, the outer hair cells seem to be more sensitive by a considerable margin: certain ototoxic drugs can be used to selectively destroy the outer hair

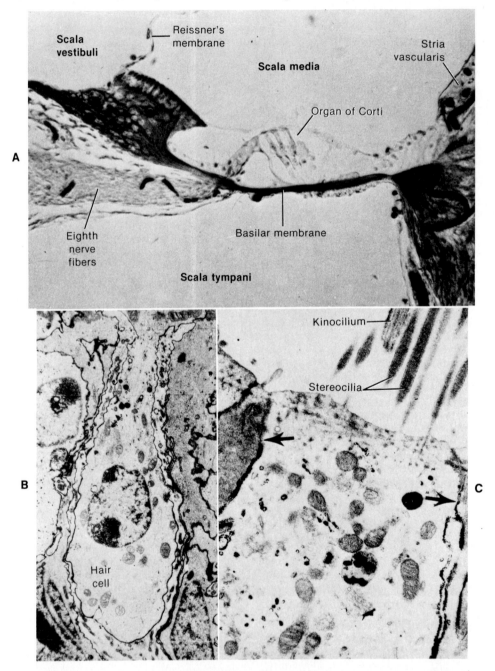

Fig. 9-28. Portions of the membranous labyrinth of a guinea pig after a tracer substance (horseradish peroxidase) had been injected into the cisterna magna. **A,** Dark reaction product fills parts of the cochlea including, to some extent, the organ of Corti; the tectorial membrane cannot be seen because no tracer escaped from the organ of Corti into endolymphatic space. **B,** Electron micrograph of the saccular macula; dark reaction product outlines all the cellular elements of the macula. **C,** Higher magnification micrograph of the apical end of the hair cell shown in **B**; reaction product fills extracellular space up to, but not beyond, junctional complexes (arrows) that separate the perilymphatic from endolymphatic space. (Courtesy of Dr. David Asher, University of Colorado Medical Center.)

cells, causing the auditory threshold to increase by a factor of 10^3 to 10^4. What this implies about the relative roles of the two populations in normal hearing is more or less unknown.

In Figs. 9-26 and 9-27, *A*, it looks as though the organ of Corti is bathed in the endolymph of the scala media. However, it has long been reasoned that this is unlikely, since it would mean (among other things) that auditory afferents traversing the tunnel of Corti would be passing through endolymph. Endolymph has such a high potassium concentration that standard nerve fibers would not be expected to work in its presence. Recent evidence is consistent with this reasoning and indicates that the perilymphatic space of the scala tympani continues through the basilar membrane and into the organ of Corti. The real barrier between endolymph and perilymph is a series of tight junctions between hair cells and supporting cells at the surface of the organ of Corti so that only the stereocilia and upper surfaces of the hair cells are exposed to endolymph. Since perilymph is continuous with the cerebrospinal fluid of subarachnoid space, marker substances introduced into the cisterna magna will infiltrate the organ of Corti and surround its hair cells, stopping only at the array of tight junctions (Fig. 9-28).

Central connections. Auditory primary afferents, whose cell bodies are located in the spiral ganglion of the modiolus, enter the brainstem at the pontomedullary junction. There each fiber bifurcates and sends one branch to the *dorsal cochlear nucleus* and one branch to the *ventral cochlear nucleus.* These cochlear nuclei form a continuous band of cells that covers the dorsal and lateral aspects of the inferior cerebellar peduncle.

Second order fibers arising in the cochlear nuclei may proceed in several different ways, but the following general principles apply:

1. Second and higher order auditory fibers are distributed bilaterally in their path toward the auditory cortex, so unilateral damage at levels rostral to the cochlear nuclei does not cause deafness of either ear.
2. More fibers, and fibers following more direct paths, travel contralateral to the ear they represent; therefore the subtle hearing loss that follows unilateral damage rostral to the cochlear nuclei involves principally the contralateral ear.
3. Some second and higher order auditory fibers cross the midline at almost every possible site along the auditory pathway.

In order to introduce the nuclei and pathways involved in the central auditory projections, a relatively direct pathway from cochlear nuclei to auditory cortex will be described first. This will be followed by a discussion of alternative pathways.

Most second order fibers pass inferior to the inferior cerebellar peduncle and cross the midline with a slight rostral inclination (although some pass dorsal to the peduncle and cross with a ventral and rostral inclination). When they reach the vicinity of the *superior olivary nucleus* just rostral to the facial motor nucleus in the caudal pons, some turn sharply rostrally and enter a bundle of fibers called the *lateral lemniscus.* The lateral lemniscus is somewhat diffuse through much of the pons, but at rostral pontine levels it forms a flattened band (Latin, lemniscus = ribbon) on the lateral surface of the tegmentum. Most fibers of the lateral lemnis-

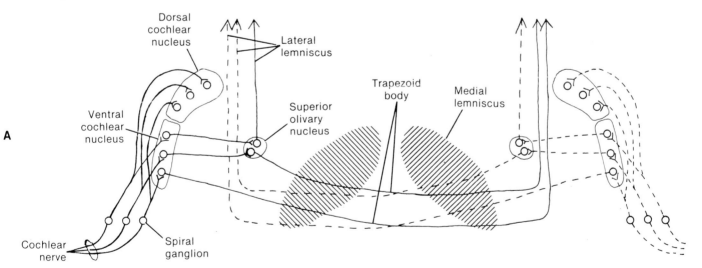

A

Fig. 9-29. Components of the ascending auditory pathway in the pons. **A,** Initial synapses and some of the initial crossings of the midline by auditory fibers; the connections of the dorsal cochlear nucleus are not shown, but they are similar to those of the ventral cochlear nucleus. The figure had to be drawn schematically, since the cochlear nuclei are located slightly caudal to the superior olivary nucleus, and they cannot all be seen in a single section. *Continued.*

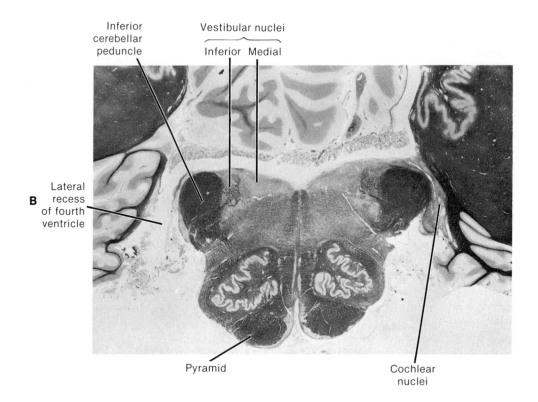

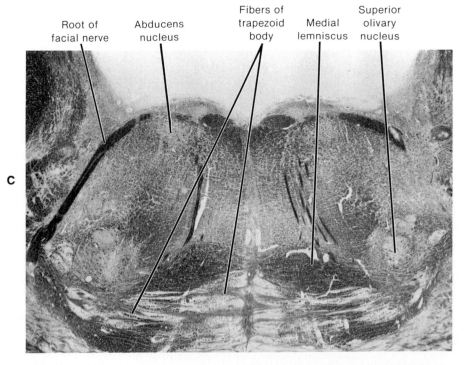

Fig. 9-29, cont'd. B, Section through the pontomedullary junction showing the cochlear nuclei. **C,** Section through the caudal pons showing the superior olivary nuclei and the trapezoid body.

cus terminate in the inferior colliculus. The inferior colliculus then gives rise to the *brachium* (Latin = arm) *of the inferior colliculus* (or *inferior brachium*), which assumes a superficial position and terminates in the *medial geniculate nucleus*, a portion of the thalamus that protrudes in a posterior direction, overlapping the mid-

brain. Fibers from the medial geniculate nucleus project to the primary auditory cortex, which is a portion of the superior temporal gyrus buried in the lateral fissure (Fig. 9-30).

Many variations on this basic pathway are found (Figs. 9-29 and 9-30). Second order fibers from the cochlear

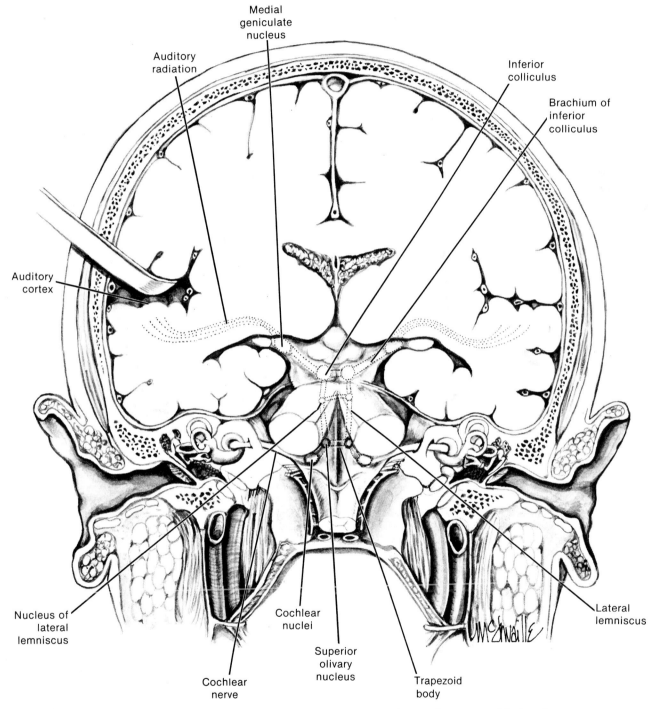

Fig. 9-30. The ascending auditory pathway. (Modified from a drawing by Max Brödel in Rothman, L., and Crowe, S.J., editors: The 1940 year book of eye, ear, nose, and throat, Chicago, 1940, Year Book Medical Publishers, Inc.)

nuclei may synapse in the ipsilateral or contralateral superior olivary nucleus. Fibers from a superior olivary nucleus may join the ipsilateral or the contralateral lateral lemniscus. The large collection of crossing second and higher order fibers between the superior olivary nuclei, passing through and ventral to the medial lemnisci, is called the *trapezoid body* (Fig. 9-29). Additional auditory synapses are possible in scattered groups of cell bodies collectively called the *nucleus of the trapezoid body* and the *nucleus of the lateral lemniscus*. Finally, recent evidence indicates that in the auditory system of chimpanzees (and probably humans) a significant number of fibers may proceed from the cochlear nuclei through the contralateral lateral lemniscus and contralateral brachium of the inferior colliculus directly to the medial geniculate nucleus.

It should be apparent that there are ample possibilities for information from the cochlear nuclei of one side to reach the medial geniculate nucleus of the same side. For example, a path exists from the cochlear nuclei via the ipsilateral superior olivary nucleus, lateral lemniscus, and inferior colliculus to the ipsilateral medial geniculate body (Fig. 9-30). There are numerous other ipsilateral paths. As a general rule in the auditory system, fibers cross wherever they have an opportunity. Thus in addition to the crossing fibers of the trapezoid body, fibers cross from each nucleus of the lateral lemniscus and each inferior colliculus. As indicated previously, the result is that auditory pathways at all levels rostral to the cochlear nuclei contain information from both ears, and damage at any of these rostral locations causes little hearing loss.

Some functional aspects of the vestibulocochlear nerve

Nystagmus. *Nystagmus* refers to involuntary rhythmic movements of one or both eyes; it can be of considerable diagnostic importance. The movements may be horizontal, vertical, or rotatory; they may have a faster component in one direction, or the movements in both directions may have the same speed. We will briefly discuss a typical example, horizontal nystagmus with a fast component in one direction, that can be induced in normal individuals. In this case the nystagmus is named for the direction of rapid movement (that is, if the eyes move slowly to the left and then rapidly back to the right, it would be called *nystagmus to the right*). Consider the reflex eye movements that occur when a person sits in a rapidly moving train, vaguely watching regularly spaced telephone poles fly by. The person's eyes tend to slowly follow a particular pole toward the rear of the train and then flick back toward the front of the train to find a new pole to fix on. In the case of an individual seated on the right side of the train, this would consti-

tute *nystagmus to the left* (Fig. 9-31). Because it is induced by moving visual stimuli, it is called *optokinetic nystagmus (OKN)*. Fortunately it is not necessary to use trains and telephone poles to demonstrate optokinetic nystagmus clinically; a rotating striped drum or a moving striped piece of cloth usually suffices.

Nystagmus can also be induced by rotating a subject. It occurs at both the onset and termination of rotation, even if the subject's eyes are closed (if the eyes are open, it may occur throughout the rotation). At the onset of rotation the nystagmus is in the direction of rotation, and at the termination of rotation it is in the opposite direction. This makes reasonable sense if you consider what these movements correspond to in terms of reflexly trying to track visual stimuli during rotation (Fig. 9-31). Since this nystagmus at the onset and termination of rotation occurs in the absence of visual stimuli, it is called *vestibular nystagmus*. It corresponds to deflection of the cupula in one direction at the onset of rotation and in the opposite direction at the end of rotation.

The same movement of endolymph that underlies vestibular nystagmus can be produced by instilling cool or warm water into a subject's ear, causing endolymphatic convection currents that, in turn, induce nystagmus. Consider an individual whose head is tilted back about 60°, bringing the horizontal semicircular canals into a vertical plane. Cool water instilled into the right ear will cause the endolymph in the right horizontal canal to cool and sink, causing a convection current of endolymph in a clockwise direction (viewed from the top of the head). This movement of endolymph relative to the canal is the same movement that is produced at the onset of rotation of the individual to the left (Fig. 9-31), and the response of this single semicircular canal is sufficient to cause nystagmus to the left. This is called *caloric nystagmus*, and its mechanism is the same as that of rotationally induced vestibular nystagmus.

The pathway involved in vestibular nystagmus includes the MLF, at least for the slow phase. The fast phase may utilize routes through the brainstem reticular formation, in addition to the MLF. The basic mechanisms for both phases of vestibular nystagmus seem to be present in the brainstem, but under normal circumstances cortical participation is probably involved in triggering the fast phase. One consequence of this is that a comatose patient with an intact brainstem, after caloric stimulation, usually shows only a tonic deviation of the eyes in the direction of the slow phase of the expected nystagmus. This can be of some utility in localizing the region of damage in a comatose patient. Similar conjugate lateral eye movements can be induced in a comatose individual with an intact brainstem by turning his head from side to side. The movements in this case are those appropriate to keep both eyes pointed in the same

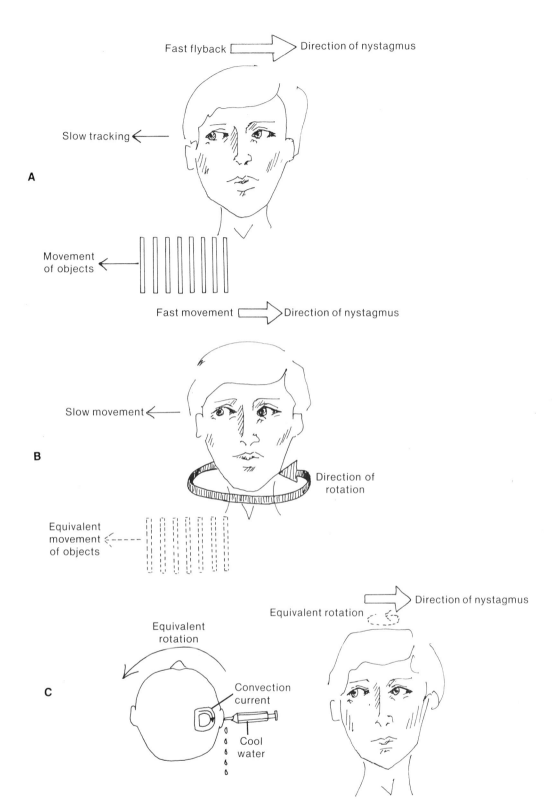

Fig. 9-31. Three different ways to cause nystagmus with its fast phase to the left. **A,** Movement of a series of objects to an individual's right causes slow tracking eye movements to the right followed by rapid "reset" movements to the left. **B,** Rotation to the left is equivalent, as far as visual movement is concerned, to movement of objects around to the right. The result is nystagmus to the left, as in **A.** If the individual's eyes are open, visual movement continues throughout the rotation, and the nystagmus may persist. If the eyes are closed, the nystagmus is mediated by the vestibular system and is transient; its direction reverses at the end of rotation. **C,** Cool water instilled into the right ear causes the same movement of endolymph in the right horizontal semicircular duct as does the rotation in **B.** The result again is nystagmus to the left.

forward direction with respect to the patient's trunk (that is, head movement to the right causes contraversive eye movements to the left). These are called *doll's head eye movements* (or the *oculocephalic reflex*) and are thought to represent a brainstem mechanism that is inhibited by signals from the cerebral cortex in normal conscious subjects. The afferent limb of the oculocephalic reflex probably includes proprioceptors from the neck, since the reflex can be elicited in comatose patients with no demonstrable labyrinthine function.

At the termination of rotation to the left, nystagmus with its fast phase to the right is seen in a normal individual, as discussed above. In addition, if the individual tries to point at something with his eyes closed, his arm will deviate to the left; this is called *past pointing*. He will also tend to fall to the left when walking. The lateral and medial vestibulospinal tracts ordinarily are quite important in directing the changes in muscle tone that correspond to the postural changes involved in balance; postrotatory past pointing and a tendency to fall demonstrate exaggerated activity in these tracts.

Stapedius reflex. As noted earlier, contraction of the stapedius stiffens the ossicular chain and hampers the transmission of vibrations. When a loud sound enters one ear, both stapedius muscles contract in a reflex fashion; an individual with a damaged facial nerve may complain that sounds are too loud in the ipsilateral ear (a condition known as *hyperacusis*). The pathway involved is from one ventral cochlear nucleus to both superior olivary nuclei and from there to both facial motor nuclei. It is possible to test this reflex arc, and this can be a useful clinical procedure. When the stapedius contracts, less sound energy incident on the eardrum is transferred along the ossicular chain, and more is reflected back from the eardrum. By measuring changes in the amount of a test sound reflected back from one eardrum when a loud sound is introduced into the contralateral ear, the stapedius reflex can be quantitatively analyzed.

The physiological function of the stapedius reflex is a matter of some dispute. The most common view is that it protects the inner ear from damage caused by excessively loud sounds. Clearly this could only work for chronic noise, since a brief loud sound would be over before the stapedius could contract. A second view of the reflex is that it helps the inner ear extract meaningful sounds from noisy backgrounds. Stapedial contraction impedes the transmission of low frequencies more than high frequencies and so could selectively reduce the effects of low-frequency noise.

The function of the tensor tympani in auditory processes is also unclear. This muscle too is activated bilaterally in some individuals in response to a loud sound in one ear, but only if the sound is extremely loud. Thus for most individuals in most physiological situations, only the stapedius is active. On the other hand, bilateral contraction of the tensor tympani is a normal component of the complex of reflexes involved in the startle response.

Brainstem auditory responses. In recent years it has been found that a brief sound causes a series of electrical waves, in the nanovolt range, that can be recorded from the surface of the head. The signals are so small that they are normally buried in background electrical noise, but by presenting the same brief stimulus many times and averaging the responses, the waves can be reproducibly measured. It is thought that the peaks of the waveform represent electrical activity at successive sites in the auditory pathway. Since this pathway extends from the pontomedullary junction to the temporal lobes, abnormalities in the *brainstem auditory response* can be helpful in localizing lesions.

ADDITIONAL READING

Adatia, A.K., and Gehring, E.N.: Proprioceptive innervation of the tongue, J. Anat. **110**:215, 1971.

Ash, P.R., and Keltner, J.L.: Neuro-ophthalmic signs in pontine lesions, Medicine **58**:304, 1979.

Beckstead, R.M., Morse, J.R., and Norgren, R.: The nucleus of the solitary tract in the monkey: projections to the thalamus and brain stem nuclei, J. Comp. Neurol. **190**:259, 1980.

Beckstead, R.M., and Norgren, R.: An autoradiographic examination of the central distribution of the trigeminal, facial, glossopharyngeal and vagal nerves in the monkey, J. Comp. Neurol. **184**:455, 1979.

Bender, M.B., and Feldman, M.: Visual illusions during head movement in lesions of the brain stem, Arch. Neurol. **17**:354, 1967. *An interesting discussion of what happens if a patient's vestibular apparatus is damaged, so that he cannot tell if movement of a visual image is caused by motion of his head or motion in the outside world.*

Borg, E.: On the neuronal organization of the acoustic middle ear reflex: a physiological and anatomical study, Brain Res. **49**:101, 1973.

Brandt, T., and Daroff, R.B.: The multisensory physiological and pathological vertigo syndromes, Ann. Neurol. **7**:195, 1980. *Stimulation or dysfunction of the vestibular, visual, or somatosensory systems can cause illusions of movement.*

Bredberg, G., Ades, H.W., and Engström, H.: Scanning electron microscopy of the normal and pathologically altered organ of Corti, Acta Otolaryngol. suppl. **301**:3, 1972. *Pretty pictures from a variety of mammals.*

Brindley, G.S.: How does an animal that is dropped in a nonupright posture know the angle through which it must turn in the air so that its feet point to the ground? J. Physiol, **180**:20P, 1965. *Briefly, it remembers which way was up when you let go of it. The paper isn't much longer than its title.*

Brodal, A.: Central course of afferent fibers for pain in facial, glossopharyngeal and vagus nerves, Arch. Neurol. Psychiatr. **57**:292, 1947.

Brodal, A.: Neurological anatomy in relation to clinical medicine, 3rd ed., New York, 1981, Oxford University Press.

Clark, D.L., Kreutzberg, J.R., and Chee, F.K.W.: Vestibular stimulation influence on motor development in infants, Science **196**:1228, 1977.

Cohen, L.A.: Role of eye and neck proprioceptive mechanisms in body orientation and motor coordination, J. Neurophysiol. **24**:1, 1961.

Dallos, P., et al.: Cochlear inner and outer hair cells: functional differences, Science **177**:356, 1972.

Darian-Smith, I.: The trigeminal system. In Iggo, A, editor: Handbook of sensory physiology, vol. II: somatosensory system, New York, 1973, Springer-Verlag, Inc.

Dewson, J.H., III: Efferent olivocochlear bundle: some relationships to stimulus discrimination in noise. J. Neurophysiol. **31**:122, 1968.

Evans, E.F., and Wilson, J.P., editors: Psychophysics and physiology of hearing, New York, 1977, Academic Press, Inc.

Fernández, C., Goldberg, J.M., and Abend, W.K.: Response to static tilts of peripheral neurons innervating otolith organs of the squirrel monkey, J. Neurophysiol. **35**:978, 1972.

Frederickson, J.M., et al.: Vestibular nerve projection to the cerebral cortex of the rhesus monkey, Exp. Brain Res. **2**:318, 1966.

Fukushima, T., and Kerr, F.W.L.: Organization of trigeminothalamic tracts and other thalamic afferent systems of the brainstem in the rat: presence of gelatinous neurons with thalamic connections, J. Comp. Neurol. **183**:169, 1979.

Goldberg, J.M., and Fernández, C.: Efferent vestibular system in the squirrel monkey: anatomical location and influence on afferent activity, J. Neurophysiol. **43**:986, 1980.

Goodwin, G.M., and Luschei, E.S.: Effects of destroying spindle afferents from jaw muscles on mastication in monkeys, J. Neurophysiol. **37**:967, 1974.

Henkin, R.I., and Christiansen, R.L.: Taste localization on the tongue, palate and pharynx of normal man, J. Applied Physiol. **22**:316, 1967.

Highstein, S.M., and Baker, R.: Excitatory termination of abducens internuclear neurons on medial rectus motoneurons: relationship to syndrome of internuclear ophthalmoplegia, J. Neurophysiol. **41**: 1647, 1978.

Hockman, C.H., Bieger, D., and Weerasuriya, A.: Supranuclear pathways of swallowing, Prog. Neurobiol. **12**:15, 1979.

Johnstone, B.M., and Sellick, P.M.: The peripheral auditory apparatus, Q. Rev. Biophys. **5**:1, 1972.

Kerr, F.W.L.: The divisional organization of afferent fibers of the trigeminal nerve, Brain **86**:721, 1963.

Kerr, F.W.L.: Evidence for a peripheral etiology of trigeminal neuralgia, J. Neurosurg. **26**:168, 1967.

King, R.B.: Evidence for a central etiology of tic douloureux, J. Neurosurg. **26**:175, 1967.

Klinke, R., and Schmidt, C.L.: Efferent influence on the vestibular organ during active movements of the body. Pflüg. Arch. **318**:325, 1970. *Clever experiments giving a hint about a goldfish's use for the efferent fibers in its vestibular nerve.*

Korte, G.E.: The brainstem projection of the vestibular nerve in the cat, J. Comp. Neurol. **184**:279, 1979.

Kunc, Z.: Treatment of essential neuralgia of the 9th nerve by selective tractotomy, J. Neurosurg. **23**:494, 1965.

Lee, D., and Lishman, R.: Vision in movement and balance, N. Scientist **65**:59, 1975. *A popularized but fascinating account of how easy it is to confuse one's position sense by presenting conflicting visual and vestibular inputs.*

Lidén, G., Peterson, J.L., and Harford, E.R.: Simultaneous recording of changes in relative impedance and air pressure during acoustic and non-acoustic elicitation of the middle-ear reflexes, Acta Otolaryngol. suppl. **263**:208, 1970.

Life without a balancing mechanism, N. Engl. J. Med. **246**:458, 1962. *A first-hand account of the remarkable compensation we can achieve after bilateral damage to the vestibular apparatus.*

Mahoney, T., Vernon, J., and Meikle, M.: Function of the acoustic re-

flex in discrimination of intense speech, Arch. Otolaryngol. **105**:119, 1979.

Martin, M.R., and Mason, C.A.: The seventh cranial nerve of the rat: visualization of efferent and afferent pathways by cobalt precipitation, Brain Res. **121**:21, 1977.

McIntyre, A.K., and Robinson, R.G.: Pathway for the jaw-jerk in man, Brain **82**:468, 1959.

Møller, A.R.: Coding of sounds in lower levels of the auditory system, Q. Rev. Biophys. **5**:59, 1972.

Norgren, R., and Leonard, C.M.: Ascending central gustatory pathways, J. Comp. Neurol. **150**:217, 1973.

Olszewski, J.: On the anatomical and functional organization of the spinal trigeminal nucleus, J. Comp. Neurol. **92**:401, 1950.

Ongerboer de Visser, B.W., and Kuypers, H.G.J.M.: Late blink reflex changes in lateral medullary lesions, Brain **101**:285, 1978.

Osterhammel, P., Terkildsen, K., and Zilstorff, K.: Vestibular habituation in ballet dancers, Adv. Otorhinolaryngol. **17**:158, 1970. *How do people who rotate for a living do it?*

Raphan, T., and Cohen, B.: Brainstem mechanisms for rapid and slow eye movements, Ann. Rev. Physiol. **40**:527, 1978.

Ryan, A., and Dallos, P.: Effect of absence of cochlear outer hair cells on behavioral auditory threshold, Nature **253**:44, 1975.

Smith, R.L.: Axonal projections and connections of the principal sensory trigeminal nucleus in the monkey, J. Comp. Neurol. **163**:347, 1975.

Spoendlin, H.: The innervation of the organ of Corti, J. Laryngol. Otol. **81**:717, 1967.

Steiger, H.-J., and Büttner-Ennever, J.: Relationship between motoneurons and internuclear neurons in the abducens nucleus: a double retrograde tracer study in the cat, Brain Res. **148**:181, 1978.

Stewart, W.A., and King, R.B.: Fiber projections from the nucleus caudalis of the spinal trigeminal nucleus, J. Comp. Neurol. **121**:271, 1963.

Stockard, J.J., Stockard, J.E., and Sharbrough, F.W.: Detection and localization of occult lesions with brainstem auditory responses, Mayo Clin. Proc. **52**:761, 1977.

Strominger, N.L., Nelson, L.R., and Dougherty, W.J.: Second order auditory pathways in the chimpanzee, J. Comp. Neurol. **172**:349, 1977.

Torvik, A.: The ascending fibers from the main trigeminal sensory nucleus, Am. J. Anat. **100**:1, 1957.

Toshikatsu, Y., and Nishikawa, N.: Somatotopic organization of trigeminal neurons within caudal medulla oblongata. In Anderson, D.J., and Matthews, B., editors: Pain in the trigeminal region, New York, 1977, American Elsevier Publishers, Inc. *A possible explanation for the "onion-skin" pattern of sensory loss often found after damage to the spinal trigeminal system.*

Von Békésy, G.: Experiments in hearing, New York, 1960, McGraw-Hill, Inc. *A large collection of clever and skillful experiments by the grand master of auditory physiology.*

Warwick, R.: Representation of the extra-ocular muscles in the oculomotor nuclei of the monkey, J. Comp. Neurol. **98**:449, 1953.

Wilson, V.J., and Jones, G.M.: Mammalian vestibular physiology, New York, 1979, Plenum Press.

Wilson, V.J., and Peterson, B.W.: Peripheral and central substrates of vestibulospinal reflexes, Physiol. Rev. **58**:80, 1978.

Younge, B.R.: Analysis of trochlear nerve palsies: diagnosis, etiology and treatment, Mayo Clin. Proc. **52**:11, 1977.

CHAPTER 10

DIENCEPHALON

The diencephalon, mostly hidden from view between the cerebral hemispheres, constitutes only about 2% of the central nervous system by weight. Nevertheless it has extremely widespread and important connections, and the great majority of sensory, motor, and limbic pathways involve one or more relays in the diencephalon. Since most motor and limbic pathways also involve telencephalic structures that are discussed in later chapters, this chapter provides only a general overview of the connections of diencephalic nuclei. A more detailed consideration of these connections in terms of functional systems is provided in subsequent chapters.

The diencephalon is conventionally divided into four parts, each of which includes the term "thalamus" (Greek = inner chamber) as part of its name. These parts are (1) the *epithalamus*, which includes the *pineal gland* and a few nearby neural structures, (2) the *dorsal thalamus*, which is usually referred to simply as the *thalamus;* (3) the *subthalamus,* and (4) the *hypothalamus.*

EXTENT OF THE DIENCEPHALON

The only part of the diencephalon that can be seen on an intact brain is the inferior surface of the hypothalamus (Figs. 2-12 and 2-13), which includes the *mammillary bodies* and the *infundibular stalk.* However, the entire medial surface of the diencephalon, much of which forms each wall of the third ventricle, can be seen on a hemisected brain (Fig. 10-1). Superiorly the diencephalon borders the subarachnoid space of the transverse cerebral fissure; inferiorly, as previously noted, it is also exposed to subarachnoid space. Laterally it is bounded by the internal capsule (Figs. 2-17 to 2-19). The caudal boundary of the diencephalon is a plane through the posterior commissure and the caudal edge of the mammillary bodies; the rostral boundary is a plane through the interventricular foramina and the optic chiasm. These rostral and caudal boundaries are approximate and semiarbitrary and are used only for purposes of dis-

cussion. Functionally continuous neural tissue extends through both boundaries; in addition (as noted in earlier chapters), certain thalamic nuclei extend through the posterior boundary to a position alongside the midbrain.

As a consequence of the cephalic flexure, the axis of the diencephalon is inclined about 100° with respect to the axis of the brainstem (Fig. 2-1). This means that sections cut in a plane similar to that used in the last few chapters (that is, perpendicular to the axis of the brainstem) would be at a peculiar angle to the diencephalon. Therefore in this and subsequent chapters, sections cut in horizontal and coronal planes are shown (Fig. 10-2). It should be noted that horizontal sections are oriented with the posterior portion at the top of the picture. This was done for reasons of internal consistency: horizontal sections are not very different from the transverse sections shown in Chapters 8 and 9, and the transverse sections were also oriented with the posterior portion at the top of the picture. However, the reader should be aware that clinical studies such as CT scans are commonly studied in the reverse fashion (that is, with the anterior portion at the top of the picture, as in, for example, Fig. 4-12).

EPITHALAMUS

The epithalamus includes the *pineal gland* and the *habenular nuclei* and their connections.

Pineal gland

The pineal gland is a midline, unpaired structure situated just rostral to the superior colliculi. Since each of us has only one pineal gland, which is located deep within the brain, it was thought for a time that this organ might be the seat of the soul. This now seems unlikely, since pineal tumors do not cause the changes one would expect to find associated with distortion of the soul; rather, these tumors compress the midbrain and cause the changes one would expect to find associated with distortion of this part of the brainstem. Early findings may

Fig. 10-1. Closeup photograph of the medial surface of the brain shown in Figs. 2-11 and 10-2 illustrating parts of the diencephalon and some surrounding structures.

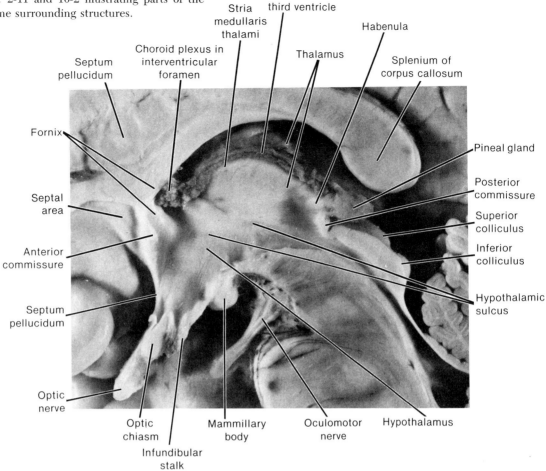

Septum pellucidum

Choroid plexus in interventricular foramen

Stria medullaris thalami

Choroid plexus of roof of third ventricle

Thalamus

Habenula

Splenium of corpus callosum

Fornix

Septal area

Anterior commissure

Septum pellucidum

Optic nerve

Optic chiasm

Infundibular stalk

Mammillary body

Oculomotor nerve

Hypothalamus

Pineal gland

Posterior commissure

Superior colliculus

Inferior colliculus

Hypothalamic sulcus

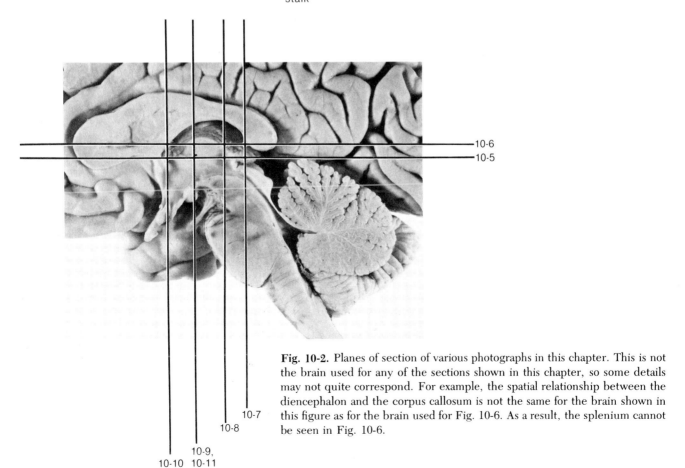

10-6
10-5

10-7

10-8

10-9,
10-10 10-11

Fig. 10-2. Planes of section of various photographs in this chapter. This is not the brain used for any of the sections shown in this chapter, so some details may not quite correspond. For example, the spatial relationship between the diencephalon and the corpus callosum is not the same for the brain shown in this figure as for the brain used for Fig. 10-6. As a result, the splenium cannot be seen in Fig. 10-6.

include hydrocephalus (because of the squeezing shut of the aqueduct) and various defects of eye movements and pupillary reactions (because of damage to the oculomotor and trochlear nuclei and pathways ending on them). In addition, pineal tumors may cause changes in sexual development, giving a clue to at least one of its functions. The pineal arises as an evagination from the roof of the diencephalon; in fish, amphibians, and many reptiles, it contains photoreceptor cells similar to those of the eye. In these species, it is suspected of monitoring day length and season and participating in the regulation of circadian and circumannual rhythms (although there are other probable functions as well). The pineal gland of birds and mammals contains no photoreceptors and consists of a collection of secretory cells (*pinealocytes*), some glial cells, and a rich vascular network. Nevertheless it still receives a light-regulated input by way of a circuitous pathway that begins in the retina and, after one or more relays in the hypothalamus, reaches the intermediolateral cell column of the spinal cord. Preganglionic sympathetic fibers from the spinal cord then synapse on postganglionic neurons of the superior cervical ganglion, which in turn send their axons to the pineal.

The mammalian pineal is an endocrine gland involved in reproductive cycles and has no known neural output. It secretes an antigonadotropic hormone called *melatonin* at relatively high rates during darkness. Light, by way of the neural pathway just described, causes a decrease in melatonin production. Thus increasing day lengths cause a decrease in melatonin production, which in turn causes an increase in gonadal function. This system is of considerable importance in mammals with prominent seasonal sexual cycles, but its effects in humans are not clear. It is known, however, that nonparenchymal pineal tumors, which presumably destroy pinealocytes, tend to be associated with precocious puberty, as though the production of some antigonadotropic substance had been halted. The converse is true as well: parenchymal pineal tumors tend to be associated with hypogonadism. These tumors are quite rare, however, and the routine clinical importance of the pineal arises from the fact that after the age of 17 calcareous concretions accrue in it. This makes it opaque to x rays and hence a useful radiological landmark, since it normally lies in the midline, and slight shifts in its position can be indicative of expanding masses of various types.

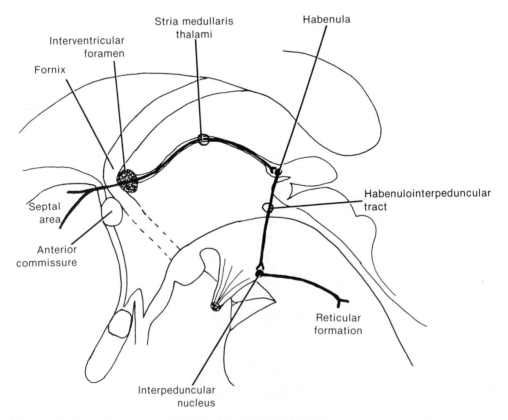

Fig. 10-3. Pathway through the habenula. The stria medullaris thalami is depicted as arising in the septal area, a part of the limbic system; as discussed in Chapter 16, other limbic structures contribute as well.

Habenula

The pineal gland is attached to the dorsal surface of the diencephalon by a stalk. Caudally at the base of the stalk is the posterior commissure; rostrally is a small swelling on each side called a *habenula* (Fig. 10-1 and 10-5). Underlying each habenula are the *habenular nuclei*. The two habenulae are interconnected by the small *habenular commissure*. The habenula receives one major input bundle, the *stria medullaris thalami*, and gives rise to one major output bundle with the awesome name of *habenulointerpeduncular tract* (or *fasciculus retroflexus*). The stria medullaris thalami (Figs. 10-1, 10-3, and 10-8) underlies a horizontal ridge on the dorsomedial surface of the thalamus to which the roof of the third ventricle is attached. The habenulointerpeduncular tract, as its name implies, extends from the habenula to the *interpeduncular nucleus*, which is located between the cerebral peduncles in the reticular formation of the rostral midbrain (Figs. 10-3 and 10-8). The fibers of the stria medullaris thalami originate in various limbic structures, so the pathway through the habenula is one route through which the limbic system can influence the brainstem reticular formation.

SUBTHALAMUS

The midbrain tegmentum continues into the diencephalon as the *subthalamus*, or *subthalamic region*. This area is completely surrounded by neural tissue and is located inferior to the thalamus, lateral to the hypothalamus, and medial to the basis pedunculi and internal capsule (Figs. 10-9 and 10-11). The subthalamus contains rostral portions of the red nucleus and substantia nigra and is traversed by somatosensory pathways on their way to the thalamus as well as by several pathways involving the cerebellum and basal ganglia (the latter pathways are discussed in Chapters 13 and 14). In addition, the subthalamus contains the *subthalamic nucleus* and *zona incerta* (Fig. 10-11). The subthalamic nucleus (occasionally called the nucleus of Luys) is biconvex in shape and is located just medial and superior to portions of the basis pedunculi and internal capsule. This nucleus is a component of the extrapyramidal motor system, and its connections are discussed in Chapter 13. The zona incerta is a small mass of gray matter intervening between the subthalamic nucleus and the thalamus. It appears to be a rostral continuation of the midbrain reticular formation, but its connections and functions are largely unknown.

THALAMUS

The thalamus is a large egg-shaped nuclear mass, making up about 80% of the diencephalon. It extends anteriorly to the interventricular foramen, superiorly to the transverse cerebral fissure, and inferiorly to the hypothalamic sulcus; posteriorly it overlaps the midbrain (Fig. 10-1). The thalamus is part of a remarkably large number of pathways: all sensory pathways (except olfactory) relay in the thalamus, and many of the anatomical loops comprising cerebellar, basal ganglionic, and limbic pathways also involve thalamic relays. These various systems utilize more or less separate portions of the thalamus, which has therefore been subdivided into a series of nuclei. These nuclei can be distinguished from each other both by their topographical locations within the thalamus and by the patterns of their connections with the cerebral cortex.

Topographical subdivisions

The general organization of the thalamus is shown in Fig. 10-4. A thin, curved sheet of myelinated fibers, the *internal medullary lamina*, divides most of the thalamus into medial and lateral groups of nuclei. Anteriorly the internal medullary lamina bifurcates and encloses an anterior group of nuclei. In the human thalamus, the medial group contains a single large nucleus, the *dorsomedial nucleus (DM)*; for this reason, the DM is sometimes referred to simply as the *medial nucleus* (Figs. 10-5, 10-6, 10-8, and 10-9). The only large nucleus in the anterior group in humans is the *anteroventral nucleus (AV)*. This is an unfortunate name, since the nucleus is anterior but not particularly ventral (Figs. 10-6, 10-9, and 10-10). The smaller nuclei of the anterior group are thought to have connections similar to those of the AV, so the whole complex is sometimes referred to simply as the *anterior nucleus*.

The lateral group of nuclei composes the bulk of the thalamus and is further subdivided into a dorsal tier and a ventral tier. The dorsal tier consists of the very large *pulvinar* (Figs. 10-5, 10-6, and 10-7), the *lateral posterior nucleus (LP)* (Fig. 10-8), and the *lateral dorsal nucleus (LD)* (Fig. 10-8). The lateral posterior nucleus is continuous with the pulvinar; both nuclei have somewhat similar connections, so the two together are sometimes referred to as the pulvinar/LP complex. The ventral tier of the lateral nuclear group consists of three nuclei arranged along an anterior-posterior line: (1) the *ventral anterior (VA)* (Figs. 10-6 and 10-10), (2) the *ventral lateral (VL)* (Fig. 10-9), and (3) the *ventral posterior (VP)* (Fig. 10-8) nuclei. The ventral posterior nucleus is customarily subdivided into the *ventral posterolateral (VPL)* and *ventral posteromedial (VPM)* nuclei. The VPL is the somatosensory relay nucleus for the body and the VPM for the head. The VA and VL are involved in motor control circuits that include the cerebellum and basal ganglia.

There are several other thalamic nuclei that do not fit conveniently into the framework given above.

1. The *lateral geniculate nucleus* (visual system) and *medial geniculate nucleus* (auditory system) are located

Text continued on p. 174.

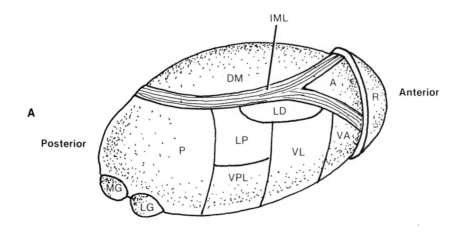

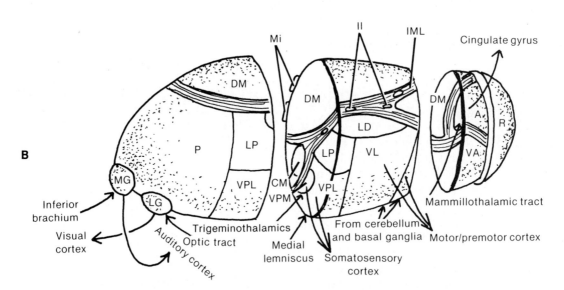

Fig. 10-4. Diagrammatic illustration of the way in which the thalamus is subdivided. **A,** Lateral view of the right thalamus as seen from slightly above and behind. Most of the reticular nucleus has been removed; ordinarily it would cover the entire lateral surface. **B,** Same as **A,** but exploded into three pieces to show certain aspects of the internal organization of the thalamus. Tracts ending in the specific relay nuclei are indicated, as are the destinations of the outputs from these nuclei. The more posterior sliced surface corresponds approximately to Fig. 10-8; the more anterior sliced surface corresponds approximately to Fig. 10-9. *A,* Anterior nucleus; *CM,* centromedian nucleus; *DM,* dorsomedial nucleus; *Il,* intralaminar nuclei; *IML,* internal medullary lamina; *LD,* lateral dorsal nucleus; *LG,* lateral geniculate nucleus; *LP,* lateral posterior nucleus; *MG,* medial geniculate nucleus; *Mi,* midline nuclei; *P,* pulvinar; *R,* reticular nucleus; *VA,* ventral anterior nucleus; *VL,* ventral lateral nucleus; *VPL,* ventral posterolateral nucleus; *VPM,* ventral posteromedial nucleus. (Modified from Brodal, A.: Neurological anatomy in relation to clinical medicine, ed. 3, New York, 1981, Oxford University Press.)

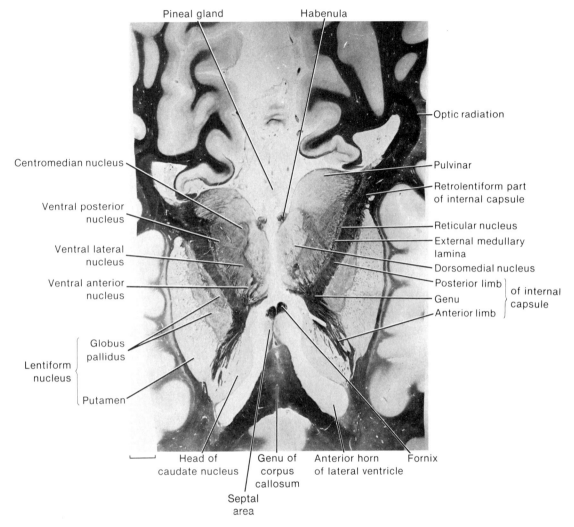

Pineal gland   Habenula

Optic radiation

Centromedian nucleus

Pulvinar

Retrolentiform part
of internal capsule

Ventral posterior
nucleus

Reticular nucleus

External medullary
lamina

Ventral lateral
nucleus

Dorsomedial nucleus

Ventral anterior
nucleus

Posterior limb ⎫
                    ⎬ of internal
Genu   ⎭ capsule

Anterior limb

Globus
pallidus

Lentiform
nucleus

Putamen

Head of   Genu of   Anterior horn   Fornix
caudate nucleus corpus   of lateral ventricle
                 callosum

Septal
area

Fig. 10-5. Horizontal section through the thalamus at the level of the centromedian nucleus. Scale mark = 5 mm. At this magnification and with this staining technique, the VPL/VPM, VL, and VA can be distinguished from one another only by location and not by appearance.

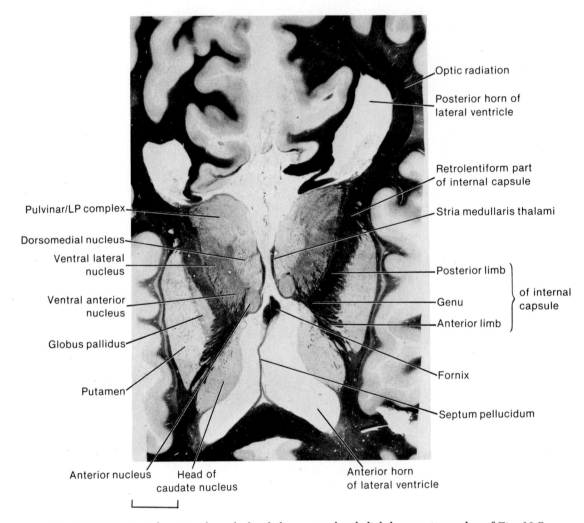

Optic radiation

Posterior horn of
lateral ventricle

Retrolentiform part
of internal capsule

Stria medullaris thalami

Posterior limb

Genu

Anterior limb

of internal
capsule

Fornix

Septum pellucidum

Pulvinar/LP complex

Dorsomedial nucleus

Ventral lateral
nucleus

Ventral anterior
nucleus

Globus pallidus

Putamen

Anterior nucleus   Head of
caudate nucleus

Anterior horn
of lateral ventricle

Fig. 10-6. Horizontal section through the thalamus at a level slightly superior to that of Fig. 10-5. Scale mark = 1 cm.

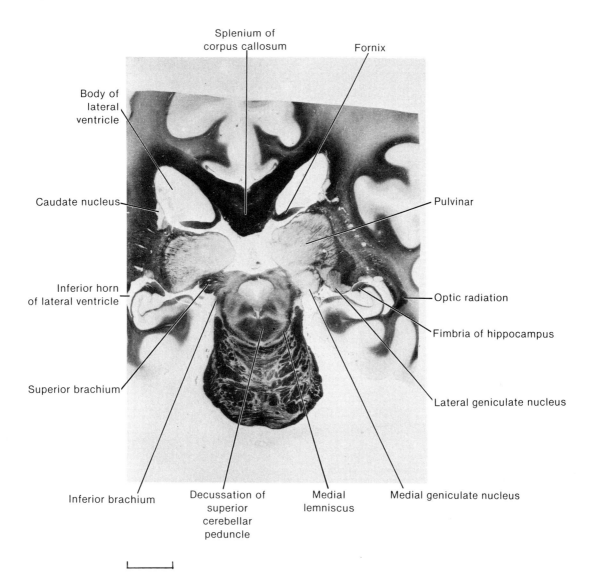

Fig. 10-7. Coronal section through the posterior thalamus. Scale mark = 1 cm. The fimbria of the hippocampus curves dorsally (following the lateral ventricle) and is continuous with the fornix.

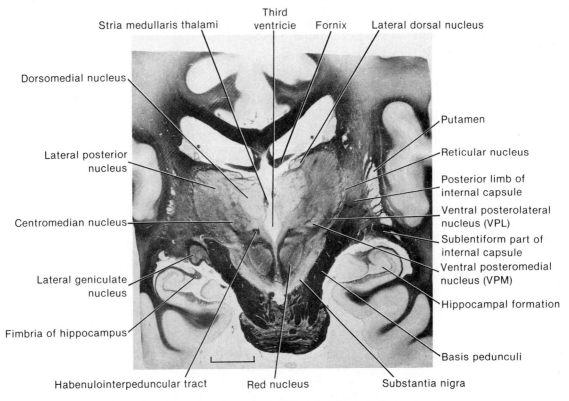

Stria medullaris thalami

Third ventricle

Fornix

Lateral dorsal nucleus

Dorsomedial nucleus

Lateral posterior nucleus

Centromedian nucleus

Lateral geniculate nucleus

Fimbria of hippocampus

Putamen

Reticular nucleus

Posterior limb of internal capsule

Ventral posterolateral nucleus (VPL)

Sublentiform part of internal capsule

Ventral posteromedial nucleus (VPM)

Hippocampal formation

Basis pedunculi

Habenulointerpeduncular tract

Red nucleus

Substantia nigra

Fig. 10-8. Coronal section through posterior thalamus. Scale mark = 1 cm.

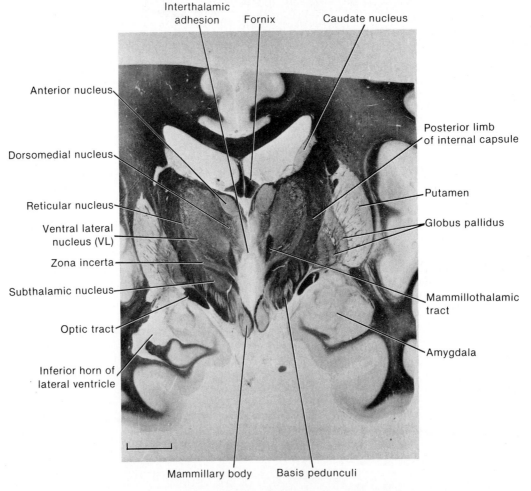

Interthalamic adhesion

Fornix

Caudate nucleus

Anterior nucleus

Dorsomedial nucleus

Reticular nucleus

Ventral lateral nucleus (VL)

Zona incerta

Subthalamic nucleus

Optic tract

Inferior horn of lateral ventricle

Posterior limb of internal capsule

Putamen

Globus pallidus

Mammillothalamic tract

Amygdala

Mammillary body

Basis pedunculi

Fig. 10-9. Coronal section through anterior thalamus. Scale mark = 1 cm.

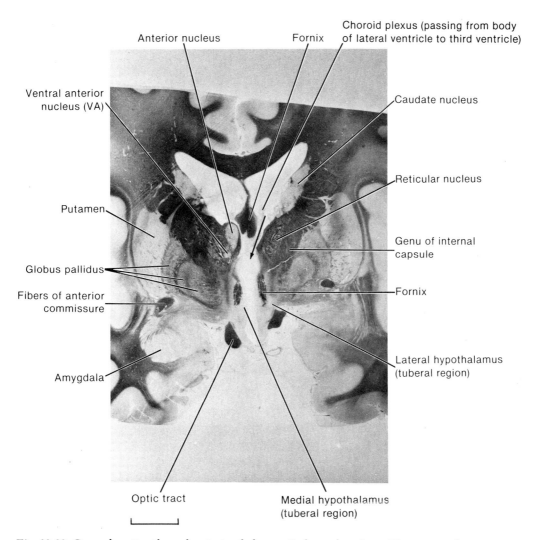

Anterior nucleus

Fornix

Choroid plexus (passing from body of lateral ventricle to third ventricle)

Ventral anterior nucleus (VA)

Caudate nucleus

Putamen

Reticular nucleus

Globus pallidus

Genu of internal capsule

Fibers of anterior commissure

Fornix

Amygdala

Lateral hypothalamus (tuberal region)

Optic tract

Medial hypothalamus (tuberal region)

Fig. 10-10. Coronal section through anterior thalamus. Scale mark = 1 cm. The arrow is shown passing from the lateral ventricle to the third ventricle through the interventricular foramen.

posterior and a bit ventral to the VPL/VPM and protrude posteriorly alongside the midbrain (Fig. 10-7). These two nuclei are sometimes considered as a separate thalamic group called the *metathalamus*.

2. At certain locations within the thalamus the internal medullary lamina splits and encloses groups of cells. These nuclei are collectively called the *intralaminar nuclei*, the two largest of which are the *centromedian (CM)* and *parafascicular (PF) nuclei* (Figs. 10-5 and 10-8). The centromedian nucleus is a large, round nucleus located medial to the VPL/VPM; the VPM conforms to the rounded shape of the centromedian nucleus, and for this reason the VPM was once called the semilunar or arcuate nucleus. The parafascicular nucleus is located medial

to the centromedian nucleus and received its name from the fact that the habenulointerpeduncular tract (fasciculus retroflexus) passes through it.

3. The lateral surface of the thalamus is covered by a second curved sheet of myelinated fibers called the *external medullary lamina*. The thin shell of cells that intervenes between the external medullary lamina and the internal capsule is the *reticular nucleus* of the thalamus (Figs. 10-5, 10-6, 10-8, and 10-11). The reticular nucleus is continuous inferiorly with the zona incerta (Fig. 10-11), but this is of no apparent functional significance.

4. A thin layer of cells, essentially a rostral continuation of parts of the periaqueductal gray, covers portions of the medial surface of the thalamus. These cells con-

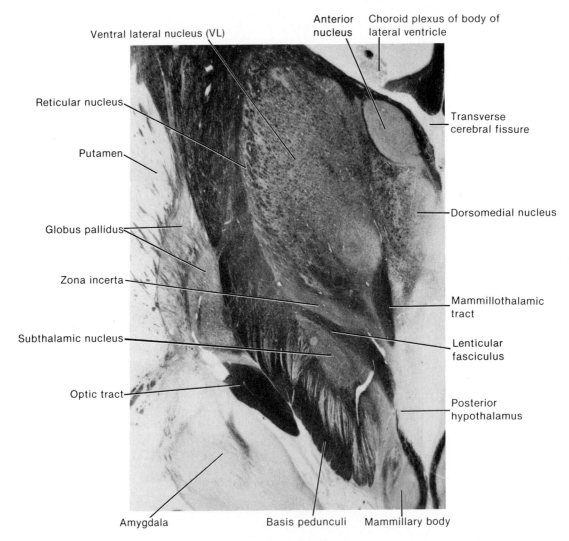

Fig. 10-11. Enlargement of part of Fig. 10-9 to demonstrate subthalamic region more clearly. The lenticular fasciculus is an output bundle from the basal ganglia on its way from the globus pallidus to the VL and VA.

stitute the *midline nuclei* of the thalamus (not to be confused with the medial, or dorsomedial, nucleus). The midline nuclei of the two sides fuse in the interthalamic adhesion, when it is present.

Functional subdivisions

Thalamic nuclei are interconnected with the cerebral cortex in various ways. Some receive well-defined bundles of fibers and project very specifically to particular functional areas of the cerebral cortex; these are called *specific relay nuclei*. A good example of a specific relay nucleus is the medial geniculate nucleus, which receives the inferior brachium and projects to auditory cortex in the temporal lobe. Other nuclei receive their inputs from a variety of places (especially from other thalamic nuclei) and project to fairly broad areas of association cortex (explained in Chapter 15); these are appropriately called *association nuclei*. Still other nuclei, called *nonspecific nuclei*, project to extremely widespread areas of the cortex, frequently via fibers that are collaterals of fibers on their way to someplace else. Finally, some nuclei have no projections to the cerebral cortex at all. They are naturally called *subcortical nuclei*.

The cortical connections of thalamic nuclei are often described as though they were one-way affairs (for example, inferior brachium → medial geniculate nucleus → auditory cortex). However, as a general rule these connections are reciprocal. In addition, thalamic nuclei may receive inputs from cortical areas to which they do not project. Some of these descending cortical projections are exactly analogous to the now-familiar descending inputs to sensory relay nuclei and to sensory receptors themselves. Thus the cortex is able to exert some feedback control over the information that reaches it. Beyond this, however, little can be said about the function of these connections.

Specific relay nuclei. The specific relay nuclei and their connections are indicated in Fig. 10-4 and Table 5. They include the sensory relay nuclei (the VPL/VPM and the geniculate nuclei) and several others as well, since parts of the motor and limbic systems also have thalamic relays. The VL and VA are the motor relay nuclei, receiving the superior cerebellar peduncle and various outputs from the basal ganglia and projecting to motor and premotor cortex. The anterior nucleus is the principal relay nucleus for the limbic system, receiving the *mammillothalamic tract* and projecting to the cingulate gyrus. The mammillothalamic tract, as its name implies, arises in the mammillary body (Fig. 10-9). The cingulate gyrus is a prominent component of the limbic lobe (Fig. 2-5). The way in which this pathway fits into the limbic system as a whole is detailed in Chapter 16. It was thought for a time that the lateral dorsal nucleus (LD) was an association nucleus connected to association cortex in the parietal lobe. However, recent evidence indicates that it closely resembles the anterior nucleus in projecting to the cingulate gyrus. Therefore, in spite of the fact that a discrete input tract does not end in it,

TABLE 5
Thalamic nuclei

Type	Name of nucleus	Major input*	Major output
Specific relay	Lateral geniculate	Optic tract	Visual cortex
	Medial geniculate	Inferior brachium	Auditory cortex
	Ventral posterolateral (VPL)	Medial lemniscus, spinothalamic tract	Somatosensory cortex
	Ventral posteromedial (VPM)	Trigeminothalamic tracts	Somatosensory cortex
	Ventral lateral, ventral anterior (VL/VA)	Cerebellum, basal ganglia	Motor/premotor cortex
	Anterior (anteroventral) (AV)	Mammillothalamic tract	Cingulate gyrus
Association	Pulvinar	Other thalamic nuclei, superior colliculus	Parietal-occipital-temporal association cortex
	Lateral posterior (LP)	Other thalamic nuclei	Parietal association cortex
	Lateral dorsal (LD)	Unknown	Cingulate gyrus
	Dorsomedial (DM)	Other thalamic nuclei, amygdala, hypothalamus	Prefrontal cortex
Nonspecific	Part of VA	Other thalamic nuclei	Collaterals to prefrontal cortex
	Intralaminar	Other thalamic nuclei, reticular formation, basal ganglia	Collaterals to widespread cortical areas
Subcortical	Reticular	Thalamus	Thalamus

*Inputs from cerebral cortex not included.

some authors have begun to refer to the LD as a relay nucleus. As might be expected from the uncertainty surrounding its connections, the function of this nucleus is unknown.

Association nuclei. There are two great areas of association cortex in the human brain (Fig. 15-13). One is the prefrontal cortex, anterior to the motor areas of the frontal lobe. The second is the parietal-occipital-temporal association cortex occupying the area surrounded by the primary somatosensory, visual, and auditory cortices. Corresponding to these two areas are two large association nuclei or nuclear complexes. The dorsomedial nucleus is reciprocally interconnected with the prefrontal cortex and is involved in prefrontal functions such as affect and foresight, as described further in chapters 15 and 16. Bilateral damage to the dorsomedial nucleus or to its connections with the frontal lobe has effects similar to those of prefrontal lobectomy. Major inputs to the dorsomedial nucleus, in addition to those from prefrontal cortex, come from other thalamic nuclei and from various elements of the limbic system, such as the hypothalamus and the amygdala.

The pulvinar/LP complex is reciprocally interconnected with the parietal-occipital-temporal association cortex. The major inputs to this complex, aside from those arising in association cortex, come from other thalamic nuclei, especially the sensory relay nuclei. In addition, the pulvinar receives visual inputs from the superior colliculus. The pulvinar is the largest nucleus in the human thalamus and is better developed in humans than in any other mammal. One would expect that a nucleus this large and this highly developed in humans would have an important, well-defined function. Unfortunately the role of the pulvinar (and of the LP) is almost entirely unknown at this time. There are hints that it may be involved in some aspects of visual perception, and there are occasional reports of language deficits following damage to it, but in general no particular syndrome and no obvious sensory deficits follow damage to the pulvinar/LP complex.

Nonspecific nuclei. The midline and intralaminar nuclei and a portion of the VA form a nonspecific system that projects to widespread areas of the cerebral cortex. The precise connections of individual nuclei vary, but with the exception of the centromedian nucleus, they will be treated as a group in the following account. Inputs to these nuclei are from diverse sources, including other thalamic nuclei, basal ganglia, the brainstem reticular formation, and spinothalamic and spinoreticulothalamic fibers carrying information about dull, aching pain. The efferent projections have long been a matter of controversy. For a time they were regarded as having projections to other thalamic nuclei and to the basal ganglia but none to the cerebral cortex, since retrograde

degeneration was not seen in them following removal of large areas of cortex. This finding was at odds with physiological studies showing that stimulation of the nonspecific nuclei causes changes in the electrical activity of broad cortical areas. Recent anatomical studies using newer tracing techniques appear to have resolved the problem. The major output projections of the nonspecific nuclei are to noncortical targets such as the basal ganglia, but these efferents also send collaterals to the cerebral cortex. The damage caused by destruction of these collaterals during cortical removal in the older anatomical experiments was presumably insufficient to cause retrograde degeneration.

The broad extent of the cortical connections of the nonspecific nuclei make them suitable for general roles such as regulating the level of cortical excitability; they are considered to be the route through which the ascending reticular activating system affects the cortex.

Although the centromedian nucleus is one of the intralaminar nuclei, it has a special relationship with the basal ganglia and probably has a role different from that of the other nonspecific nuclei. The centromedian nucleus, like the pulvinar, is disproportionately large in primates, and its growth parallels the increase in size of the caudate nucleus and putamen. As discussed further in Chapter 13, its major connections are with the basal ganglia and motor areas of the cortex.

Subcortical nuclei. With the cortical projections of the nonspecific nuclei confirmed, the reticular nucleus became the principal representative of the subcortical thalamic nuclei. Inspection of Figs. 10-5 and 10-6 will reveal that most of the fibers reciprocally connecting the thalamus and cortex must traverse the reticular nucleus. As they do so, these fibers give off collaterals to the reticular nucleus. Thus, for example, the portion of the reticular nucleus adjacent to the VPL/VPM receives convergent inputs from somatosensory fibers on their way to the postcentral gyrus, and from descending fibers on their way from the postcentral gyrus to the VPL/VPM. The output of each portion of the reticular nucleus goes to that thalamic nucleus from which it receives its input. This leads to the interesting hypothesis that the reticular nucleus compares cortical afferent and efferent activity and then modulates thalamic activity accordingly.*

Blood supply

Inspection of a hemisected brain (Fig. 5-4) will reveal that the anterior and middle cerebral arteries and their

---

*The meaning of "accordingly" in this instance is thoroughly unclear. Experiments appropriate for clarifying the role of the reticular nucleus are difficult or impossible to perform, since destruction of the reticular nucleus is accompanied by destruction of the thalamocortical and corticothalamic fibers that traverse it. Likewise these same fibers would be stimulated by stimulation of the reticular nucleus.

branches near the circle of Willis are anterior to most of the thalamus. The blood supply of the thalamus is therefore mostly from branches of the posterior cerebral artery. Specifically branches of the posterior choroidal artery supply some dorsomedial regions, and most of the rest of the thalamus is supplied by small ganglionic or perforating arteries arising from the posterior cerebral and posterior communicating arteries. These ganglionic arteries are sometimes divided into two groups: a *posteromedial* group arising within the circle of Willis and a *posterolateral* group arising distal to the circle. The posteromedial group tends to supply medial and anterior portions of the thalamus as well as the subthalamus. The posterolateral group (sometimes also called *thalamogeniculate arteries*) supplies most of the posterior and lateral thalamus. Finally, the anterior choroidal artery often sends a few small branches to the subthalamus and to ventral regions of the thalamus, particularly the lateral geniculate nucleus.

Some functional aspects of the thalamus

As a general rule, the cerebral cortex is more important for the proper functioning of sensory systems in humans than it is in other mammals. For example, cats deprived of somatosensory cortex or visual cortex retain a significant portion of their previous somatosensory or visual capabilities, and rats treated similarly retain even more. Nevertheless it is often claimed that sensory stimuli, particularly somatosensory stimuli, "enter consciousness" in humans at the level of the thalamus. When the somatosensory cortex in humans is destroyed, the remaining awareness of stimuli is very crude, consisting mainly of an ability by the individual to recognize the fact that he or she has been touched or has received a painful stimulus. The individual's ability to localize the stimulus or to discriminate its intensity is severely impaired. These conclusions are based mainly on studies of humans who have sustained damage to one parietal lobe, and it is not yet entirely clear if the remaining sensory capabilities are in fact a result of consciousness at the level of the thalamus ipsilateral to the lesion. In most cases, it appears that the remaining capabilities could be a result of slight bilaterality in the function of the contralateral thalamus and parietal lobe.

Damage to the thalamus most often occurs as a result of vascular accidents, particularly involving the thalamogeniculate arteries. Occasionally tumors may involve the thalamus. The damage almost always involves other structures in addition to the thalamus (for example, the adjacent internal capsule), and a large collection of deficits with far-reaching consequences may result from relatively small lesions in this area. Characteristically a type of dysesthesia results from damage more or less restricted to the posterior thalamus. The condition is somewhat similar to trigeminal neuralgia in that paroxysms of intense pain may be triggered by somatosensory stimuli. This pain may spread to involve one entire half of the body. It is usually resistant to pain-killing drugs and is called *thalamic pain.* In addition, those stimuli that do not cause a pain attack may be perceived abnormally: their intensity (and even their modality) may be distorted, and they may seem unusually uncomfortable or pleasant. As mentioned previously, some pain syndromes following damage to more caudal levels of the nervous system are thought to result from an imbalance between the activities of the fast-pain and slow-pain systems. A similar mechanism may be involved in thalamic pain, since the fast-pain spinothalamic fibers end in the VPL/VPM, whereas many of the slow-pain spinothalamic and spinoreticulothalamic fibers end in the intralaminar nuclei (excluding the centromedian nucleus). Thus it would be possible for a posterior thalamic lesion to preferentially damage the fast-pain system, just as mesencephalic tractotomy does (see Chapter 8).

Extensive damage to the posterior thalamus also causes total (or nearly total) loss of somatic sensation in the contralateral head and body. After a period of time, some appreciation of painful, thermal, and gross tactile stimuli usually returns. Functions customarily associated with the medial lemniscus tend to be more severely and permanently impaired. Discriminative tactile sensibility may be abolished, position sense may be greatly impaired, and a sensory type of ataxia (resulting from the loss of priorioception) may persist. The combination of thalamic pain, hemianesthesia, and sensory ataxia, all contralateral to a posterior thalamic lesion, is called the *thalamic syndrome.* It is often accompanied by mild and transient paralysis (a result of damage to corticospinal fibers in the adjacent internal capsule) and by various types of residual involuntary movements (a result of damage to nearby basal ganglia).

INTERNAL CAPSULE

The large collection of thalamocortical and corticothalamic fibers just described need a route by which to travel from their origins to their destinations. This route is provided by the *internal capsule,* a compact bundle of fibers through which almost all the neural traffic to and from the cerebral cortex passes. As Figs. 10-5 and 10-6 indicate, the internal capsule is in a convenient location for fibers entering or leaving the thalamus. In addition to these, other fibers descend from the cortex through the internal capsule and then through the cerebral peduncle to reach pontine nuclei (*corticopontine fibers*), motor nuclei of cranial nerves (*corticobulbar fibers*), and spinal cord motor neurons and interneurons (*corticospinal fibers*). Still other fibers project from the cerebral cortex

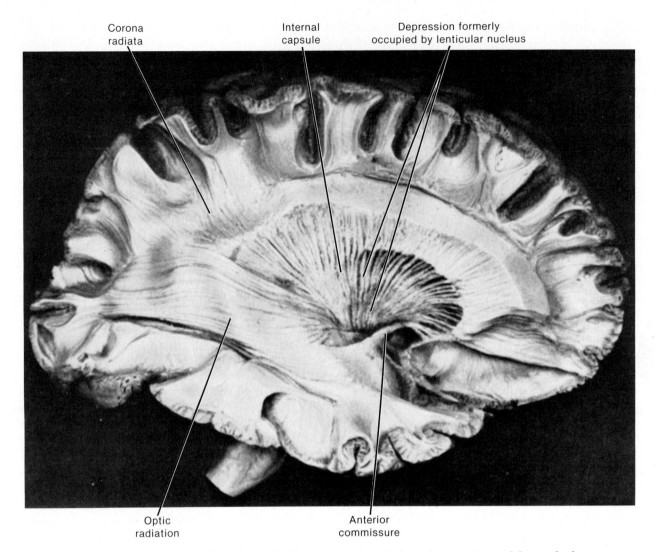

Corona radiata   Internal capsule   Depression formerly occupied by lenticular nucleus

Optic radiation   Anterior commissure

Fig. 10-12. Dissection of the right cerebral hemisphere from its lateral aspect. Most of the cerebral cortex, including that of the insula, was removed. The lenticular nucleus (putamen and globus pallidus) was then removed, revealing the internal capsule. The internal capsule outlines the former location of the lenticular nucleus, and its fibers then continue into the corona radiata. The fibers of the anterior commissure can also be seen collecting from the temporal lobe and projecting toward the midline. (From Ludwig, E., and Klingler, J.: Atlas cerebri humani, Boston, 1956, Little, Brown and Co.)

through the internal capsule to additional subcortical targets, such as various nuclei of the extrapyramidal system (for example, the putamen and the caudate nucleus).

The three-dimensional shape of the internal capsule is a bit difficult to visualize, but the beautiful dissections shown in Figs. 10-12 and 10-13 should help. The internal capsule is a continuous sheet of fibers that forms the medial boundary of the lenticular nucleus (Fig. 10-12) and then continues around posteriorly and inferiorly to partially envelop this nucleus (Fig. 10-13). Inferiorly many of the fibers in the internal capsule funnel down

into the cerebral peduncle. Superiorly they all fan out into the *corona radiata* (Figs. 10-12 and 10-13), in which they travel through the cerebral white matter to reach their cortical origins or destinations. Thus the entire fiber system is shaped like a trumpet with a large notch cut out of its bell (Fig. 10-13): the flared-out bell corresponds to the region where the fibers of the internal capsule spread out to form the corona radiata, and the notch corresponds to the location where this continuous sheet of fibers is interrupted in an intact brain by the lateral fissure. The narrowest part of the trumpet corresponds

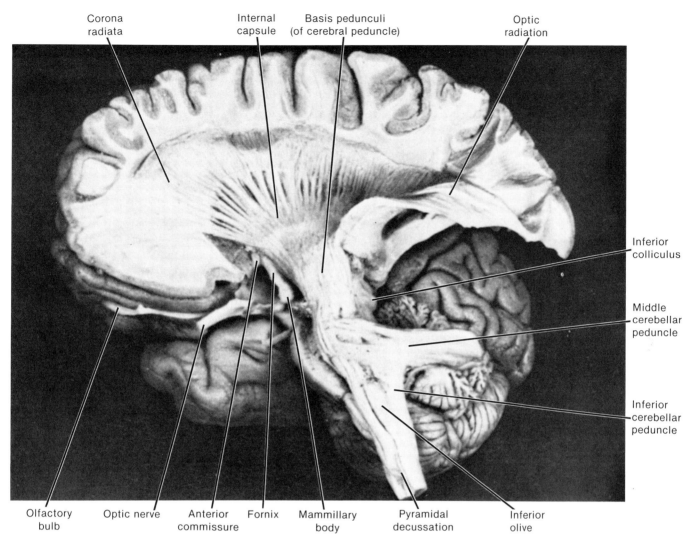

Corona radiata | Internal capsule | Basis pedunculi (of cerebral peduncle) | Optic radiation

Inferior colliculus

Middle cerebellar peduncle

Inferior cerebellar peduncle

Olfactory bulb | Optic nerve | Anterior commissure | Fornix | Mammillary body | Pyramidal decussation | Inferior olive

Fig. 10-13. Dissection of the left cerebral hemisphere from its lateral aspect. This dissection is similar to that of Fig. 10-12 except that the temporal lobe has also been removed so that the continuity of the internal capsule and the cerebral peduncle can be seen. The flared-out, trumpet-shaped progression from the cerebral peduncle, through the internal capsule, and into the corona radiata is shown here about as well as it can be. The entire course of the pyramidal tract from the corona radiata through the medullary pyramid can also be seen, as can the origin of the middle cerebellar peduncle in the basal part of the pons. (From Ludwig, E., and Klingler, J.: Atlas cerebri humani, Boston, 1956, Little, Brown and Co.)

to the cerebral peduncle, and in an intact brain, the lenticular nucleus sits where a mute would sit in a trumpet.

The internal capsule is divided into five regions on the basis of the relationship of each part to the lenticular (lentiform) nucleus (Figs. 10-5 and 10-6). The *anterior limb* is the portion between the lenticular nucleus and the head of the caudate nucleus. The *posterior limb* is the portion between the lenticular nucleus and the thalamus. The *genu* is the portion at the junction of the anterior and posterior limbs; since this junction occurs at

the anterior end of the thalamus, the genu is adjacent to the interventricular foramen (Figs. 10-5 and 10-10) and to the venous angle (Fig. 5-13). The *retrolenticular part* is the portion posterior to the lenticular nucleus. The *sublenticular part* is the portion inferior to the lenticular nucleus. The demarcation of the anterior and posterior limbs is distinct at the genu, but the transition from the posterior limb to the retrolenticular part to the sublenticular part is gradual, and dividing lines between these portions are somewhat arbitrary. Since the internal capsule is a continuous, curved sheet of fibers, it is not possible to see all of its parts in any one section, no matter what the plane of the section is. It is possible to see the first four parts mentioned above in a single horizontal section (Figs. 10-5 and 10-6), but to get a clear idea of the sublenticular part, it is usually necessary to use coronal sections (Fig. 10-8).

By and large, the contents of each portion of the internal capsule can be inferred from its anatomical location. Major components are as follows:

1. The anterior limb contains the fibers interconnecting the anterior nucleus and the cingulate gyrus and those interconnecting the dorsomedial nucleus and prefrontal cortex. Also included are some of the fibers projecting from the frontal lobe to ipsilateral pontine nuclei (*frontopontine fibers*).

2. The posterior limb contains fibers interconnecting the VA and VL with the motor and premotor cortex. It also contains the corticospinal and corticobulbar fibers and the somatosensory fibers projecting from the VPL/VPM to the postcentral gyrus. It was thought for many years that the corticospinal and corticobulbar fibers were located in the anterior portion of the posterior limb near the genu. However, recent evidence indicates that these fibers are actually located in the posterior third of the posterior limb adjacent to the somatosensory projections.

3. The genu is a transition zone between the anterior and posterior limbs and contains some frontopontine fibers as well as many of the fibers interconnecting the VA and VL with the motor and premotor cortex.

4. The retrolenticular part of the internal capsule contains most of the fibers interconnecting the thalamus with posterior portions of the cerebral hemisphere. These include the fibers passing in both directions between the parietal-occipital-temporal association cortex and the pulvinar/LP complex. They also include part of the *optic radiation*. The optic radiation is the large collection of visual system fibers projecting from the lateral geniculate nucleus to the banks of the calcarine sulcus. The portion in the retrolenticular part of the internal capsule ends in the superior bank of the calcarine sulcus. As explained in the next chapter, these are the fibers conveying information from inferior portions of the visual fields. Finally, the retrolenticular part also contains additional corticopontine fibers, principally from the parietal lobe.

5. The sublenticular part of the internal capsule is continuous with the retrolenticular part and contains the remainder of the optic radiation (that is, those fibers ending in the inferior bank of the calcarine sulcus and carrying information about superior visual fields). The sublenticular part also contains the *auditory radiation*, whose fibers pass laterally from the medial geniculate nucleus under the lenticular nucleus and lateral fissure

and then turn superiorly to end in the superior temporal gyrus (Figs. 9-30 and 10-8).

Blood supply

The blood supply of the internal capsule is from two principal sources, the *lateral striate arteries* and the *anterior choroidal artery*. The lateral striate (or *lenticulostriate*) arteries are the collection of fine ganglionic branches of the proximal portion of the middle cerebral artery and supply most of the anterior limb, genu, and posterior limb. The anterior limb and genu also receive part of their supply from ganglionic branches of the anterior cerebral and anterior communicating arteries, particularly from a relatively large one called the *recurrent artery (artery of Heubner)*, or *medial striate artery*. The anterior choroidal artery supplies inferior and posterior regions of the internal capsule. It overlaps the lateral striate arteries in supplying the posterior limb and provides most of the supply of the retrolenticular and sublenticular parts. Ganglionic branches of the posterior cerebral artery also help supply the retrolenticular and sublenticular parts.

Small strokes in the internal capsule could obviously have major consequences. Hemorrhage of a lateral striate artery in the vicinity of the posterior limb can result in contralateral spastic paralysis and hemianesthesia. If the retrolenticular and sublenticular parts are also involved, visual deficits would be added to the symptoms (and would indicate that the damage was almost certainly in the internal capsule). The auditory radiations would be damaged as well, but this would produce relatively minor deficits because of the bilateral nature of the central auditory pathways.

HYPOTHALAMUS

The hypothalamus is a small portion of the diencephalon (weighing only about 4 grams) but is important as a nodal point in pathways concerned with autonomic, endocrine, emotional, and somatic functions. As examples, stimulation of appropriate hypothalamic areas in experimental animals can cause vasodilatation, rage, feeding behavior, or alterations of pituitary function. Accordingly the connections of the hypothalamus are rather widespread and complex, but they fall into three principal categories: (1) interconnections with various components of the limbic system, (2) outputs that influence the pituitary gland, and (3) interconnections with various visceral and somatic nuclei, both motor and sensory, of the brainstem and spinal cord. The hypothalamus is divided into a number of nuclei and areas, as described shortly. Each of these different nuclei and areas has more or less distinctive connections, but for the sake of simplicity these connections are discussed here as though the hypothalamus were by and large a uniform structure.

Extent and subdivisions of the hypothalamus

The inferior surface of the hypothalamus (Figs. 2-12 and 2-13), exposed directly to subarachnoid space, is bounded by the optic chiasm, the optic tracts, and the posterior edge of the mammillary bodies. This area, exclusive of the mammillary bodies, is called the *tuber cinereum* (Fig. 10-14). The *median eminence*, a swelling on the surface of the tuber cinereum, is continuous with the infundibular stalk, which in turn is continuous with the posterior lobe of the pituitary. The median eminence, infundibular stalk, and posterior lobe together constitute the *neurohypophysis*.

The medial surface of the hypothalamus (Fig. 10-1) extends anteriorly to the lamina terminalis, superiorly to the hypothalamic sulcus, and posteriorly to the caudal edge of the diencephalon. As mentioned previously, the longitudinal boundaries are semiarbitrary. For example, the anterior border of the hypothalamus technically is the plane through the anterior edge of the optic chiasm and the posterior edge of the anterior commissure. However, the neural tissue immediately in front of this formal boundary is structurally and functionally continuous with the hypothalamus. Therefore this region (the *preoptic area*), technically part of the telencephalon, is usually treated as part of the hypothalamus.

The hypothalamus is subdivided from anterior to posterior into three zones (in addition to the preoptic area)

on the basis of the features of its inferior surface. These logically named zones are the *supraoptic region* (above the optic chiasm), the *tuberal region* (above and including the tuber cinereum), and the *mammillary region* (above and including the mammillary bodies). In addition, the entire hypothalamus of each side is divided into *medial* and *lateral* zones by a parasagittal plane through the fornix as this fiber bundle traverses the hypothalamus (Figs. 10-10 and 10-15). Thus the hypothalamus proper consists of six parts on each side: the medial and lateral zones of the supraoptic, tuberal, and mammillary regions. The principal nuclei of each of these areas are indicated in Table 6 and Fig. 10-15.

The lateral zone consists mainly of scattered cells interspersed among longitudinally running fibers. Anteriorly it is continuous with the lateral portion of the preoptic area, and caudally it is continuous with the midbrain tegmentum. Part of the supraoptic nucleus intrudes into it, as do clumps of cells called *lateral tuberal nuclei*, but otherwise it is undivided.

The medial zone, on the other hand, contains a number of nuclei. The supraoptic region contains two distinctive groups of neurosecretory cells, the *supraoptic* and *paraventricular nuclei*. The supraoptic nucleus sits astride the optic tract, extending into the lateral hypothalamic zone; the paraventricular nucleus is higher up in the wall of the third ventricle, adjacent to the anterior

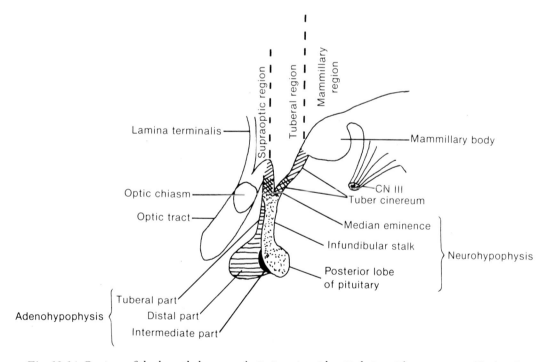

Fig. 10-14. Regions of the hypothalamus and pituitary in midsagittal view. The entire area filled with diagonal lines is the tuber cinereum. The crosshatched portion of the tuber cinereum is the median eminence.

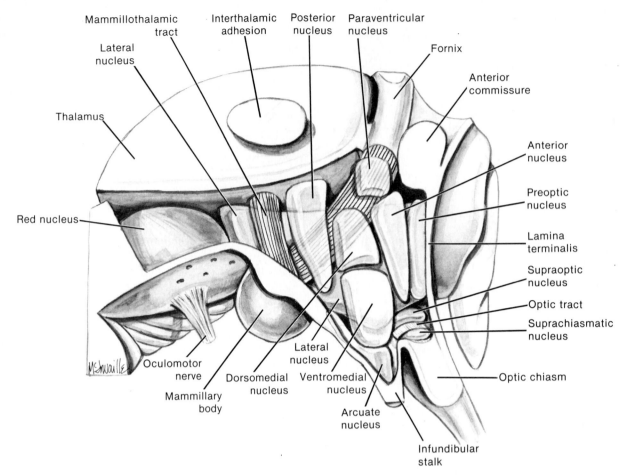

Fig. 10-15. Principal nuclei of the hypothalamus. (Modified from Nauta, W.J.H., and Haymaker, W.: The hypothalamus, Springfield, Ill., 1969, Charles C Thomas, Publisher.)

TABLE 6

Hypothalamic nuclei

Region	Medial area	Lateral area
Supraoptic	Supraoptic nucleus	Lateral nucleus
	Paraventricular nucleus	Part of supraoptic
	Anterior nucleus	nucleus
	Suprachiasmatic nucleus	
Tuberal	Dorsomedial nucleus	Lateral nucleus
	Ventromedial nucleus	Lateral tuberal nuclei
	Arcuate (infundibular) nucleus	
Mammillary	Mammillary body	Lateral nucleus
	Posterior nucleus	

commissure. The cells of both nuclei secrete hormones that travel down the axons of these cells and are released in the neurohypophysis. The hormones involved and the pathway traversed by them are discussed later in this chapter (Fig. 10-18). The supraoptic region also contains a small *suprachiasmatic nucleus* and a larger *anterior nucleus.* The suprachiasmatic nucleus, as described in the next chapter, receives direct projections from the retina and is thought to be important in the regulation of diurnal rhythms. The anterior nucleus is continuous anteriorly with the medial portion of the preoptic area.

The medial tuberal region is subdivided into dorsal and ventral portions called the *dorsomedial* and *ventromedial nuclei,* respectively. In addition, cells in the floor of the infundibular recess of the third ventricle constitute the *arcuate* (or *infundibular*) *nucleus.*

The medial mammillary region contains the mammillary body (actually a complex of several nuclei) and the *posterior hypothalamic nucleus,* which is continuous with the periaqueductal gray of the midbrain.

Afferents to the hypothalamus

Hypothalamic inputs arise in two general areas (Fig. 10-16): (1) various parts of the diencephalon and telencephalon, particularly components of the limbic system, and (2) the brainstem, particularly portions of the reticular formation and periaqueductal and periventricular

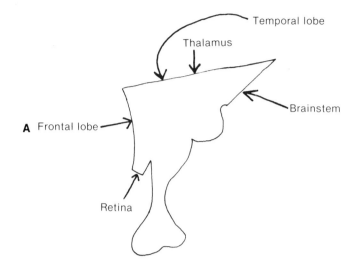

Fig. 10-16. Major inputs to the hypothalamus. **A,** Schematic indication of the directions from which these inputs come. Those labeled "frontal lobe" arise in the orbital cortex of the frontal lobe and also from limbic structures near the hypothalamus such as the septal area. Inputs from the temporal lobe arise in the hippocampal formation and amygdala. **B,** More detailed depiction of hypothalamic afferents. The medial forebrain bundle includes afferents arising in both the septal area and the brainstem. Some inputs from the amygdala travel through the stria terminalis, which follows a path parallel to the lateral ventricle; others take a more direct route (indicated but unlabeled in this figure) under the lenticular nucleus, referred to as the *ventral amygdalofugal pathway. AM,* Amygdala; *DLF,* dorsal longitudinal fasciculus; *DM,* dorsomedial nucleus (of thalamus); *F,* fornix; *H,* hippocampus; *MFB,* medial forebrain bundle; *MP,* mammillary peduncle; *O,* orbital cortex of frontal lobe; *OT,* optic tract; *R,* retina; *S,* septal area; *ST,* stria terminalis.

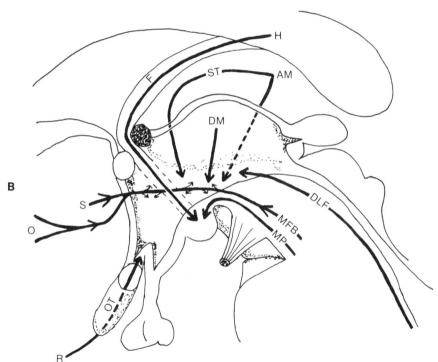

gray. Afferents from the brainstem convey visceral and somatic sensory information, while those from limbic structures convey information relevant to the role of the hypothalamus in mediating many of the autonomic and somatic aspects of affective states. The connections of limbic components with each other and with the hypothalamus are discussed in Chapter 16 and will only be mentioned briefly here.

Afferents from the forebrain. Major diencephalic and telencephalic afferents to the hypothalamus arise in (1) the septal area, (2) the hippocampus, (3) the amygdala, (4) the orbital cortex of the frontal lobe, (5) the thalamus, and (6) the retina. The *septal area,* a prominent component of the limbic system located adjacent to the sep-

tum pellucidum, projects fibers to the hypothalamus through the *medial forebrain bundle.* The medial forebrain bundle is built like a frayed rope, with fibers entering and leaving it at all levels as it traverses the lateral hypothalamic zone and extends into the midbrain tegmentum. This is a bidirectional bundle, containing afferents from the brainstem to the hypothalamus as well as hypothalamic efferents passing both rostrally and caudally and fibers interconnecting different hypothalamic levels.

The major output from the hippocampus is contained in the fornix. This fiber bundle arches around under the corpus callosum and through the hypothalamus, where most of its fibers reach the mammillary body (Fig. 16-9).

The amygdala projects fibers to the hypothalamus by two different routes. Some travel through the *stria terminalis*, a long, curved fiber bundle that accompanies the caudate nucleus. Others take a shorter course and pass under the lentiform nucleus directly to the hypothalamus.

The frontal lobe projects to the hypothalamus by both direct and indirect pathways. Some fibers originating in the orbital cortex of the frontal lobe join the medial forebrain bundle and travel to the hypothalamus. *Periventricular fibers* originating in the dorsomedial nucleus of the thalamus travel near the wall of the third ventricle to the hypothalamus. Since the dorsomedial nucleus is extensively interconnected with prefrontal cortex, the periventricular fibers are an indirect route by which the frontal lobe can influence the hypothalamus.

Afferents from the brainstem. An assortment of sensory inputs reaches the hypothalamus by routes that are poorly understood but are usually considered to involve

synapses in various portions of the reticular formation and periaqueductal gray. Some of these afferents travel in the medial forebrain bundle, while others are contained in the *dorsal longitudinal fasciculus*, a collection of thinly myelinated fibers that passes through the periventricular and periaqueductal gray of the brainstem and then fans out among the periventricular fibers of the hypothalamus. Others travel from the midbrain reticular formation to the mammillary body and other parts of the hypothalamus by way of the *mammillary peduncle;* many of these fibers join the medial forebrain bundle once they reach the hypothalamus. Still other afferents enter the hypothalamus as collaterals of fibers in other pathways such as the spinothalamic tract.

Physical inputs. In addition to receiving various types of visceral and somatic information through the brainstem pathways just mentioned, the hypothalamus contains cells that are directly responsive to physical stimuli. Some of these cells are sensitive to the temperature

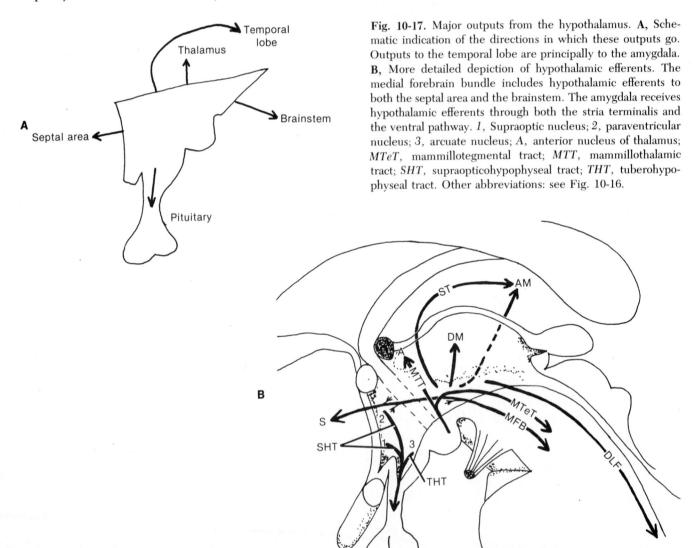

Fig. 10-17. Major outputs from the hypothalamus. **A,** Schematic indication of the directions in which these outputs go. Outputs to the temporal lobe are principally to the amygdala. **B,** More detailed depiction of hypothalamic efferents. The medial forebrain bundle includes hypothalamic efferents to both the septal area and the brainstem. The amygdala receives hypothalamic efferents through both the stria terminalis and the ventral pathway. *1,* Supraoptic nucleus; *2,* paraventricular nucleus; *3,* arcuate nucleus; *A,* anterior nucleus of thalamus; *MTeT,* mammillotegmental tract; *MTT,* mammillothalamic tract; *SHT,* supraopticohypophyseal tract; *THT,* tuberohypophyseal tract. Other abbreviations: see Fig. 10-16.

of the hypothalamus itself, while the activity of others is sensitive to such things as the concentration of glucose or certain hormones in the hypothalamus.

Efferents from the hypothalamus

Efferent pathways from the hypothalamus are, to a great extent, reciprocal to the afferent pathways (Fig. 10-17). Thus the hypothalamus projects to the septal area, the hippocampus, the amygdala, the dorsomedial nucleus of the thalamus, and the brainstem by way of the same fiber bundles that carry afferents to the hypothala-

mus (the mammillary peduncle, however, is thought to contain no hypothalamic efferents). In addition, a few pathways are totally or predominantly efferent in nature. The prominent *mammillothalamic tract* passes from the mammillary body to the anterior nucleus of the thalamus (Figs. 10-9 and 16-13). Some fibers in the mammillo-thalamic tract travel in the opposite direction as well (that is, from the anterior nucleus to the mammillary body). The *mammillotegmental tract* branches from the mammillothalamic tract near the latter's origin and projects to the midbrain reticular formation.

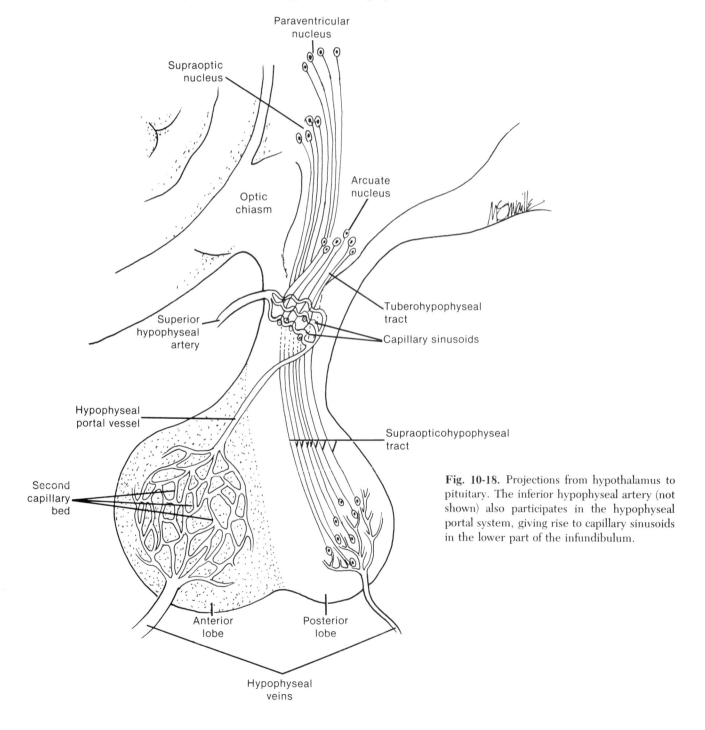

Fig. 10-18. Projections from hypothalamus to pituitary. The inferior hypophyseal artery (not shown) also participates in the hypophyseal portal system, giving rise to capillary sinusoids in the lower part of the infundibulum.

Outputs to the pituitary gland. The final efferent pathways from the hypothalamus are of great functional importance because they control the *pituitary gland* (or *hypophysis*). This control is accomplished by two means: a neural projection to the neurohypophysis and a vascular link with the adenohypophysis.

The supraoptic and paraventricular nuclei, as mentioned previously, consist of neurosecretory cells. Cells of the supraoptic nucleus produce *antidiuretic hormone* (*ADH*, or *vasopressin*), an octapeptide whose principal physiological function is to increase the reabsorption of water in the kidney and thereby decrease the production of urine. Some cells of the paraventricular nucleus also produce ADH. The others produce *oxytocin* (Greek = rapid birth), a similar octapeptide that causes contraction of uterine and mammary smooth muscle and is important in parturition and milk ejection. Both hormones travel down the axons of their parent cell bodies by axoplasmic flow, bound to a carrier protein *(neurophysin)*. These neurosecretory cells are electrically excitable, and the passage of action potentials down their axons causes release of their hormones from bulbous endings adjacent to capillaries in the median eminence, infundibular stalk, and posterior lobe of the pituitary (Fig. 10-18). Most of the axons arise in the supraoptic nucleus, so this pathway is called the *supraopticohypophyseal tract*.

The adenohypophysis secretes a multitude of hormones whose discussion is beyond the scope of this book. It has been known for some time that electrical stimulation of certain areas of the hypothalamus can modulate the rates of secretion of these hormones, but no neural connections are known that could explain this modulation. This drew attention to the *hypophyseal portal system* as a vascular connection between the hypothalamus and the adenohypophysis (Fig. 10-18). The *superior hypophyseal artery*, a branch of the internal carotid, breaks up into a capillary bed in the median eminence and proximal part of the infundibular stalk. Blood in these capillaries then re-collects into *hypophyseal portal vessels*, which travel down the infundibular stalk and break up into a second capillary bed in the adenohypophysis. Abundant evidence has now shown that small peptides, called *hypothalamic releasing factors* and *inhibiting factors*, are secreted by cells of the arcuate nucleus, travel down the axons of these cells, and are released into the bloodstream in the first capillary bed. From there the releasing and inhibiting factors travel down the hypophyseal portal vessels to the adenohypophysis, where they act. As their names imply, releasing factors promote the release of particular hormones, whereas inhibiting factors prevent this release. The entire collection of axons carrying these releasing and inhibiting factors is called the *tuberoinfundibular* or *tuberohypophyseal tract*.

A great deal of interest has been generated by the recent discovery that certain of these small hypothalamic peptides are also found in other neurons in widespread areas of the CNS and in other cells of the body as well. This is reminiscent of the situation with enkephalins and endorphins, briefly discussed in Chapter 8. Whether and in what ways hypothalamic releasing factors also serve as neurotransmitter substances for some neurons is not yet clear, but the role of this assortment of small peptides in normal neuronal function is an exciting and rapidly expanding area of current research.

Blood supply

Inspection of Fig. 5-1 will reveal that the infundibular stalk is located just about in the middle of the circle of Willis, and the inferior surface of the entire hypothalamus is more or less surrounded by the circle. The arterial supply of the hypothalamus is derived from a series of small ganglionic or perforating arteries arising from arteries in and adjacent to the circle of Willis. Specifically the *anteromedial* group of ganglionic arteries, arising from the anterior cerebral and anterior communicating arteries, supplies the preoptic and supraoptic regions; the *posteromedial* group, arising from the posterior communicating arteries and the proximal portions of the posterior cerebral arteries, supplies the tuberal and mammillary regions; the *anterolateral* group (or lateral striate arteries), arising from proximal portions of the middle cerebral arteries, helps supply the lateral hypothalamus.

Some functional aspects of the hypothalamus

The connections of the hypothalamus with the limbic system, pituitary, and brainstem make it eminently suitable for controlling various visceral functions and activities involved in drives and emotional states. Consistent with this, many hypothalamic "centers" have been described that are concerned with feeding and drinking behavior, temperature regulation, gut motility, sexual activity, and numerous other functions. In most cases, however, fragments of a behavior pattern elicited by stimulating a hypothalamic location can be elicited by stimulating appropriate sites in the brainstem. Thus many of the hypothalamic sites associated with particular behaviors may really be trigger points that, when stimulated, initiate neural activity in other parts of the CNS, which in turn causes the behavior pattern. Furthermore many parts of the hypothalamus are organized loosely enough that electrical stimulation of only a certain part of a certain nucleus is impossible. For example, the medial forebrain bundle runs through the lateral hypothalamus, so if a particular behavior were elicited by stimulating a particular site in the lateral hypothalamus, it could be the result of stimulating either a portion of the lateral hypothalamic nucleus or some fibers of the medial forebrain bundle.

Given these caveats, it has nevertheless been found that certain types of changes consistently follow stimulation of or damage to particular hypothalamic areas in experimental animals. Since the hypothalamus is so small, discrete lesions affecting individual functional areas of the human hypothalamus are quite rare; in addition, lesions must be bilateral to disrupt most hypothalamic functions. However, the clinical findings in humans with hypothalamic damage are generally consistent with what would be expected from work on experimental animals. Only a few examples will be cited.

The hypothalamus is in overall control of the autonomic nervous system in the sense that practically any type of autonomic response can be elicited by stimulating some hypothalamic site. Although the sites overlap to a considerable degree, those associated with parasympathetic responses tend to be located anteriorly, and those associated with sympathetic responses tend to be located posteriorly. Appropriate somatic motor activity accompanies these autonomic responses, as the example of hypothalamic control of temperature regulation demonstrates. Stimulation of the anterior hypothalamus and preoptic area induces panting (or sweating in humans) and cutaneous vasodilatation, which in turn causes body temperature to fall. In contrast, stimulation of the posterior hypothalamus causes cutaneous vasoconstriction and shivering, which in turn causes an increase in body temperature. The hypothalamus thus acts as a thermostat, monitoring the temperature of blood passing through it and activating heat-dissipation or heat-production mechanisms as necessary to maintain the desired value. Bilateral lesions of the anterior hypothalamus make an animal unable to dissipate heat in a warm environment. (Such lesions may also cause diabetes insipidus, in which large amounts of dilute urine are produced as a result of destruction of the supraoptic nuclei.) Bilateral lesions of the posterior hypothalamus may make an animal unable to regulate its body temperature in either a warm or a cold environment, since the destruction involves not only the area concerned with the production and conservation of heat but also the fibers descending from the more anterior heat-dissipation areas.

The role of the hypothalamus in more complex activities is demonstrated by its involvement in feeding behavior. Here again, two areas with opposing influences have been found. Bilateral destruction of the ventromedial nucleus ("satiety center") produces animals that overeat and get fat, while destruction of the lateral hypothalamus in the tuberal region ("feeding center") produces animals that do not eat and may actually starve to death unless force-fed during the postoperative weeks. The complete mechanism of these effects is not known,

but they are probably not as simple as they sound. The obesity following ventromedial lesions, for example, results not only from overeating but also from decreased physical activity and from metabolic changes favoring the accumulation of fat.

One should not get the impression that discrete lesions in the hypothalamus cause single changes such as hypothermia or obesity. The case of bilateral lesions of the ventromedial nucleus provides an instructive example not only of multiple effects from discrete lesions but also of the involvement of the hypothalamus in emotional behavior. Cats with bilateral ventromedial lesions overeat and get fat and are also extremely nasty.* They respond with full-blown, hissing rages to the most innocuous of stimuli. Similar rage responses can be elicited by stimulation of the lateral hypothalamus adjacent to the ventromedial nucleus of an intact cat. The attacks are coordinated and well directed but cease the moment the stimulus does. The ways in which such emotional responses are related, under normal circumstances, to activity in the limbic system are discussed in Chapter 16.

---

*"One of my own most striking memories is of huge, fat and extremely hostile cats with ventromedial hypothalamic lesions. When they observed laboratory visitors through the bars, thankfully strong bars, of their cages, they appeared to have a singular interest in attack. They gave every sign of dedication to the goal of destroying the visitor. Their great size made the threat something not to be taken lightly." (From Isaacson, R.L.: The limbic system, New York, 1974, Plenum Press, p. 85.)

ADDITIONAL READING

Adams, J.H., Daniel, P.M., and Prichard, M.M.L.: Observations on the portal circulation of the pituitary gland, Neuroendocrinol. 1:193, 1965/66.

Bergland, R.M., and Page, R.B.: Pituitary-brain vascular relations: a new paradigm, Science **204**:18, 1979. *Recent results that indicate that the pituitary portal system may not be so straightforward; for example, it may at times function in reverse, transporting adenohypophyseal hormones to the brain.*

Carmel, P.W.: Efferent projections of the ventral anterior nucleus of the thalamus in the monkey, Am. J. Anat. **128**:159, 1970.

Carpenter, M.B.: Ventral tier thalamic nuclei. In Williams, D., editor: Modern trends in neurology, vol. 4, New York, 1967, Appleton-Century-Crofts.

Dierickx, K.: Immunocytochemical localization of the vertebrate cyclic nonapeptide neurohypophyseal hormones and neurophysins, Int. Rev. Cytol. **62**:120, 1980.

Eisenman, J.E., and Masland, W.S.: The hypothalamus. In Goldensohn, E.S. and Appel, S.H., editors: Scientific approaches to clinical neurology, Philadelphia, 1977, Lea and Febiger. *A nice, concise review of hypothalamic anatomy and physiology.*

Groothuis, D.R., Duncan, G.W., and Fisher, C.M.: The human thalamocortical sensory path in the internal capsule: evidence from a small capsular hemorrhage causing a pure sensory stroke, Ann. Neurol. **2**:328, 1977.

Guillemin, R.: Peptides in the brain: the new endocrinology of the neuron, Science **202**:390, 1978.

Hardy, J.D., Hellon, R.F., and Sutherland, K.: Temperature-sensitive neurones in the dog's hypothalamus, J. Physiol. **175**:242, 1964.

Haymaker, W.E., Anderson, E., and Nauta, W.J.H., editors: The hypothalamus, Springfield, Ill., 1969, Charles C Thomas, Publisher.

Hayward, J.N.: Functional and morphological aspects of hypothalamic neurons, Physiol. Rev. 57:574, 1977.

Heller, H.C., Crawshaw, L.I., and Hammel, H.T.: The thermostat of vertebrate animals, Sci. Am. 239(2):102, 1978.

Jones, E.G.: Some aspects of the organization of the thalamic reticular complex, J. Comp. Neurol. 162:285, 1975.

Jones, E.G., and Leavitt, R.Y.: Retrograde axonal transport and the demonstration of non-specific projections to the cerebral cortex and striatum from thalamic intralaminar nuclei in the rat, cat, and monkey, J. Comp. Neurol. 154:349, 1974.

Kievit, J., and Kuypers, H.G.J.M.: Organization of the thalamo-cortical connections to frontal lobe in the rhesus monkey, Exp. Brain Res. 29:299, 1977. *An indication, based on experiments using newer anatomical tracing techniques, that thalamocortical projections are highly ordered topographically but not necessarily in the traditionally accepted pattern: strips of cortex receive inputs from thalamic slabs that sometimes run right through conventional nuclear boundaries.*

Krieger, D.T., and Liotta, A.S.: Pituitary hormones in brain: Where, how, and why? Science 205:366, 1979.

Langworthy, O.R., and Fox, H.M.: Thalamic syndrome. Syndrome of the posterior cerebral artery: a review, Arch. Intern. Med. 60:203, 1937.

Ludwig, E., and Klingler, J.: Atlas cerebri humani, Boston, 1956, Little, Brown and Co. *A collection of remarkable dissections of human brains. Formalin-fixed brains were frozen and thawed once or twice, which for some reason makes dissection much easier. (This accounts for the spongy appearance of the cortex in Figs. 10-12 and 10-13.) The actual dissections were done with jeweler's forceps and wooden probes.*

Mikol, J., et al.: Connections of laterodorsal nucleus of the thalamus, II: experimental study in *Papio papio*, Brain Res. 138:1, 1977.

Mosko, S.S., and Moore, R.Y.: Neonatal suprachiasmatic nucleus lesions: effects on the development of circadian rhythms in the rat, Brain Res. 164:17, 1979.

Mountcastle, V.B., and Henneman, E.: The representation of tactile sensibility in the thalamus of the monkey, J. Comp. Neurol. 97:409, 1952. *An early physiological demonstration of the mapping of the body surface onto the VPL/VPM.*

Plets, C., et al.: The vascularization of the human thalamus, Acta Neurol. Belg. 70:687, 1970. *Long and detailed.*

Purpura, D.P., and Yahr, M.D., editors: The thalamus, New York, 1966, Columbia University Press.

Raisman, G., and Brown-Grant, K.: The "suprachiasmatic syndrome": endocrine and behavioural abnormalities following lesions of the suprachiasmatic nucleus in the female rat, Proc. R. Soc. Lond. B198: 297, 1977.

Reeves, A.G., and Plum, F.: Hyperphagia, rage and dementia accompanying a ventromedial hypothalamic neoplasm, Arch. Neurol. 20: 616, 1969.

Reichlin, S., Baldessarini, R.J., and Martin, J.B.: The hypothalamus, Res. Pub. Assoc. Res. Nerv. Ment. Dis., vol. 56, 1978. *A volume principally about hypothalamic involvement in neuroendocrine function but including an interesting chapter by Fred Plum on human hypothalamic disorders.*

Reiter, R.J., editor: The pineal and reproduction: progress in reproductive biology, vol. 4., Basel, 1978, S. Karger.

Rinvik, E.: The corticothalamic projection from the pericruciate and coronal gyri in the cat: an experimental study with silver-impregnation methods, Brain Res. 10:79, 1968.

Ross, E.D.: Localization of the pyramidal tract in the internal capsule by whole brain dissection, Neurology 30:59, 1980.

Saper, C.B., et al.: Direct hypothalamo-autonomic connections. Brain Res. 117:305, 1976. *Recent evidence that at least some hypothalamic efferents reach their target nuclei directly rather than via relays in the reticular formation.*

Schally, A.V., Kastin, A.J., and Arimura, A.: Hypothalamic hormones: the link between brain and body, Am. Sci. 65:712, 1977.

Singer, W.: Control of thalamic transmission by corticofugal and ascending reticular pathways in the visual system, Physiol. Rev. 57: 386, 1977.

Sugitani, M.: Electrophysiological and sensory properties of the thalamic reticular neurones related to somatic sensation in rats, J. Physiol. 290:79, 1979.

Swaab, D.F., Nijveldt, F., and Pool, C.W.: Distribution of oxytocin and vasopressin in the rat supraoptic and paraventricular nucleus, J. Endocr. 67:461, 1975.

Walker, A.E.: The primate thalamus, 1938, University of Chicago Press. *An early (and historically very important) exposition of the thalamic terminology commonly used today.*

Wasman, M., and Flynn, J.P.: Directed attack elicited from hypothalamus, Arch. Neurol. 6:220, 1962.

Whitsel, B.L., et al.: Thalamic projections to S-I in macaque monkey, J. Comp. Neurol. 178:385, 1978. *The microarchitecture of the projection from the VPL/VPM to the cortex, giving some idea of how remarkably detailed this projection is.*

Wilkins, R.H., and Brody, I.A.: The thalamic syndrome, Arch. Neurol. 20:560, 1969. *A brief introduction to (and excerpted translation of) the original work (Dejerine, J., and Roussy, G.: Le Syndrome Thalamique, Rev. Neurol. 14:521, 1906).*

Wurtman, R.J., Axelrod, J., and Kelly, D.E.: The pineal, New York, 1968, Academic Press, Inc.

CHAPTER 11

VISUAL SYSTEM

It is clear from everyday experience that we are a visually oriented species. While it is arguable which of our senses is the most important, loss of the visual sense is certainly a greater handicap for humans than loss of, for example, the olfactory or gustatory sense. Partly because of its importance (and partly for anatomical and technical reasons to be discussed later), a great deal of research has been done on the visual system. At the present time, we probably know more about the visual system than about any other sensory system, and there is considerable promise that with further study we will be able to understand in some detail how this portion of the central nervous system actually works.

Some lizards, fish, and amphibians have a photosensitive pineal organ that constantly stares up at the sky as a sort of "third eye." In mammals, however, all photic information originates in the *rods* and *cones* of the retina and is then conveyed to the brain by way of the axons of the output cells (called *ganglion cells*) of the retina. These axons, together with the axons of higher order cells on which they synapse, form a visual pathway that begins in the eyes anteriorly and ends in the occipital lobes posteriorly. Throughout this course a precise *retinotopic* arrangement of fibers is maintained, so that particular small regions of the retina are represented in particular small regions of more central parts of the pathway. Damage at many different locations within this system can result in visual deficits, and a knowledge of the anatomy involved makes it possible to understand these deficits. Conversely, the same knowledge is frequently helpful in deducing the site of a lesion.

RETINAL HISTOLOGY

The retina is a two-part structure, reflecting its origin from the two layers of infolded optic cup (Fig. 11-1). The outer portion, adjacent to the choroid, is the *retinal pigment epithelium*, while the inner portion, adjacent to the vitreous, is the *neural retina*. Under normal conditions, no space exists between the pigment epi-

thelium and the neural retina in the adult. However, the mechanical connections between the two are not very strong, and under certain circumstances this potential space opens, constituting *retinal detachment.* Retinal receptors are metabolically dependent on pigment epithelial cells, so detached areas stop working.

Cell types

One reason so much research has been done on the visual system is the overall anatomical simplicity of the neural retina relative to other parts of the nervous system. Although it contains hundreds of millions of cells, there are only five basic types involved in the processing of visual information, and their patterns of interconnections are fundamentally the same throughout the retina.

The five cell types have their somata neatly arranged in three layers and make most of their synapses in two additional layers. In each synaptic zone, one cell type brings visual information in, another type carries information out, and a third type serves as a laterally interconnecting (association) element.

A simplified, schematic illustration of these basic connection patterns is shown in Fig. 11-2, *B*. Starting peripherally, the photoreceptor cells, stimulated by light, project to the first layer of synapses, where they terminate on the aptly named *bipolar* and *horizontal cells*. The bipolar cells then project to the next layer of synapses, while the horizontal cells spread laterally and interconnect receptors, bipolar cells, and other horizontal cells. In the second layer of synapses, bipolar cells terminate on ganglion cells and *amacrine cells*. Axons of the ganglion cells leave the eye as the *optic nerve*, while processes of the amacrine cells spread laterally and interconnect bipolar cells, ganglion cells, and other amacrine cells.

Retinal layers

The entire retina is conventionally described as a ten-layered structure, beginning with the pigment epi-

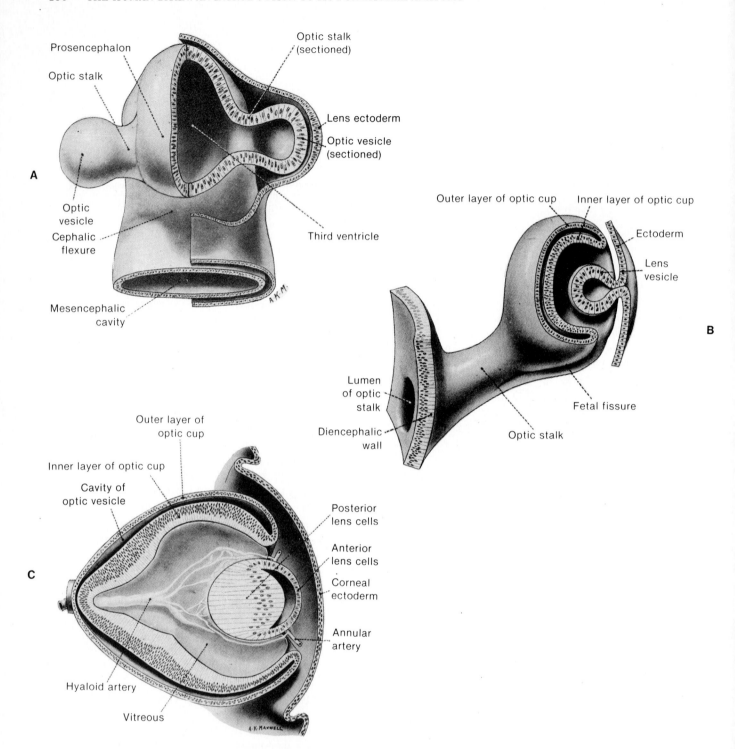

Fig. 11-1. Embryological development of the eye. **A,** At about 4 weeks, the optic vesicle of each side has evaginated from the diencephalon. **B,** At about 5 weeks, the initially spherical optic vesicle has folded in on itself to form the two-layered optic cup; the optic cup partially envelops the lens vesicle, which is derived from surface ectoderm. **C,** At about 6 weeks, the lens vesicle has pinched off, and additional surface ectoderm has begun to form the cornea. The outer layer of the two-layered optic cup will go on to form the retinal pigment epithelium; the inner layer will form the neural retina. Anteriorly both layers will grow around farther in front of the lens and participate in the formation of the iris. (From Hamilton, W.J.: Textbook of human anatomy, ed. 2, St. Louis, 1976, The C.V. Mosby Co. By permission of Macmillan Press, London and Basingstoke.)

A

B

PE

Direction of
information flow

Direction
of light

Outer
segment

Inner
segment

R

Outer
limiting
membrane

R

Layer of
rods and cones

Outer nuclear layer

H

B

B

B

Outer plexiform layer

A

A

H

B

A

Inner nuclear layer

G

G

G

A

G

Inner plexiform layer

Ganglion cell layer

G

Nerve fiber
layer

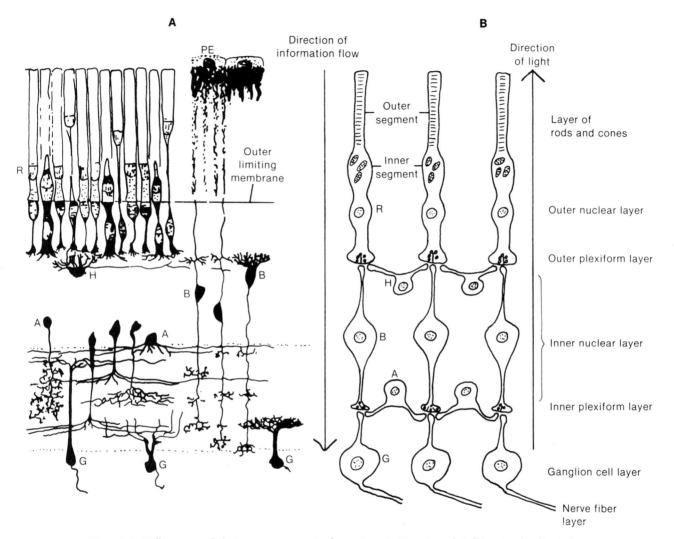

Fig. 11-2. Cell types and their arrangement in the retina. **A,** Drawing of Golgi-stained cells of the frog retina. (Modified from Ramón y Cajal, S.: Histologie du système nerveux, vol. 2, Paris, 1911, Libraire Maloine.) **B,** Schematic illustration of a generalized vertebrate retina showing retinal layers. *A,* Amacrine cell; *B,* bipolar cell; *G,* ganglion cell; *H,* horizontal cell; *PE,* pigment epithelium; *R,* receptor cell (rod or cone).

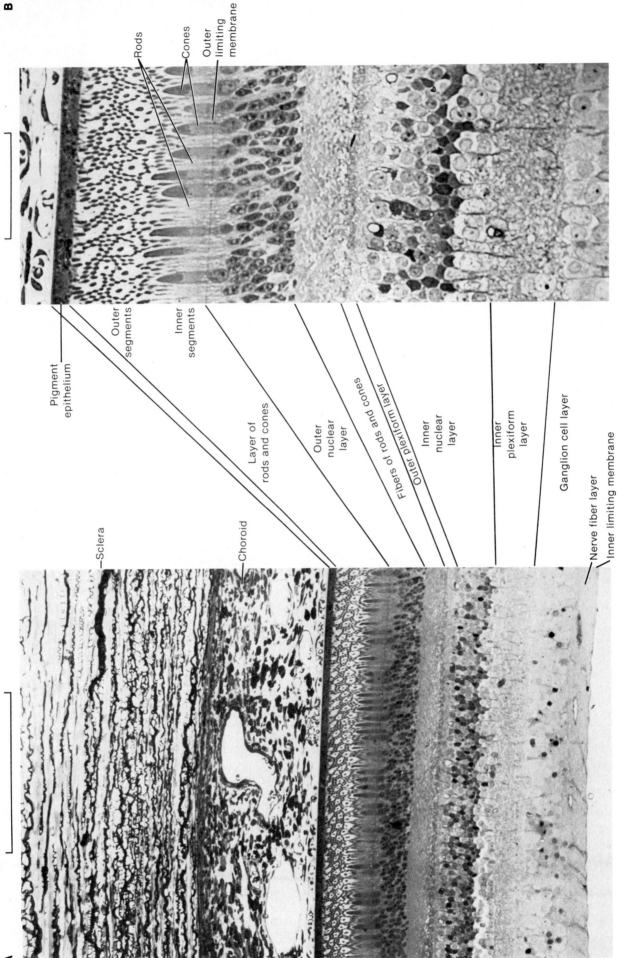

B

Rods

Cones

Outer limiting membrane

Pigment epithelium

Outer segments

Inner segments

Layer of rods and cones

Outer nuclear layer

Fibers of rods and cones

Outer plexiform layer

Inner nuclear layer

Inner plexiform layer

Ganglion cell layer

Nerve fiber layer

Inner limiting membrane

Sclera

Choroid

A

Fig. 11-3. A, Section through the entire wall of an eye of a rhesus monkey near the fovea, showing the sclera, choroid, and retina; scale mark = 200 μm. **B,** Enlarged view of part of **A,** showing the retina; the plane of section is not quite parallel to the outer segments of the rods and cones, so they are cut transversely and appear as dots. Scale mark = 50 μm. (Courtesy of Fay Eldred and Virginia Frank, University of Colorado Health Sciences Center.)

thelium (Fig. 11-3); five of these layers are the layers of cell bodies and synapses mentioned above. In naming these layers, the term "nuclear" refers to cell bodies and the term "plexiform" to synaptic zones. "Inner" and "outer" refer to the number of synapses by which a structure is separated from the brain, so that, for example, receptors are "outer" with respect to bipolar cells. The ten layers of the retina are as follows.

1. The *pigment epithelium* is a single layer of polygonal, pigmented cells. One side of each cell adjoins the choroid, whose capillaries supply the avascular first two layers of the retina. The other side of each cell forms numerous fine processes that partially surround the outer portions of the receptor cells and obliterate the space that existed embryonically within the wall of the optic cup. Pigment epithelial cells are intimately involved metabolically with the receptors. They also play a role in absorbing light that has passed through the retina.

2. *Rods* and *cones* are the two different types of vertebrate photoreceptor. Each consists of several regions (Fig. 11-4): an *outer segment*, an *inner segment*, a cell body, and a synaptic terminal. Strictly speaking, "rod" or "cone" refers to only the outer segment plus the

inner segment of a photoreceptor cell, but in common usage these terms are often used to refer to entire receptors.

The outer segment of a rod is relatively long and cylindrical, while that of a cone is shorter and tapered (Figs. 11-4 and 11-5). Each type of outer segment is filled with flattened membranous sacs, or *disks*. In cones, the interior of many of these disks is continuous with extracellular space, but in rods, almost all of the disks have pinched off from the external membrane and are wholly intracellular. The major protein constituent of the outer segment membranes of both rods and cones is the visual pigment, which is called *rhodopsin* in rods. (There is no universally accepted name for the visual pigments of cones, and they are often called rhodopsins as well, or simply *cone pigments*). As one might expect from this localization of visual pigment, the outer segment is the site of visual transduction: photons absorbed here cause a receptor potential that then spreads to the rest of the cell. Note that the photosensitive portion of the receptor cells is located in the part of the neural retina that is farthest removed from incoming light (that is, the retina is inverted with respect to the path of light through it). This curious situation is universally

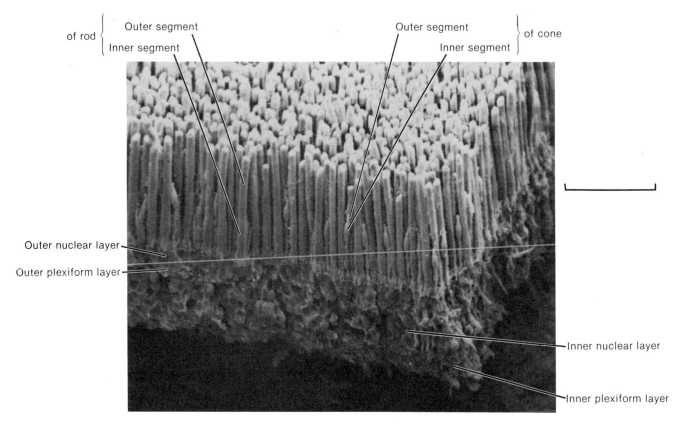

Fig. 11-4. Scanning electron micrograph of the retina of a bullfrog. Scale mark = 50 μm. (Courtesy of Dr. Roy H. Steinberg, University of California at San Francisco. From Steinberg, R.H.: Scanning electron microscopy of the bullfrog's retina and pigment epithelium, Z. Zellforsch. **143:**451, 1973.)

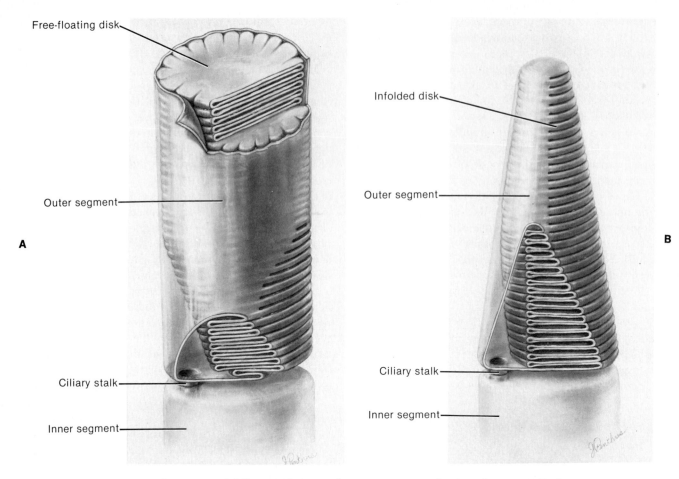

Free-floating disk

Outer segment

A

Ciliary stalk

Inner segment

Infolded disk

Outer segment

B

Ciliary stalk

Inner segment

Fig. 11-5. Ultrastructural differences between the outer segment of rods and cones. **A,** Rod outer segment (cut off toward the top in order to be the same length as the cone outer segment in **B**); note that some disks toward the base of the outer segment are open to the outside world but that most disks are pinched off and completely surrounded by cytoplasm. **B,** Cone outer segment; note that this outer segment tapers towards its apex (hence its name) and that all of its disks are infoldings of the plasma membrane with their interiors still continuous with extracellular space. (Courtesy of Dr. Richard W. Young, University of California at Los Angeles.)

true among vertebrates. However, this does not detract from visual sensitivity or acuity, since the retina is thin and transparent and since other anatomical modifications (discussed shortly) are found in the retinal area of greatest acuity.

Each outer segment is connected to an inner segment by a narrow ciliary stalk. The inner segments contain, among other organelles, a very prominent collection of mitochondria. These mitochondria are thought to supply the energy necessary for processes associated with transduction and for the synthesis of visual pigments. These pigments are continually renewed, being synthesized in the inner segment, transported through the ciliary stalk, and incorporated into disk membranes. "Old" disks at the apical ends of the outer segments of rods (and probably cones) are then phagocytosed by the pigment epithelium. There is good evidence that certain

types of retinal degeneration are caused by a defect in this renewal-phagocytosis process.

Rods are considerably more sensitive than cones and are the receptors used in dim light. However, there is a great deal of convergence in rod pathways, so the spatial acuity mediated by them is relatively poor. In addition, there is only one type of rod in the human retina, so color vision is not possible when only rods are active. On the other hand, we have three types of cones (red-, yellow-, and blue-sensitive), so information about the colors of objects can be extracted by the cone system if the illumination is bright enough. There is also relatively little convergence in the cone pathway, so spatial acuity is good.

3. The *outer limiting membrane* was so named because it has the appearance of a distinct line when viewed with a light microscope. However, electron

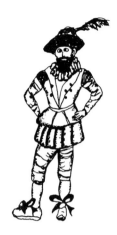

Fig. 11-6. How to demonstrate your right eye's blind spot to yourself. Close your left eye, hold the book at arm's length, stare fixedly at the spot on the left side of the figure, and slowly move the book toward you. At some point about a foot from your face, the bearded gentleman will lose his head. (Based on a technique of King Charles II, as recounted by Rushton, W.A.H.: King Charles II and the blind spot, Vision Res. **19**:225, 1979.)

microscopy has revealed it to be a row of intercellular junctions. Elongated specialized glial cells called *Müller cells* span almost the entire retina, ending distally at the bases of the inner segments of the rods and cones. Here adjacent Müller processes and inner segments are joined by junctional complexes, which collectively form the outer limiting membrane.

4. The *outer nuclear layer* consists of the cell bodies of the rods and cones.

5. The *outer plexiform layer* is the relatively thin synaptic zone in which receptors terminate on horizontal and bipolar cells and processes of horizontal cells spread laterally. The actual pattern of interconnections is somewhat more complex than that shown in Fig. 11-2, *B*. For example, there are differences between the synaptic complexes of rods and cones, and there are several subpopulations of bipolar cells. Other types of junctions are either known or inferred. For example, there is evidence for receptor-receptor connections and for feedback synapses of horizontal cells onto receptors.

6. The *inner nuclear layer* contains the cell bodies of all the retinal interneurons as well as those of the Müller cells. The nuclei of horizontal cells are found near its distal edge, those of bipolar cells in the middle, and those of amacrine cells near its proximal edge. Bipolar cells conduct visual information through this layer, projecting to the second synaptic zone.

7. The *inner plexiform layer* is the relatively thick synaptic zone in which bipolar cells terminate on amacrine and ganglion cells, and processes of amacrine cells spread laterally. Here again, the actual pattern of interconnections is somewhat more complex than that shown in Fig. 11-2, *B*.

8. The *ganglion cell layer* contains the cell bodies of

the ganglion cells, whose dendrites ramify in the inner plexiform layer, and whose axons leave the eye as the optic nerve. This cell layer is considerably thinner than either the outer or the inner nuclear layer in most retinal locations, reflecting the fact that there are 6 to 7 million cones and more than 100 million rods in a human retina but only about 1 million ganglion cells. Clearly a good deal of convergence is involved in retinal processing, but the convergence is not uniform across the retina. As discussed shortly, some regions are specialized for high acuity and have little convergence, while other regions are specialized for high sensitivity and have a great deal of convergence.

9. The *nerve fiber layer* is the collection of axons of ganglion cells, which radiate like spokes toward the *optic disk* or *optic papilla* (located posteriorly and slightly medial to the midline of the eye), where they form the optic nerve.

10. The *inner limiting membrane* is a thin basal lamina that intervenes between the vitreous and the proximal ends of the Müller cells.

RETINAL TOPOGRAPHY

Cross sections through the retina do not have the same appearance at all locations. For example, no photoreceptors, interneurons, or ganglion cells are present at the optic disk, where the axons of ganglion cells leave the eye to form the optic nerve. These axons originate near the vitreous, so they must turn posteriorly and traverse the retina before passing through the sclera. Since there are no photoreceptors or interneurons at the optic disk, we are blind to any object whose image falls on this part of the retina. Although the *blind spot* can easily be demonstrated (Fig. 11-6), we have no awareness as we walk around of a blank spot in visual space. One might think this is because the left eye can see the part of the visual field that falls on the right eye's blind spot, and vice versa. This cannot be the explanation, though, since we are unaware of the blind spot even with one eye closed. The real reason is that our nervous system simply "fills it in." We are actually quite skillful at this, and patients with damage to their visual systems can become blind in surprisingly large areas of their visual fields without being aware of it.

Beginning at about the lateral edge of the optic disk is a circular portion of the retina in which many of the cells contain a yellow pigment. This gives the area a yellowish color when examined with appropriate illumination and has led to its being called the *macula lutea* (Latin = yellow spot), often shortened to *macula*. In the center of the macula is a small depression called the *fovea centralis* (often shortened to *fovea*), which contains only elongated cones (no rods) and is directly in line with the visual axis (Fig. 11-7). The fovea is specialized for vision of the highest acuity; all the neurons and capillaries that are present elsewhere (and that light would otherwise traverse before reaching the receptors) are collected around the edges of the fovea. Specialized interneurons called *midget bipolar cells* contact individual foveal cones. These bipolars in turn contact indi-

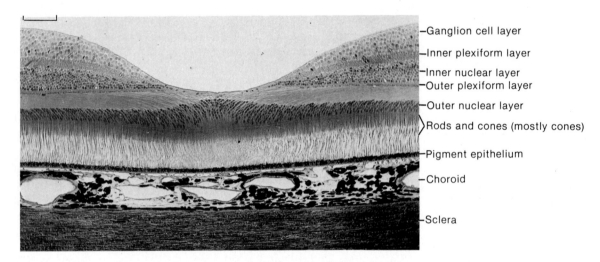

Ganglion cell layer
Inner plexiform layer
Inner nuclear layer
Outer plexiform layer
Outer nuclear layer
Rods and cones (mostly cones)
Pigment epithelium
Choroid
Sclera

Fig. 11-7. Fovea of a rhesus monkey. Note that all retinal elements (except the photoreceptors, which are all cones in the center of the fovea) are displaced to either side, so that light only needs to pass through the outer nuclear layer before reaching the cones. The nerve fiber layer is scanty in this region because the axons of more laterally placed ganglion cells arc around the fovea on their way to the optic disk. Scale mark = 100 μm. (From Fine, B.S., and Yanoff, M.: Ocular histology, ed. 2, New York, 1979, Harper and Row, Publishers, Inc.)

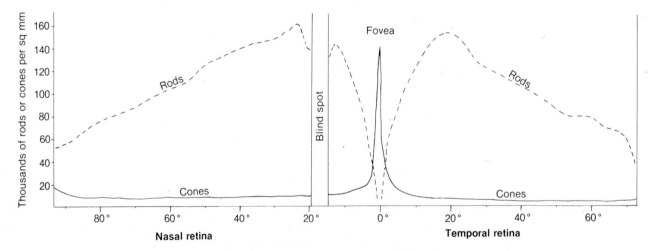

Fig. 11-8. Packing densities of rods and cones in the human retina along a horizontal band passing through the fovea. (Modified from Østerberg, G.A.: Acta Ophthal., suppl. 6, 1935.)

vidual *midget ganglion cells*, so that an anatomical basis for highly detailed foveal vision is maintained.

The fovea is one extreme in a changing rod/cone distribution across the retina. The packing density of cones decreases sharply outside the fovea while that of the rods increases, reaching a maximum just outside the macula. From here to the edge of the retina, the cone density remains at a low level, and the rod density slowly declines as well (Fig. 11-8). Given the known properties of rods and cones, it follows from these distributions that the fovea is used for high-acuity color vision in reasonably bright light, while extrafoveal regions function at lower light levels.

CENTRAL VISUAL PATHWAYS

Ganglion cell axons travel in the optic nerve to the *optic chiasm*, where they undergo a partial decussation and enter one or the other *optic tract*. Most of the fibers in each optic tract then terminate in the *lateral geniculate nucleus*, which is the thalamic relay nucleus for vision. Geniculate fibers travel through the internal capsule and corona radiata to the primary visual cortex in the banks of the calcarine fissure. In addition, a considerable number of optic tract fibers project to the midbrain and a few to the hypothalamus. Throughout this pathway, the numbers of fibers and areas of representation for the macula are disproportionately large for the macula's actual size. This reflects the relatively small amount of convergence in the macula, which in turn reflects its specialization for high acuity.

Optic nerve, chiasm, and tract

The unmyelinated axons of ganglion cells collect at the optic disk, pierce the sclera in a region called the *lamina cribrosa*, and acquire myelin sheaths, forming the optic nerve. The optic nerve is, by embryology and adult anatomy, actually a tract of the CNS and as such has meningeal coverings much like other areas. The sclera continues as its dural sheath, lined in turn by arachnoid and pia. The subarachnoid space around the optic nerve communicates with subarachnoid space generally; increases in intracranial pressure are transmitted to the optic nerve. Such an increase in pressure can cause detectable swelling of the optic disk. This swelling, called *papilledema*, can be a very valuable diagnostic sign.

Just anterior to the infundibular stalk, the two optic nerves partially decussate in the optic chiasm. All fibers from the nasal half of each retina cross to the contralateral optic tract; all fibers from the temporal half of each retina pass through the lateral portions of the chiasm without crossing and enter the ipsilateral optic tract. The result is that each optic tract contains the fibers arising in the temporal retina of the ipsilateral eye and the nasal retina of the contralateral eye. As indicated in Fig. 11-9, this apparently curious partial

decussation is exactly appropriate for delivering all the information from the contralateral visual field to each optic tract. Also since much of the basis for depth perception involves a comparison of the slightly different views seen by our two eyes, it is necessary to bring together information from comparable areas of the two retinas, which the optic chiasm accomplishes.

In the optic tract, fibers arising in corresponding areas of the two retinas (that is, fibers carrying information about the same area in the visual field) travel together. This relationship holds throughout the remain-

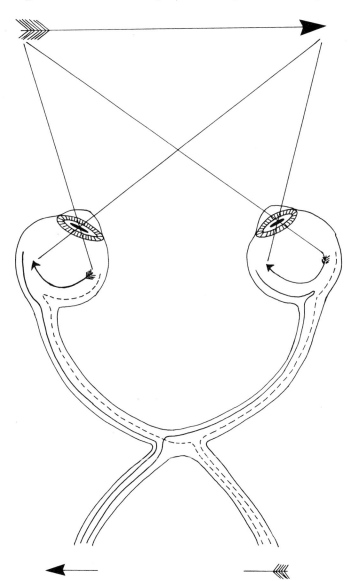

Fig. 11-9. Schematic diagram illustrating the formation of the optic chiasm and tracts. All information from the temporal side of a vertical line passing through a given fovea enters the ipsilateral optic tract; all information from the nasal side crosses in the chiasm and enters the contralateral optic tract. The result, as indicated, is that each optic tract "looks" at the contralateral visual field.

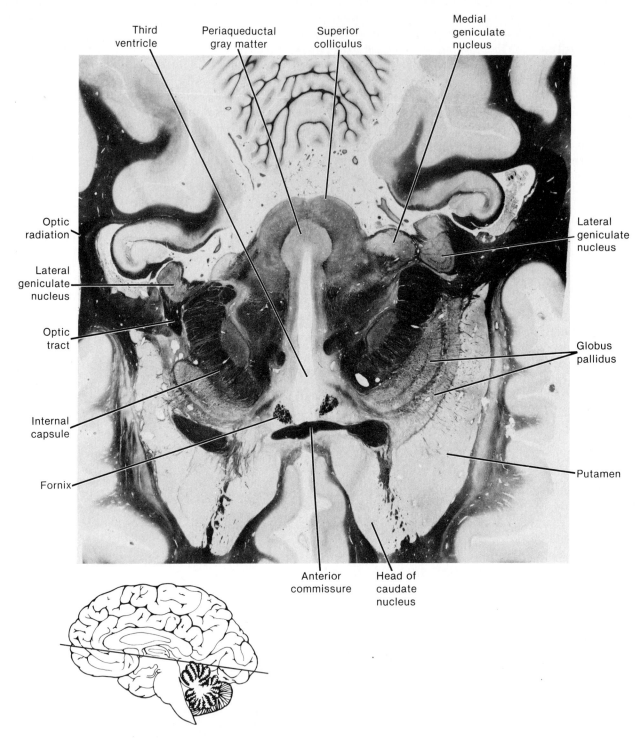

Fig. 11-10. Horizontal section showing the optic tract entering the lateral geniculate nucleus on one side. The continuity of the cerebral aqueduct (surrounded by periaqueductal gray) and the third ventricle is shown nicely in this section.

der of the visual pathway, so that damage to the optic tract or more central parts of the pathway tends to cause comparable visual deficits in both eyes.

Lateral geniculate nucleus

The optic tract curves posteriorly around the cerebral peduncle, and most of its fibers terminate in the lateral geniculate nucleus (Fig. 11-10). This is a six-layered, dome-shaped nucleus in which the optic fibers terminate in a precise retinotopic pattern. The pattern is about the same in each layer, so that a given point in the visual field is represented in a column of cells extending through all six layers. However, each layer receives input from only one eye: layers 1 (most inferior), 4, and 6 (most superior) from the contralateral eye and layers 2, 3, and 5 from the ipsilateral eye. Consistent with this anatomical arrangement, electrical recordings from the lateral geniculate nucleus reveal very few cells that can be activated by both eyes.

Optic radiation

Fibers arising in the lateral geniculate nucleus project through the retrolentiform and sublentiform parts of the internal capsule, curve around the lateral wall of the lateral ventricle (Fig. 11-10 and 11-11), and terminate in the cortex adjacent to the calcarine fissure. The optic radiation is often called the *geniculocalcarine tract*, reflecting its origin and termination. Not all of these fibers pass directly backward to the occipital lobe. Rather, they form a broad sheet covering much of the posterior and inferior horns of the ventricle. Fibers representing superior visual quadrants (that is, those representing inferior retinal quadrants) loop out into the temporal lobe *(Meyer's loop)* before turning posteriorly (Fig. 11-11, *A*). As a result, temporal lobe damage can produce a somewhat surprising visual deficit.

A retinotopic organization is maintained in the optic radiation. Fibers representing inferior visual fields are most superior, while those representing superior visual

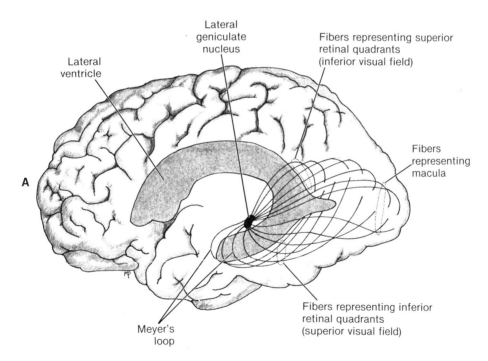

Lateral geniculate nucleus

Lateral ventricle

Fibers representing superior retinal quadrants (inferior visual field)

Fibers representing macula

A

Meyer's loop

Fibers representing inferior retinal quadrants (superior visual field)

Fig. 11-11. Three different views of the optic radiation. **A,** Schematic illustration of the course of geniculocalcarine fibers as they loop over the lateral aspect of the lateral ventricle and then turn posteriorly to end in the banks of the calcarine fissure on the medial surface of the hemisphere; note that the fibers representing inferior visual fields end in the upper bank, fibers representing superior visual fields end in the lower bank, and fibers representing areas near the visual midline (macula) end most posteriorly. (**B** from Ludwig, E., and Klingler, J.: Atlas cerebri humani, Boston, 1956, Little, Brown and Co.; **C** courtesy of Dr. John T. Willson, University of Colorado Health Sciences Center.)   *Continued.*

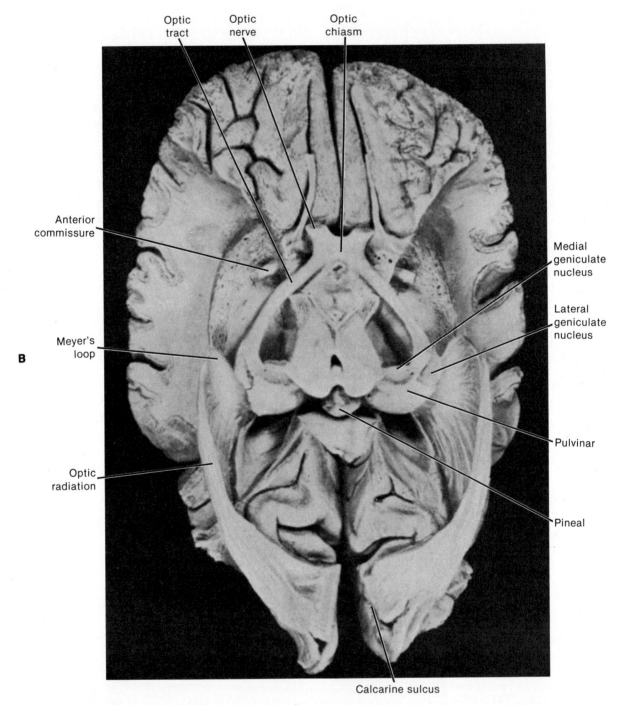

Fig. 11-11, cont'd. B, Inferior aspect of a brain dissected to show the entire visual pathway from optic nerve to striate cortex.

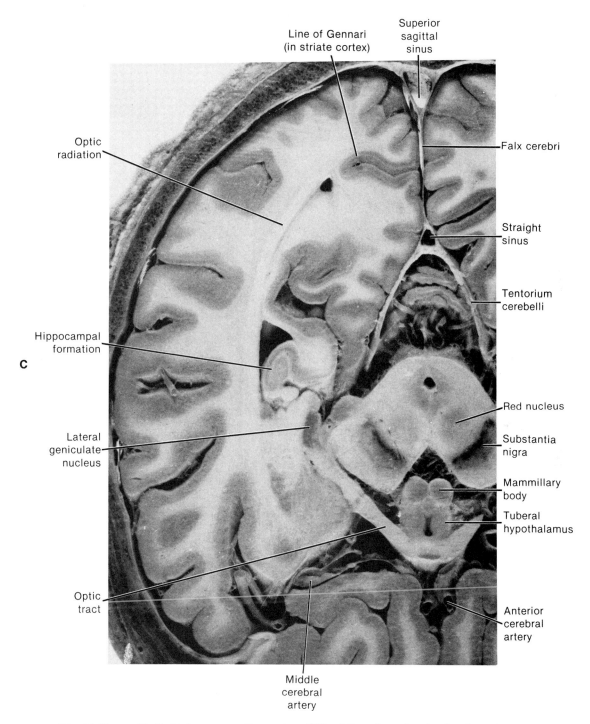

Line of Gennari
(in striate cortex)

Superior
sagittal
sinus

Optic
radiation

Falx cerebri

Straight
sinus

Tentorium
cerebelli

Hippocampal
formation

Lateral
geniculate
nucleus

Red nucleus

Substantia
nigra

Mammillary
body

Tuberal
hypothalamus

Optic
tract

Anterior
cerebral
artery

C

Middle
cerebral
artery

Fig. 11-11, cont'd. C, Enlargement of a portion of Fig. 3-3 to show the visual pathway in a section approximately perpendicular to the long axis of the brainstem.

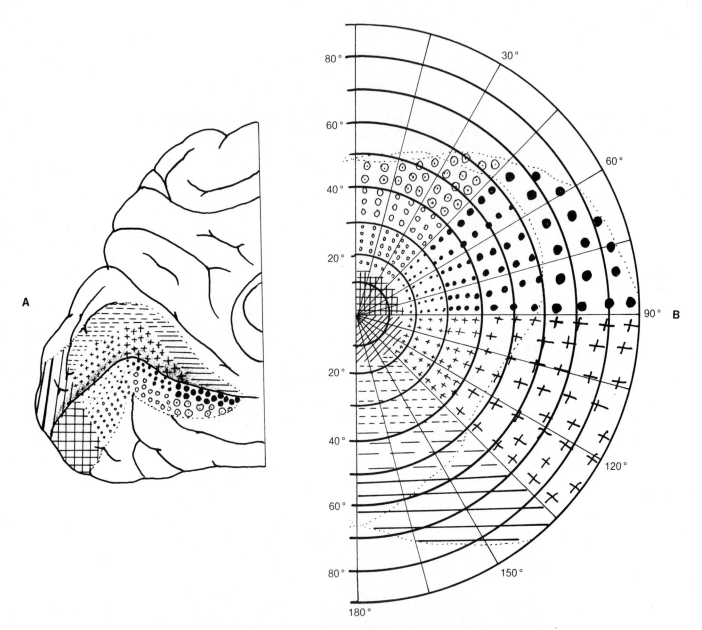

Fig. 11-12. Mapping from the right visual field (**B**) to the striate cortex of the left hemisphere (**A**). In **A**, imagine that the calcarine sulcus has been pried open, so that the map extends into its depths. In **B**, the inner dotted line outlines the area seen by both eyes; the right eye can see to the edge of the area outlined by the outer dotted line (compare Fig. 11-15). Note the disproportionately large area of striate cortex devoted to the representation of the macula (hatched and cross-hatched regions). (Redrawn from Holmes, G.: The organization of the visual cortex in man, Proc. R. Soc. Lond. **B132**:348, 1945.)

fields loop farthest out into the temporal lobe. Macular fibers occupy a broad middle area. The visual pathway is more dispersed in the optic radiation than elsewhere, and individual fibers still carry information from only one eye, so damage here sometimes results in deficits that are slightly different for the two eyes.

The visual pathway ends retinotopically in the cortex above and below the calcarine fissure (*area 17;* this numerical nomenclature, with which the cerebral cortex is divided into a series of areas called *Brodmann's areas,* is discussed in Chapter 15). Inferior visual fields project to the cortex above the calcarine fissure and superior fields to the cortex below the fissure. The macula is represented more posteriorly and peripheral fields more anteriorly (Fig. 11-12). Numerous myelinated fibers ramify within this cortex in a discrete layer that can be seen as a thin white stripe (the *line of Gennari*) with the naked eye. Hence primary visual cortex is also called *striate cortex.*

The striate cortex parallels the calcarine fissure and extends for a very short distance onto the posterior surface of the occipital lobe. It is surrounded by *area 18,* which in turn is surrounded by *area 19,* the two together comprising almost all the rest of the occipital lobe. Areas 18 and 19 are commonly referred to as the *visual association cortex* and are heavily interconnected with area 17.

Superior colliculus

All vertebrates possess two parallel visual pathways, one involving the lateral geniculate nucleus (or its equivalent) and the other involving the superior colliculus (or its equivalent). In lower vertebrates, the collicular (or tectal) pathway is the more important, but in primates, it is much less so. Nevertheless the major inputs to the primate superior colliculus are still visual, one arising in the retina and the second in the striate cortex. The retinal input consists of a substantial number of fibers in each optic tract that bypass the lateral geniculate nucleus, pass over the medial geniculate nucleus in a bundle called the *brachium of the superior colliculus* (or simply *superior brachium*) (Fig. 10-7), and terminate retinotopically in the superior colliculus. Many of these fibers (possibly all of them in primates) are collaterals of axons that also terminate in the lateral geniculate nucleus. The cortical input consists of cells in area 17 that project to the superior colliculus (again via its brachium) and end in a pattern that coincides with the retinotopic map in the colliculus.

In addition to visual inputs, the superior colliculus receives (1) somatosensory inputs (sometimes referred to as the *spinotectal tract*), chiefly consisting of collaterals of fibers in somatosensory pathways ascending to the thalamus, (2) auditory inputs, chiefly by way of pro-

jections from the inferior colliculus, and (3) additional inputs from widespread areas of the cortex.

Efferent connections of the superior colliculus include projections to the reticular formation, the inferior colliculus, and the cervical spinal cord (the *tectospinal tract*). Of interest with respect to the visual system, the superior colliculus also projects to the posterior thalamus, notably to the lateral geniculate nucleus and the pulvinar. The pulvinar, in turn, projects to cortical areas 18 and 19, the visual association cortex.

The function of the superior colliculus in humans is almost completely unknown. It is commonly stated that it mediates a variety of reflexes such as turning the head toward a moving visual stimulus, but in fact there is no known clinical condition in humans that can be attributed specifically to damage to the superior colliculus. On the other hand, monkeys have been shown, with careful training, to have considerable visual capacity after extensive lesions of the striate cortex, particularly when dealing with moving stimuli. In a few rare cases of selective damage to the striate cortex, humans too have been found to have residual visual capacities that are strange and paradoxical: for example, despite having no conscious awareness of visual stimuli in the "blind" portions of their visual fields, they may be able to point to such stimuli quite accurately. There are a number of alternatives for the anatomical basis for this residual visual capacity; an example is the pathway to areas 18 and 19 via the superior colliculus and pulvinar. The relative importance of the various possible pathways is poorly understood at present, as is the function of these paths in the intact nervous system.

Retinohypothalamic fibers

Photic input is involved in many neuroendocrine functions, and it has long been speculated that there are projections from the retina to the hypothalamus. It has now been shown directly that such fibers exist in a variety of mammals (including monkeys); these fibers end in a small hypothalamic nucleus above the optic chiasm called the *suprachiasmatic nucleus.* It seems likely that there are similar connections in humans (even though the suprachiasmatic nucleus is not particularly prominent).

PROCESSING OF VISUAL INFORMATION

The visual system can be viewed as a series of synapses beginning in the outer plexiform layer and extending to and beyond the visual association cortex of areas 18 and 19. At each level a certain amount of information processing takes place, so that cortical neurons respond best to stimuli that are quite different from those best able to stimulate individual rods and cones. A cell at any given level in the visual system is conventionally characterized by its *receptive field,* which refers to that area of the retina in which changing conditions of illumination produce an alteration of the cell's activity. By extension, receptive fields can also be defined in terms of the particular part of the outside world whose image falls on this region of the retina. One initially surprising observation about the receptive fields of the bipolar cells and more proximal neurons is that the intensity of illumination is relatively unimportant in determining a cell's level of activity. Rather the important parameter is the contrast between different areas of the receptive field. That is, the visual system is especially attuned to the detection of borders between light and dark areas.

Recordings from individual ganglion cells show that their receptive fields are composed of two concentric, roughly circular zones. Illumination of the central area (the *center*) causes either an increase or a decrease in the background firing rate, whereas illumination of the peripheral area (the *surround*) has the opposite effect. Simultaneous illumination of both center and surround causes relatively little change in firing rate, since the antagonistic effects of the two areas tend to cancel each other. Thus even at the level of the ganglion cell, the contrast between two different areas of the receptive fields is of paramount importance.

The properties of the center of such a receptive field reflect the "straight-through" receptor-bipolar-ganglion cell path. The properties of the surround result at least partially from the influence of receptors in the surround on bipolar cells in the center by way of horizontal cells. Thus the basic spatial organization of ganglion cell receptive fields occurs in the outer plexiform layer. Further lateral interactions in the inner plexiform layer, mediated by amacrine cells, are thought to modify such things as the temporal characteristics of the ganglion cell response. For example, some ganglion cells respond only transiently to a change in illumination, whereas others show a maintained change in discharge rate. Many lower vertebrates have much more complex ganglion cell receptive fields, and there is a corresponding increase in the thickness of the inner plexiform layer and a proliferation of amacrine cell synapses.

Receptive fields of cells in the lateral geniculate nucleus are generally similar to those of ganglion cells. The contrast detection mechanism is somewhat more efficient, so that uniform illumination causes less response than in the case of ganglion cells.

The receptive fields of cortical neurons are rather more complicated, and names such as "simple," "complex," and "hypercomplex" have been coined to describe these cells. Simple cells respond best to either a dark bar on a light background or to a light bar on a dark background; uniform illumination has essentially no effect. In addition, the bar must be oriented at a particular angle. It has been hypothesized that the receptive fields of simple cells result from the convergence of a large number of geniculate axons onto a single cortical neuron: if the receptive fields of these axons fell along a straight line, then a bar-shaped receptive field with flanking antagonistic areas could result. Complex and hypercomplex cells respond best to edges, bars, and corners and have particular orientation and movement properties. Many of their properties, like those of the simple cells, can be explained by the convergence of more peripheral neurons onto a single cell.

This account of visual processing is obviously highly simplified. It is selective as well in that data dealing with color vision and binocular interactions have not been discussed. It is known, for example, that many cells in the primate visual system have wavelength-specific properties and that there are cortical neurons that are sensitive to the location of an object in three-dimensional space as well as to its size and shape.

PLASTICITY

The visual system has provided a unique opportunity to study the extent to which connections within the CNS are genetically determined and unchangeable and the extent to which they can be influenced by the environment.

Recordings from neurons in the visual cortex of newborn cats and monkeys never previously exposed to light reveal that the basic properties of these neurons are similar to those of adults. This indicates that the wiring pattern of the visual system is, to a great extent, genetically determined and does not depend on visual input for its formation.

If, however, one eye of a newborn animal is covered for the first few months of its life, that eye will be permanently blind (in a perceptual sense) when uncovered. At the same time, cortical neurons are found to respond only to stimulation of the eye that had not been covered. Whether this is a result of degeneration of idle synapses or replacement of idle synapses by connections reflecting activity in the uncovered eye is not completely known, but it appears that a replacement process is at least partially involved.

This effect of covering an eye is specific to the first few months of life, and no deficit results if it occurs later. Also it is not simply a result of the eye not being exposed to light. If the eye is covered with translucent rather than opaque material so that the retina is exposed to light but not patterns, the same functional blindness results. This is consistent with the fact that normal cortical neurons respond as poorly to diffuse illumination as they do to no illumination at all. This also corresponds to the finding that infantile cataracts (and even more subtle defects) in humans can result in permanent blindness (called *amblyopia*), unless they are corrected at a very early age.

VISUAL REFLEXES
Pupillary light reflex

Light directed into one eye causes both pupils to constrict. The response of the pupil of the illuminated eye is called the *direct pupillary light reflex,* while that of the other eye is called the *consensual pupillary light reflex.* The afferent limb of the reflex arc consists of optic tract axons that enter the brachium of the superior colliculus and terminate in the *pretectal area,* which is directly rostral to the superior colliculus at the junction between midbrain and diencephalon. Pretectal neurons project bilaterally to the Edinger-Westphal nucleus, with fibers crossing both through the posterior commissure and through the periaqueductal gray matter ventral to the aqueduct. Axons of cells in the Edinger-Westphal nucleus travel in the third nerve as preganglionic parasympathetic fibers to the ciliary ganglion, where they synapse. Postganglionic fibers in the short ciliary nerves complete the reflex arc, synapsing on the smooth muscle cells of the pupillary sphincter.

Since one optic tract contains axons from ganglion cells in both eyes, and since each pretectal area projects bilaterally to the Edinger-Westphal nucleus, light directed into one eye causes the same amount of activity in the Edinger-Westphal nucleus on each side. This is the basis of the consensual light reflex.

The pathways of the pupillary light reflex are utilized clinically in a procedure known as the *swinging flashlight test* for damage to one retina or optic nerve (Fig. 11-13). With the patient seated in a dimly lit room, a light source is quickly moved back and forth from one eye to the other, while the examiner observes the behavior of each pupil in turn. For example, assume the right optic nerve is damaged. When the left eye is illuminated, both pupils will constrict. When the right eye is illuminated, the light reflex arc will be less effectively activated, and both pupils will dilate. Therefore when the light is moved from the left eye to the right, the right pupil will be seen to dilate, indicating damage to the right retina or optic nerve.

Near reflex (accommodation reflex)

When visual attention is directed to a nearby object, three things happen in a reflex manner: (1) *convergence* of the two eyes, so that the image of the object falls on both foveas, (2) contraction of the ciliary muscle and a resultant thickening of the lens (*accommodation*), so that the image of the object is in focus on the retina,

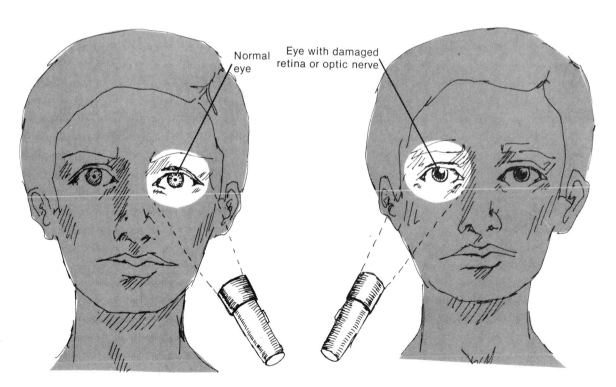

Fig. 11-13. Swinging flashlight test with the results expected from an individual with a damaged right retina or optic nerve.

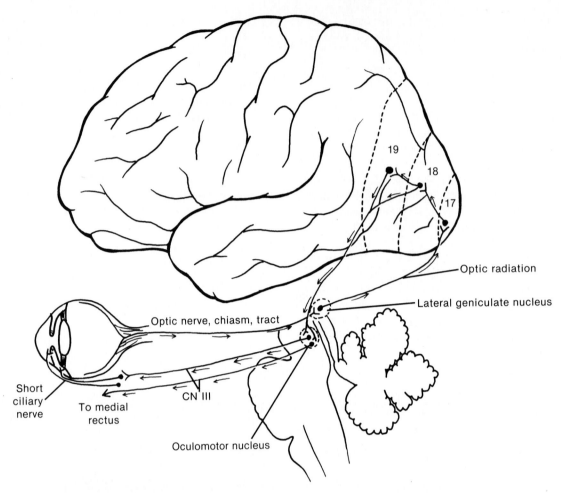

Fig. 11-14. Pathway of the near reflex. Although the efferent projections from the occipital lobe to the oculomotor nucleus are usually spoken of as arising in area 19, this is not known with certainty, and possible involvement of area 18 is also indicated. (Modified from Nolte, J.: Iris and pupil. In Records, R.E., editor: Physiology of the human eye and visual system, New York, 1979, Harper and Row, Publishers, Inc.)

and (3) pupillary *constriction*, which improves the optical performance of the eye by reducing certain types of aberration and by increasing its depth of field.

Unlike the pupillary light reflex, the *near reflex* requires the participation of the cerebral cortex. The pathway involved is poorly understood but is generally considered to follow the normal visual pathway to the striate cortex, project to the visual association cortex, and go from there to the superior colliculus and/or pretectal area (Fig. 11-14). Impulses are then relayed to the oculomotor nucleus, stimulating medial rectus motor neurons and preganglionic motor neurons of the Edinger-Westphal nucleus.

Although the same preganglionic parasympathetic fibers are thought to mediate the pupillary constriction of both the light reflex and the near reflex, these two types of constriction can nevertheless be dissociated in certain pathological conditions. An *Argyll Robertson pupil* refers to a condition (usually bilateral and usually a manifestation of neurosyphilis) in which the pupil constricts during the near reflex but not in response to light. The site of the lesion involved is not known with certainty, but it is often assumed to be in that portion of the pretectal area subserving the light reflex.

SOME FUNCTIONAL ASPECTS OF THE VISUAL SYSTEM
Visual deficits

Visual fields are tested by moving a small object in from the periphery until the patient, with one eye cov-

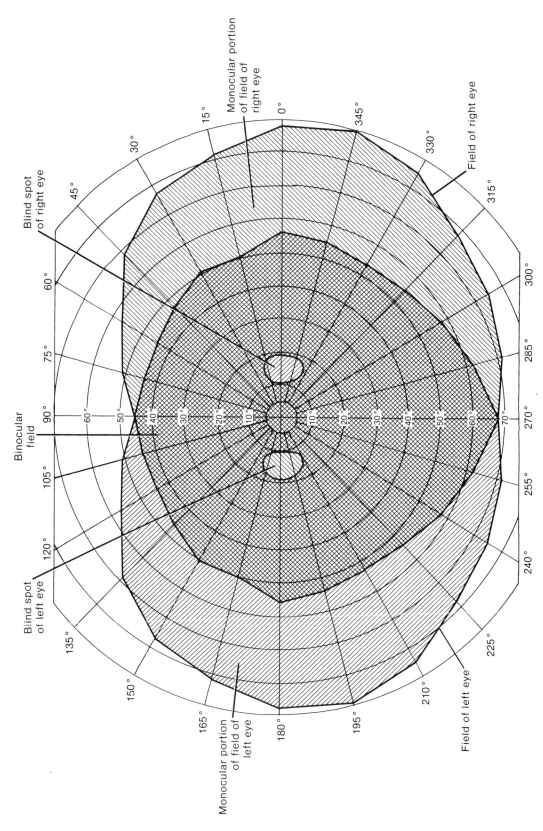

Fig. 11-15. Normal visual fields for the two eyes, superimposed on each other. (Courtesy of Dr. Bruce Wilson and Marilyn Haner, Denver General Hospital.)

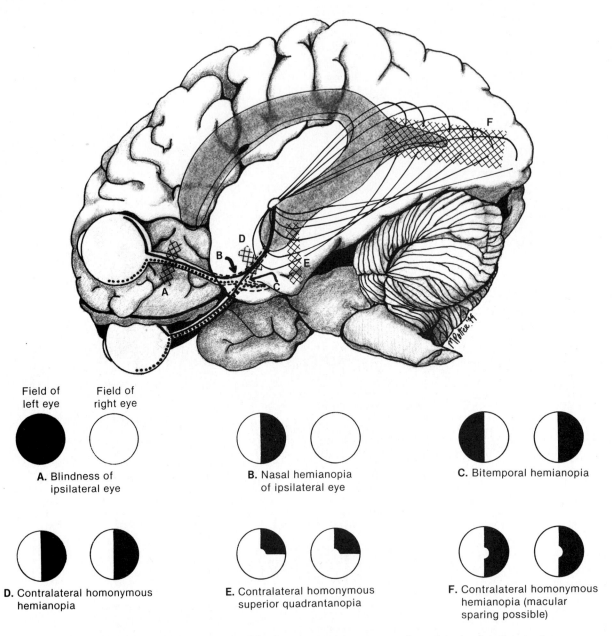

Field of   Field of
left eye   right eye

A. Blindness of
ipsilateral eye

B. Nasal hemianopia
of ipsilateral eye

C. Bitemporal hemianopia

D. Contralateral homonymous
hemianopia

E. Contralateral homonymous
superior quadrantanopia

F. Contralateral homonymous
hemianopia (macular
sparing possible)

Fig. 11-16. Visual field deficits caused by lesions at various points along the visual pathway. **A,** Destruction of one optic nerve causes blindness of the eye in which that nerve arises. **B,** Damage to one side of the optic chiasm destroys the noncrossing fibers from the ipsilateral eye; these fibers arise in the temporal retina, so a nasal hemianopsia of the ipsilateral eye results. **C,** Pressure on the middle of the optic chiasm, typically from a pituitary tumor, destroys the crossing fibers from both eyes, causing a bitemporal hemianopsia (one type of heteronymous hemianopsia). **D,** Destruction of one optic tract causes contralateral homonymous hemianopsia. **E,** Damage to one temporal lobe could destroy part of the optic radiation, specifically the fibers representing the contralateral superior quadrant of each visual field; since the optic radiation is rather spread out at this point, some fibers are likely to be spared (for example, in this case the macular fibers remain intact). **F,** Massive damage to one occipital lobe (such as might be caused by occlusion of one posterior cerebral artery) causes contralateral homonymous hemianopsia; the macular representation is quite large, and some of it is likely to survive, resulting in macular sparing.

ered, reports seeing it. By repeating this for many different directions of motion, a chart of the visual field can be made (Fig. 11-15). Each eye can normally see a surprising 90° from the visual axis in a temporal direction, but the field is less extensive in other directions. The area of overlap of the two visual fields is the area in which binocular vision is possible.

Deficits resulting from damage to various parts of the visual pathways are named according to certain conventions. Most importantly, visual defects are always named according to the visual field loss and not according to the area of the retina that is nonfunctional. Since the retinal image is inverted and reversed, damage to temporal areas of the retina would cause nasal field losses, and damage to superior areas of the retina would cause inferior field losses. The combining form "-anopsia" (or "-anopia") is used to denote loss of one or more quadrants of a visual field; *hemianopsia* would refer to loss of half of a visual field, *quadrantanopsia* to loss of one quarter of a visual field. Finally the term *homonymous* denotes a condition in which the visual field losses are the same for both eyes, and *heteronymous* denotes a condition in which the two eyes have nonoverlapping field losses.

Using this terminology, it is possible to name the deficits resulting from damage at most locations in the visual pathway (Fig. 11-16); some of the names are quite spectacular. A lesion of one optic nerve causes blindness of that eye. Damage in the central region of the optic chiasm, affecting the crossing fibers, causes a heteronymous hemianopsia (or in this case, a *bitemporal hemianopsia*). This can result from midline pressure exerted by a tumor of the pituitary, which lies very close to the chiasm (compare Fig. 2-13). Lateral pressure on one side of the chiasm, affecting the noncrossing fibers on that side, would cause an ipsilateral *nasal hemianopsia*. This occasionally results from an aneurysm of the internal carotid artery, which lies adjacent to the chiasm (Fig. 5-1). In the rare event of aneurysms of both internal carotid arteries, a *binasal hemianopsia* could result. Destruction of one optic tract would interrupt all the fibers carrying information from the contralateral visual fields, causing a contralateral *homonymous hemianopsia*.

Damage to the optic radiation is rarely extensive enough to cause complete hemianopsia, and roughly quadrantic deficits are more often the result. For example, a large destructive lesion of the left temporal lobe, interrupting the fibers of Meyer's loop (which represent inferior retinal quadrants), would produce a *right homonymous superior quadrantanopsia*. Lesions in either the optic radiation or visual cortex leave the pupillary light reflex undisturbed, as would be predicted from the anatomical pathways involved in this reflex.

In cases of massive damage to the visual cortex of one occipital lobe (as, for example, after occlusion of one posterior cerebral artery), a contralateral homonymous hemianopsia would be the expected result. In fact, it is frequently observed clinically that vision is preserved over much of the macula. This phenomenon is called *macular sparing*, and its existence, extent, and basis have been a topic of debate for many years. Part of its origin may lie in the disproportionately large representation of the macula in the striate cortex: even very large cortical lesions may leave part of the macular region undamaged. In addition, the distributions of the middle and posterior cerebral arteries overlap near the occipital pole. Therefore even total occlusion of the posterior cerebral artery allows for supply of part of the macular region by the middle cerebral artery.

ADDITIONAL READING

Altman, J., and Carpenter, M.B.: Fiber projections of the superior colliculus in the cat, J. Comp. Neurol. **116:**157, 1961.

Brouwer, B., and Zeeman, W.P.C.: The projection of the retina in the primary optic neuron in monkeys, Brain **49:**1, 1926. *A description of the retinotopic organization of the optic nerve, chiasm, and tract, and of the pattern of termination of the optic tract in the lateral geniculate nucleus.*

Denny-Brown, D., and Chambers, R.A.: Physiological aspects of visual perception, I: functional aspects of visual cortex, Arch. Neurol. **33:**219, 1976.

Denny-Brown, D., and Fischer, E.G.: Physiological aspects of visual perception, II: the subcortical visual direction of behavior, Arch. Neurol. **33:**228, 1976.

Dowling, J.E.: Organization of vertebrate retinas, Invest. Ophthalmol. **9:**655, 1970. *A nice, concise review of the cellular and synaptic organization and basic neurophysiology of the retina.*

Holmes, G.: The organization of the visual cortex in man, Proc. R. Soc. Lond. **B132:**348, 1945.

Hoyt, W.F., and Luis, O.: The primate chiasm, Arch. Ophthalmol. **70:**69, 1963.

Hubel, D.H., and Wiesel, T.N.: Functional architecture of macaque monkey visual cortex, Proc. R. Soc. Lond. **B198:**1, 1977. *A detailed discussion of the elegant experiments on the primate visual system done by these two investigators over the past 20 years.*

Humphrey, N.K., and Weiskrantz, L.: Vision in monkeys after removal of the striate cortex, Nature **215:**595, 1967.

Jampel, R.S.: Representation of the near-response on the cerebral cortex of the macaque, Am. J. Ophthalmol. **48:**573, 1959.

Kupfer, C.: The projection of the macula in the lateral geniculate nucleus in man, Am. J. Ophthalmol. **54:**597, 1962.

Lowenstein, O., and Loewenfeld, I.E.: The pupil. In Davson, H., editor: The eye, vol. 3, Muscular mechanisms, New York, 1969, Academic Press, Inc.

Magoun, H.W., et al.: The afferent path of the pupillary light reflex in the monkey, Brain **59:**234, 1936.

Mohler, C.W., and Wurtz, R.H.: Role of striate cortex and superior colliculus in visual guidance of saccadic eye movements in monkeys, J. Neurophysiol. **40:**74, 1977.

Moore, R.Y.: Retinohypothalamic projection in mammals: a comparative study, Brain Res. **49:**403, 1973.

Nguyen-Legros, J.: Fine structure of the pigment epithelium in the vertebrate retina, Int. Rev. Cytol. (Suppl.) **7:**287, 1978.

Pearlman, A.L., Birch, J., and Meadows, J.C.: Cerebral color blindness: an acquired defect in hue discrimination, Ann. Neurol. **5**:253, 1979. *One example of the notion that the primary visual cortex and visual association cortex are not like a screen on which the retinal image is projected; rather, a number of different subareas deal selectively with different aspects of the visual world.*

Pettigrew, J.D., Olson, C., and Hirsh, H.V.B.: Cortical effect of selective visual experience: degeneration or reorganization? Brain Res. **51**:345, 1973.

Pollack, J.G., and Hickey, T.L.: The distribution of retinocollicular axon terminals in rhesus monkey, J. Comp. Neurol. **185**:587, 1979.

Records, R.E., editor: Physiology of the human eye and visual system, New York, 1979, Harper and Row, Publishers, Inc.

Rushton, W.A.H.: King Charles II and the blind spot, Vision Res. **19**:225, 1979.

Schneider, G.E.: Two visual systems, Science **163**:895, 1969. *Differential effects of collicular and cortical damage on a hamster's visual capabilities.*

Schwartz, W.J., and Gainer, H.: Suprachiasmatic nucleus: use of ^{14}C-labelled deoxyglucose uptake as a functional marker, Science **197**:1089, 1977.

Weiskrantz, L., et al.: Visual capacity in the hemianopic field following a restricted cortical ablation, Brain **97**:709, 1974. *Remarkable account of the visual capabilities remaining in one individual after known selective damage to his striate cortex.*

Wilson, M.E., and Cragg, B.G.: Projections from the lateral geniculate nucleus in the cat and monkey, J. Anat. **101**:677, 1967.

Wong-Riley, M.T.T.: Connections between the pulvinar nucleus and the prestriate cortex in the squirrel monkey as revealed by peroxidase histochemistry and autoradiography, Brain Res. **134**:249, 1977.

Wray, S.H.: Neuro-ophthalmologic manifestations of pituitary and parasellar lesions. In Keener, E.B., editor: Clinical neurosurgery, Baltimore, 1977, The Williams & Wilkins Co.

CHAPTER 12

CORTICOSPINAL AND CORTICOBULBAR TRACTS

Each of us has fewer than 1 million motor neurons with which to control muscles. Without them, we would be completely unable to communicate with the outside world. With them, however, we are capable of an enormous range of complex activities, from automatic and semiautomatic movements such as postural adjustments to the characteristically human movements involved in speaking and writing. The ways in which a wide variety of neural structures interact to make these activities possible is the topic of Chapters 12 to 14.

LEVELS OF ORGANIZATION OF MOTOR SYSTEMS

Determinants of activity in motor neurons may be very broadly divided into three overlapping classes:
1. *Built-in patterns* of neural connections
2. *Descending pathways* that modulate the activity of motor neurons; these effects may be direct or they may be indirect by way of influences on built-in neural subsystems
3. *Higher centers* that influence the activity of descending pathways

Built-in patterns

The stretch reflex is an obvious and simple example of a built-in pattern of neural connections that controls, to some extent, the activity of motor neurons. Stretching a muscle stimulates its muscle spindles, whose afferent fibers end on motor neurons that in turn cause the muscle to contract (Fig. 7-7). Other reflexes, such as the flexor reflex (Figs. 7-9 and 7-11), are more complex and involve a number of muscles and spinal segments. It also appears that there are networks of interneurons in the brainstem and spinal cord that can act as pattern generators for movements such as walking. The mechanism of these *central programs* (as they are often called)

is not simply a stringing together of reflexes, each one triggering the next; the principal features of these programs can persist in the absence of afferent input.

Descending pathways

Several descending pathways with effects on somatic motor neurons have already been mentioned (Fig. 7-17). The *vestibulospinal tracts* are important mediators of postural adjustments. The *corticospinal tract* classically has been considered the principal mediator of voluntary movement, although as discussed in this chapter, its real role is not so clear these days. The *reticulospinal tracts* and the *rubrospinal tract* are important alternate routes for the mediation of voluntary movement. The rubrospinal tract originates in the red nucleus, crosses to the other side of the midbrain, descends in the lateral part of the brainstem tegmentum, and travels through the lateral funiculus of the spinal cord in company with the lateral corticospinal tract. The relative importance of the rubrospinal tract and the reticulospinal tracts in humans has been a subject of debate for years, and the matter is far from settled. However, there is some evidence that the rubrospinal tract is fairly small in primates, and so, for convenience, we will treat the reticulospinal tracts as the major alternate route to the spinal cord. A *tectospinal tract* has also been described, descending from the superior colliculus through the contralateral anterior funiculus of cervical levels of the spinal cord. It is assumed to be important in reflex turning of the head in response to visual and perhaps other stimuli, but little is actually known of its function in humans.

Higher centers

Even though cortico-, rubro-, reticulo-, and vestibulospinal fibers are able to influence motor neurons and

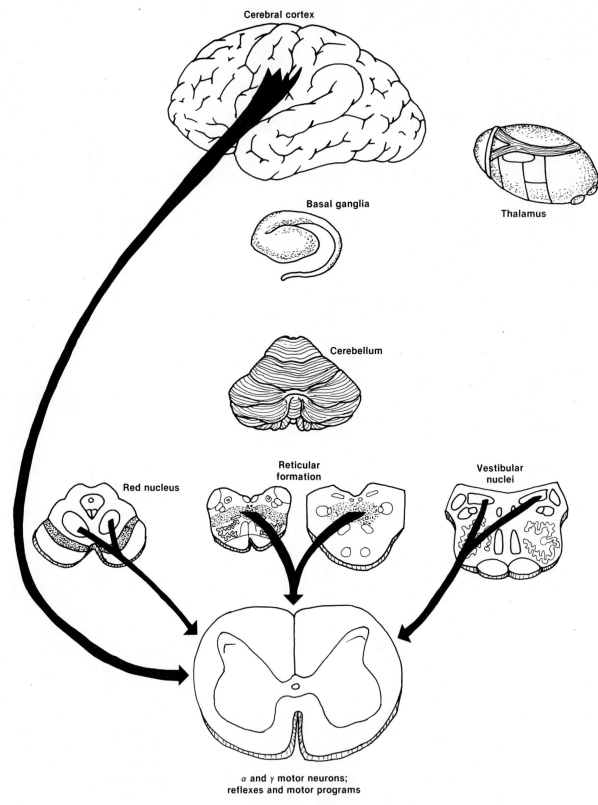

Fig. 12-1. Schematic drawing of descending motor control pathways. Note that although the cerebral cortex can influence motor neurons by both direct and indirect pathways, some other structures associated with motor control (most notably the basal ganglia and the cerebellum) have no such access to motor neurons.

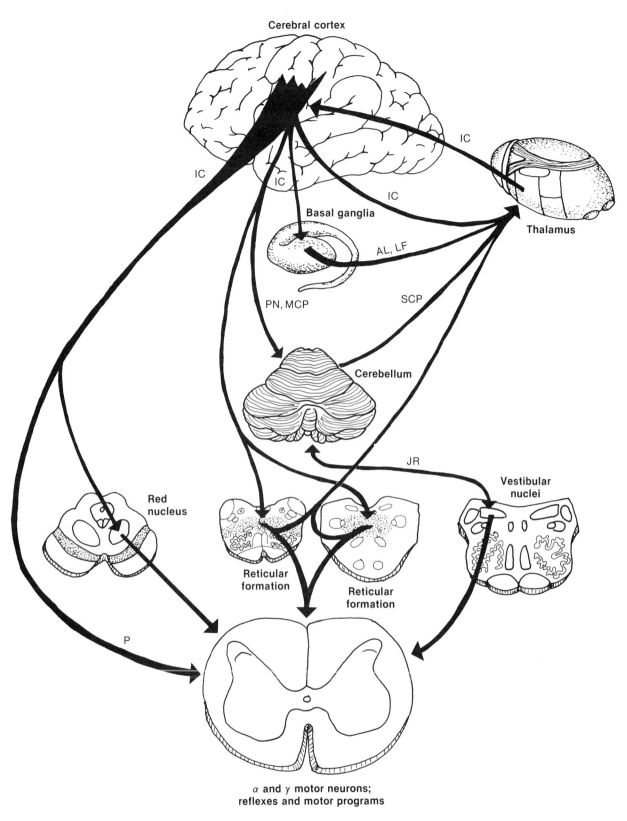

Fig. 12-2. Principal interconnections of neural structures involved in motor control, illustrating in a schematic way their arrangement in a series of interlocking loops. This is intended to be a general overview and is simplified and incomplete. For example, not all the indicated structures project to the same part of the thalamus, and by no means do all the inputs to structures like the cerebellum originate in the cerebral cortex. Abbreviations refer to the discrete anatomical structures through which these connections pass. *AL,* Ansa lenticularis (Chapter 13); *IC,* internal capsule; *JR,* juxta-restiform body (part of inferior cerebellar peduncle); *LF,* lenticular fasciculus (Chapter 13); *MCP,* middle cerebellar peduncle; *P,* pyramid of medulla (corticospinal tract); *PN,* pontine nuclei; *SCP,* superior cerebellar pendunle. The term "basal ganglia" as used in this diagram refers primarily to the caudate and lenticular nuclei. As discussed in Chapter 13, other structures with other connections are usually included with the basal ganglia.

their local connections, this still does not explain how a voluntary movement is made. At the present time we are able to say very little about the nature of the little person within the central nervous system who pulls the strings when we decide to move. We can, however, specify some of the structures and connections that must be involved in the sense that damage to these structures and connections results in defective movements. In addition to the portions of the CNS already mentioned, these structures include the basal ganglia, the cerebellum, and portions of the thalamus. The basal ganglia and the cerebellum are the subjects of Chapters 13 and 14, but the general way in which the various components of the motor system are interconnected will be briefly discussed here.

The connections already mentioned are diagrammed in Fig. 12-1. Notice that the cerebral cortex can influence motor neurons directly via the corticospinal tract and indirectly via inputs to the red nucleus and reticular formation (Fig. 12-2). This fact is of extreme importance in understanding the different deficits caused by damage to different portions of the motor system. Most of the remaining connections can be characterized as a

series of interlocking loops, as shown in Fig. 12-2. Notice that the basal ganglia and cerebellum have no outputs of their own to the spinal cord. Rather they act primarily by affecting the cerebral cortex.

This is an extremely simplified overview of the central motor apparatus and omits a number of important details. Some of these details will be mentioned in this and the next two chapters, while others are beyond the scope of this book. For example, no mention has been made of the role of sensory input to this system. Such input is clearly involved, since we are easily able to make appropriate modifications in the walking program to accommodate an increased load such as a backpack or modifications in the running program to accommodate the sight of an impending brick wall. A variety of pathological conditions reflect motor deficits resulting from sensory losses. One example already cited is the ataxia resulting from damage to the posterior columns.

CORTICOSPINAL TRACT

During the nineteenth century it was discovered that electrical stimulation of certain areas of the mammalian cerebral cortex causes movements of the contralateral

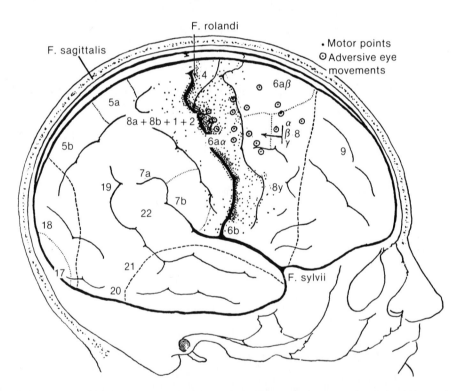

Fig. 12-3. Composite diagram of the locations that yielded discrete movements when stimulated with a very weak electrical current in a series of conscious human patients during the course of neurosurgical procedures. Note that most of the sensitive points lie on the precentral gyrus, particularly near the central sulcus, but a significant number are on the postcentral gyrus and a few anterior to the precentral gyrus. (From Penfield, W., and Boldrey, E.: Somatic motor and sensory representation in the cerebral cortex of man as studied by electrical stimulation, Brain **60**:389, 1937.)

side of the body. In humans, the area with the lowest threshold for this effect lies in the precentral gyrus (Fig. 12-3) and so has come to be called the *primary motor cortex*. Subsequent work showed that there is a distorted mapping of the body in the primary motor cortex, so that stimulation of restricted cortical areas causes contraction of small groups of muscles or even single muscles. The somatotopic map (Fig. 12-4) is distorted in such a way that the parts of the body capable of very intricate movements (such as the fingers and lips) have disproportionately large representations. The *motor homunculus* (Latin = little man) is thus similar to the sensory homunculus in the somatosensory cortex of the postcentral gyrus, and this corresponds to (among other things) the notion that detailed sensory information is required for fine motor control.

It was also known in the previous century that the primary motor cortex contains giant pyramidal cells called *Betz cells*, whose axons descend to the spinal cord through the medullary pyramids; it was further known that cerebral lesions that destroy either the area containing motor cortex or the axons of the Betz cells as they pass through the posterior limb of the internal capsule cause contralateral spastic paralysis. Therefore it became accepted neurological thinking that the cortico-

spinal tract (1) consists exclusively of large axons, (2) originates in the precentral gyrus, (3) proceeds straight to the spinal cord, (4) is necessary for voluntary movement, and (5) results in spastic paralysis if destroyed. However, it has gradually become apparent that this traditional description is incorrect in almost every way.

1. The large (up to 22 μm) axons of Betz cells are included in the corticospinal tract, but they account for only about 3% of the tract's 1 million fibers. The vast majority of corticospinal fibers are much smaller, in the 1 to 4 μm range. Whether the small fibers have a role different from that of the larger fibers is not known.

2. Betz cells reside specifically in primary motor cortex, but a total of fewer than 40% of the corticospinal fibers originate in this cortical area. The remainder come from the area anterior to primary motor cortex (the *premotor cortex*) and from the parietal lobe, particularly the somatosensory cortex of the postcentral gyrus (Fig. 12-5). In view of this fact, many investigators now refer to the cortical complex on both sides of the central sulcus as the *sensorimotor cortex*.

3. Corticospinal fibers, as their name implies, end in the spinal cord. However, in their course from cortex to cord they give rise to large numbers of collaterals that end in a wide variety of locations, including the basal

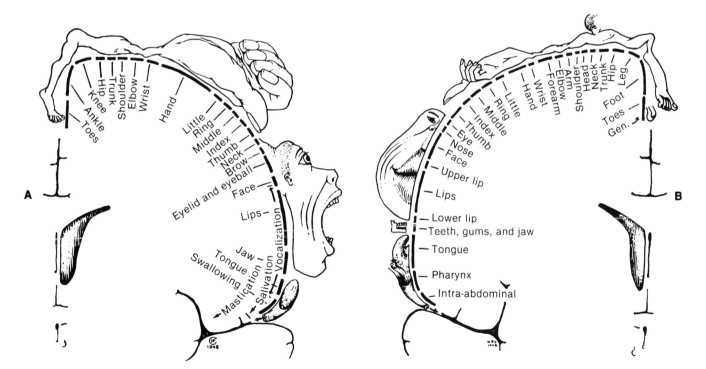

Fig. 12-4. Somatotopic mappings in human motor (**A**) and somatosensory (**B**) cortex obtained by electrical stimulation of the surface of the brains of conscious patients undergoing neurosurgery. The size of a given part of the homunculus is roughly proportional to the size of the cortical area devoted to that body part. (From The Cerebral Cortex of Man by W. Penfield and T. Rasmussen. Copyright © 1950 by Macmillan Publishing Co., Inc., renewed 1978 by T. Rasmussen.)

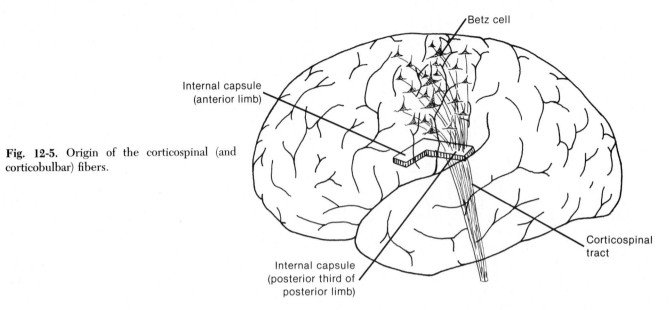

Fig. 12-5. Origin of the corticospinal (and corticobulbar) fibers.

ganglia, the thalamus, the reticular formation, and various sensory nuclei such as the posterior column nuclei. Even within the spinal cord some end in the posterior horn, others end in the intermediate gray matter, and a minority end directly on alpha and gamma motor neurons.

These numerous connections make it seem unlikely that the corticospinal tract has a single, easily specified function. The projections to sensory nuclei, for example, might serve to compensate somehow for the altered afferent activity to be caused by an impending movement.

The corticospinal tract does, of course, have a major effect on motor neurons as well, both directly and indirectly by way of interneurons. In general, both alpha and gamma motor neurons are affected similarly. The utility of this *alpha-gamma coactivation* can be seen in Fig. 6-7. If only the alpha motor neurons were activated, then during the resulting contraction, the muscle spindles would be "de-stretched" and hence inactive. Stretch reflexes thus would be inoperative and unable to help compensate for sudden changes in load during the movement. Activating the gamma motor neurons as well serves to maintain spindle sensitivity throughout the movement.

4. Studies in which both medullary pyramids of monkeys were carefully and selectively severed have demonstrated that after an initial period of flaccid paralysis, surprisingly little chronic motor deficit results from a total loss of corticospinal function. In moving about their cages, these animals are virtually indistinguishable from normal monkeys. The only behaviorally obvious deficit is a permanent inability to use their fingers individually as, for example, in picking up a small object between thumb and forefinger. This is a serious loss for creatures who use their hands as much and as skillfully as primates do, but nevertheless it falls far short of being a generalized weakness or paralysis of voluntary movements.

If lesions of medial portions of the medullary reticular formation are added to the corticospinal lesion, a severe and permanent disability of the axial muscles results. Conversely, if lesions of the lateral portions of the medullary reticular formation are added to the corticospinal lesion, a severe and permanent disability of independent use of the arms (including, of course, the fingers) results. Evidently the reticulospinal and/or rubrospinal tracts can compensate for the role normally played by the corticospinal tract in most aspects of voluntary movement.

Naturally occurring lesions in humans are never so neatly restricted as those in the monkeys just mentioned, and there are no comparable cases of humans with selective damage to the pyramids. However, there is a neurosurgical procedure (whose rationale is explained in the next chapter) in which the corticospinal tract is cut in the cerebral peduncle. In these cases, the results are quite similar to those encountered with pyramid-sectioned monkeys, and relatively little chronic deficit results.

5. Spastic paralysis, commonly the result of a stroke involving the internal capsule, is characterized by (among other things) increased muscle tone and hyperactive reflexes. However, selective damage to the corticospinal tract, as in the experiments just referred to, causes little chronic change in tone or reflexes. The reason for the apparent discrepancy can be seen in Fig. 12-2. Damage to a medullary pyramid affects a very select group of fibers, the final portions of certain axons just before they reach the spinal cord. In contrast, damage to motor/premotor cortex or to the internal capsule

affects not only corticospinal fibers but also projections from the cortex to the thalamus, basal ganglia, reticular formation, etc. Furthermore even if it were possible to selectively damage only corticospinal fibers in the internal capsule, they would be affected before they gave off their many collaterals rather than after (as in the case of damage to the pyramid). Which part of this additional damage is responsible for the appearance of spasticity is not known with certainty, but the loss of certain corticoreticular connections is a likely cause.

CORTICOBULBAR TRACT

A few corticospinal fibers, as we have seen, end directly on spinal motor neurons, while the rest end in the posterior horn, in the intermediate gray matter, or on interneurons of the anterior horn. Those not ending directly on motor neurons have a variety of effects, ranging from regulating the access of information to ascending pathways to affecting the activity of motor neurons via interneurons. In a similar manner, other fibers leave the cerebral cortex, descend through the internal capsule (immediately anterior to the corticospinal tract), and end in the brainstem on cells of sensory relay nuclei, of the reticular formation, and of motor nuclei of some cranial nerves. Strictly speaking, this entire collection of fibers is the *corticobulbar tract*. However, in common usage the term "corticobulbar tract" is often used to refer to those fibers that selectively affect the motor neurons of cranial nerves (Fig. 12-6). As in the spinal cord, some of these corticobulbar fibers end directly on motor neurons, but most act through interneurons of the reticular formation. The oculomotor, trochlear, and abducens nuclei receive no direct corticobulbar fibers; there are other peculiarities about the innervation of these nuclei, so they are treated separately in the next section. Thus the following discussion pertains to the trigeminal, facial, and hypoglossal motor nuclei, the nucleus ambiguus, and the spinal accessory nucleus.

In general, these nuclei receive a bilateral corticobulbar innervation. The fibers originate from the face portion of the motor cortex and from other areas of the frontal and parietal lobes as well. They accompany the corticospinal tract almost to the level of the nucleus they influence. Here they part company with the corticospinal tract and end in the appropriate motor nucleus on both sides or in the adjacent reticular formation. The major exception to this general pattern is in the case of the facial motor nucleus. As mentioned in Chapter 9, motor neurons to the lower facial muscles are innervated mainly by contralateral cortex, while those to upper facial muscles are bilaterally innervated. The result is that an individual with unilateral corticobulbar damage (as in a lesion of one cerebral peduncle) would be unable to smile or bare the teeth symmetrically or puff out the contralateral cheek; however, the ability to blink and wrinkle the forehead on both sides would remain. In addition, even though the hypoglossal and trigeminal motor nuclei and those neurons of the spinal accessory nucleus that innervate the trapezius receive some input from the cortex of both hemispheres, the input from the contralateral side predominates (to a degree that varies from one individual to another).

Eye movements

Our eyes do a fairly remarkable job of tracking (or moving to look at) various objects as the objects and/or we move about in three-dimensional space. Throughout this process, the two eyes stay aligned with each other to a high degree of accuracy. Two general types of movement are involved: (1) *vergence movements*, in which the two eyes move in opposite directions, as in the convergence that occurs when we look at a nearby object, and (2) *conjugate movements*, in which the two eyes move the same amount in the same direction, as in visually tracking an object that moves about at a fixed distance from us. Normally vergence and conjugate movements are smoothly integrated with one another so that images of the outside world fall on the two retinas in proper registration.

Little is known of the pathways involved in vergence movements. It is thought that the visual association cortex of the occipital lobe is important, along with projections from there to the midbrain (Fig. 11-14). The pathway ultimately influences the oculomotor nuclei (particularly the motor neurons to the two medial recti), which then converge the eyes. Consistent with this are the notions that damage to the midbrain and occasionally to the occipital lobes interferes with convergence, while damage to more caudal portions of the brainstem (including the MLF) does not.

Conjugate movements themselves are of two types, fast and slow. The fast movements are called *saccades*. They are brief, rapid movements, the kind we use to voluntarily move our eyes in any given direction, and the kind we use for the fast phase of nystagmus. The slow movements go by a variety of names but are most commonly called *smooth pursuit* or *tracking movements*. As the name implies, we use them to track slowly moving objects* and also for the slow phase of nystagmus.

---

*It comes as a surprise to most that with the head stationary, we can only move our eyes smoothly when we are tracking a slowly moving object. This is easily demonstrated, however. Watch someone's eyes as he or she tries to move them slowly and smoothly while there is nothing to track, or concentrate on your own eyes while you try to do the same thing. In either case, the result will be the same: a series of rapid, jerky movements. Some individuals can learn to have voluntary control of smooth tracking movements, but under normal circumstances and for most people, this is impossible.

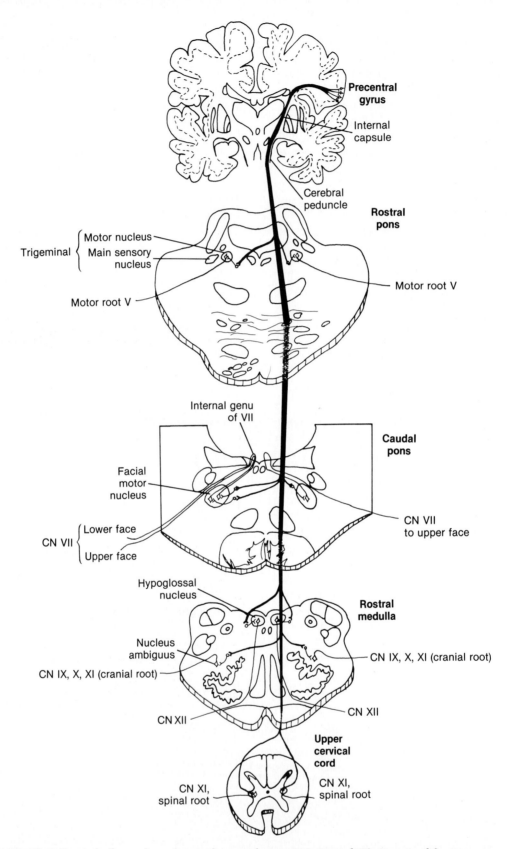

Fig. 12-6. Corticobulbar pathway (except for cranial nerves III, IV, and VI). Two simplifications were used to keep the diagram manageable. (1) Most projections are shown passing through a reticular interneuron, whereas in primates some corticobulbar fibers, like corticospinal fibers, end directly on motor neurons. (2) All corticobulbar fibers are shown accompanying the corticospinal tract, whereas many corticobulbar fibers leave this tract at various levels caudal to the cerebral peduncle and pursue a variety of aberrant courses through the brainstem.

A network of neural structures in both the brainstem and the cerebral hemispheres is involved in the initiation and coordination of conjugate eye movements. Basically it involves motor programs for these eye movements, located in the brainstem, together with cerebral centers that are able to trigger and modulate these brainstem mechanisms.

Brainstem mechanisms. The neural machinery for generating rapid horizontal movements is located in the medial reticular formation of the pons just rostral to the abducens nucleus.* Signals from this region project to the abducens/parabducens nucleus (Fig. 9-7), with each

*This particular portion of the reticular formation is now commonly referred to as the *paramedian pontine reticular formation,* or *PPRF.*

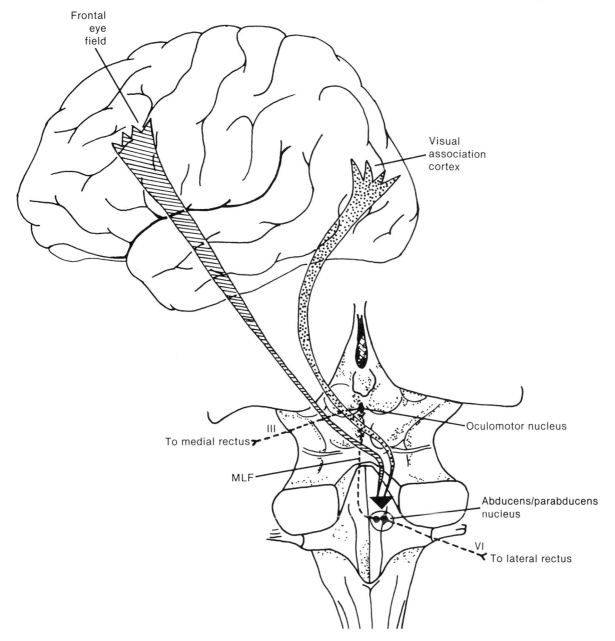

Fig. 12-7. Cortical areas concerned with conjugate deviation to the right; see text for details. Pathway for saccades originates in frontal eye fields, and pathway for slow tracking originates in occipital lobe (or possibly in adjacent parietal areas). Both pathways descend through the internal capsule, decussate in the caudal midbrain, and ultimately stimulate the right abducens/parabducens complex. Intermediate stops between the cortex and abducens/parabducens complex are not shown; they include the paramedian pontine reticular formation (and possibly the superior colliculus as well) for saccades and possibly the vestibular nuclei for slow tracking. Diagram is drawn as though one occipital lobe directs slow tracking movements to the contralateral side, but this is controversial.

side of the brainstem directing movements to the ipsilateral side (Fig. 12-7). The machinery for rapid vertical movements is located in the reticular formation of the rostral midbrain. Some recent experimental evidence and many years of clinical experience indicate that upward and downward movements are generated from slightly different locations. One of the common early effects of pineal tumors is paralysis of upward gaze (together with disturbances of convergence). Downward gaze is usually only affected later or when lesions are situated more deeply in the mesencephalic tegmentum. Both upward and downward gaze seem to be represented bilaterally in the midbrain, since unilateral lesions do not cause paralysis of vertical movements.

The neural mechanisms of the brainstem for slow eye movements are not as well known as those for rapid movements. The vestibular nuclei and the flocculus of the cerebellum seem to be important for both horizontal and vertical slow movements (whether elicited by vestibular or visual stimuli), but other structures may be involved as well.

Cortical mechanisms. Stimulation of widespread cortical areas causes eye movements. Stimuli delivered to the occipital lobe or to a restricted area of the frontal lobe are particularly effective.

The *frontal eye field*, located in the posterior portion of the middle frontal gyrus just in front of the representation of the face in the primary motor cortex (Figs. 12-3 and 12-7), is considered to be involved in the initiation of rapid eye movements. Stimulation here causes horizontal or oblique conjugate movements to the contralateral side. Damage to the frontal eye field of one hemisphere causes inability to look voluntarily to the contralateral side. It can easily be shown, however, that the appropriate muscles are not paralyzed, because the individual is able to visually track an object moving to the contralateral side. Vertical eye movements are not impaired after a unilateral lesion, and even the deficit in horizontal movements is transitory, with recovery usually occurring in a matter of days. This has led to the conclusion that rapid movements in all directions are represented in each hemisphere, that normally each hemisphere is dominant for contralateral saccades, but that in case of damage to one hemisphere, the other can substitute.

The visual association cortex of the occipital lobe is considered to be involved in the initiation of pursuit and vergence movements. Relatively little is actually known about these cortical mechanisms, and there is not even universal agreement as to whether a given occipital lobe initiates pursuit movements toward the ipsilateral or the contralateral side. Occipital damage typically causes visual deficits, so problems with eye movements may be difficult to evaluate. Here again though,

it is thought that movements in all directions are represented in each hemisphere, since the deficits that persist are not pronounced.

This localization of function seems to make good intuitive sense. The frontal eye field is adjacent to the primary motor cortex and could reasonably be expected to play a role in voluntary eye movements. Vergence, and particularly tracking, movements are usually associated with the perception of visual stimuli, so it would not be surprising if visual cortex and visual association cortex played a role in these eye movements. However, this traditional formulation has been challenged by some recent experimental evidence. With regard to the frontal eye field, it has not been possible to find any cells in this area in monkeys that increase their firing rate before the beginning of a saccade; such cells would obviously be necessary if the frontal eye field participated directly in the initiation of saccades. The actual role of this cortical area is therefore somewhat questionable at present, even though deficiencies in eye movements regularly follow damage to it. Furthermore it has been reported that extensive bilateral damage to the visual association cortex of monkeys does not interfere with smooth pursuit or vergence movements. It may be that parts of the parietal lobe just in front of the visual association cortex are more important than has been realized previously.

SOME FUNCTIONAL ASPECTS OF THE CORTICOSPINAL TRACT

The *pyramidal tract* received its name historically from the medullary pyramids and, like many other historically named neural structures, has now come to mean different things to different people. For some, it has the functional meaning of the combination of the corticospinal and corticobulbar tracts, with the emphasis on the fibers that more or less directly affect motor neurons. For others, it retains the historical-anatomical meaning and is the collection of fibers in the medullary pyramids. For still others, it means the collection of neurons whose destruction results in the clinically observed *pyramidal tract syndrome* (discussed shortly). People are sometimes misled into thinking that all three of these meanings refer to the same collection of fibers, but a major point of this chapter has been that they do not. For example, selective destruction of the medullary pyramids, though rare, is perverse enough not to cause the pyramidal tract syndrome. Also many corticospinal and corticobulbar fibers have no particular effect on motor neurons but instead modulate transmission through ascending pathways.

The pyramidal system (in the third sense, referring to fibers whose destruction causes spastic paralysis) is commonly considered in contrast to the *extrapyramidal* system. Strictly speaking, "extra-pyramidal" should mean everything except the pyramidal system (that is, at the very least, the cerebellum and basal ganglia). However, it is generally used with reference to the basal ganglia only. This pyramidal-versus-extrapyramidal terminology is rife with logical inconsistencies and opportunities for confusion. For example (as Fig. 12-2 indicates and the next chapter expands on), the principal route through which the basal ganglia are able to affect motor output is via the cerebral cortex, and from there at least partially by way of corticospinal neurons. Also, as noted previously, collaterals of at least some corticospinal fibers project to the basal ganglia; should these collaterals be considered part of the pyramidal or extrapyramidal system? Since the two systems are so thoroughly intertwined, it would probably be reasonable to abandon this pyramidal-versus-extrapyramidal terminology. This is unlikely to happen in the near future though, because the terms have been widely used for a long time and provide a convenient shorthand way to speak of two broad classes of motor disorders. As will be seen in the next chapter, the effects of damage to the basal ganglia are quite distinct from the pyramidal tract syndrome.

Spastic hemiplegia (pyramidal tract syndrome)

The most common cause of motor problems clinically attributed to the pyramidal system is a cerebrovascular accident involving the motor and premotor cortex or the posterior limb of the internal capsule. Immediately after the stroke a period of flaccid paralysis ensues, analogous to spinal shock. After a period of days to weeks, tone and reflexes return and increase, and the situation resolves into *spastic hemiplegia* or *hemiparesis*.* Muscle tone is increased in a characteristic way, such that when a muscle is stretched (as by an examiner forcibly flexing the patient's leg), its resistance to further stretch increases greatly. At some point this increased resistance suddenly melts away, and the limb collapses in flexion (or extension, if the arm is forcibly extended). This sudden collapse is called the *clasp-knife effect* and is usually attributed to inhibition of motor neurons by Golgi tendon organs; inhibitory effects of the secondary endings of muscle spindles are also likely to be important. The increased tone is especially pronounced in the flexors of the arm and fingers and in the extensors of the leg, leading to a typical hemiparetic stance and gait. Standard stretch reflexes such as the knee-jerk reflex are hyperactive. Sudden stretch of a muscle may lead to *clonus*, a rapid series of rhythmic contractions main-

tained for the duration of the stretch. This combination of hypertonia and hyperreflexia is spasticity. In addition, certain normal reflexes disappear and some abnormal reflexes appear. The best known of the latter is Babinski's sign. Interestingly, Babinski's sign is normally seen in human infants before the corticospinal tract is fully myelinated and functional and is also seen after selective damage to the corticospinal tract in the cerebral peduncle.

Some voluntary movement eventually returns, again in a characteristic pattern. Proximal muscles recover more than distal muscles, and movements of the fingers are the most severely and permanently affected. Skilled movements recover less than do coarser movements of entire limbs.

ADDITIONAL READING

Balagura, S., and Katz, R.G.: Undecussated innervation to the sternocleidomastoid muscle: a reinstatement, Ann. Neurol. 7:84, 1980.

Bender, M.B.: Brain control of horizontal and vertical eye movements, Brain **103**:23, 1980.

Brinkman, J., and Kuypers, H.G.J.M.: Cerebral control of contralateral and ipsilateral arm, hand and finger movements in the split-brain rhesus monkey, Brain **96**:653, 1973. *Complex but interesting experiments whose results indicate that each cerebral hemisphere can exercise some control over the movements of both arms but not the fingers of both hands.*

Brodal, A.: Self-observations and neuro-anatomical considerations after a stroke, Brain **96**:675, 1973. *A fascinating account by an eminent neuroanatomist of a stroke suffered by him and the pattern of his recovery. Such an individual is able to provide information about motor control and other cerebral functions that is probably impossible to obtain in any other way.*

Bucy, P., Keplinger, J.E., and Siqueira, E.B.: Destruction of the "pyramidal tract" in man, J. Neurosurg. **21**:385, 1964.

Denny-Brown, D., and Chambers, R.A.: Physiological aspects of visual perception, I: functional aspects of visual cortex, Arch. Neurol. **33**:219, 1976. *Although it is mainly concerned with visual perception, this study nevertheless provides some information about the role of the occipital cortex in eye movements.*

Desmedt, J.E., editor: Cerebral motor control in man: long loop mechanisms, Progress in clinical neurophysiology, vol. 4, Munich, 1978, S. Karger.

Endo, K., Araki, T., and Yagi, N.: The distribution and pattern of axon branching of pyramidal tract cells, Brain Res. **57**:484, 1973.

Gay, A.J., et al.: Eye movement disorders, St. Louis, 1974, The C.V. Mosby Co.

Gilman, S., Lieberman, J.S., and Marco, L.A.: Spinal mechanisms underlying the effects of unilateral ablation of areas 4 and 6 in monkeys, Brain **97**:49, 1974. *How are motor and premotor cortex related to the mechanism of spasticity?*

Goldberg, M.E., and Robinson, D.L.: Visual mechanisms underlying gaze: function of the cerebral cortex. In Baker, R., and Berthoz, A., editors: Control of gaze by brain stem neurons, Developments in neuroscience, vol. 1, New York, 1977, Elsevier North-Holland, Inc.

Grillner, S.: Locomotion in vertebrates: central mechanisms and reflex interaction, Physiol. Rev. **55**:247, 1975. *A review of what is known about central motor programs.*

Holmes, G.: The cerebral integration of the ocular movements, Brit. Med. J. **2**:107, 1938. *The now-traditional version, which is probably a serious oversimplification.*

Hoyt, W.F., and Frisén, L.: Supranuclear ocular motor control: some

---

*Hemiplegia (Greek, -plegia, = stroke), strictly speaking, means total paralysis on one side. Since some voluntary movement returns after injury to the motor cortex or internal capsule, the condition is actually a hemiparesis (Greek, paresis = slackening), indicating weakness or partial paralysis.

clinical considerations—1974. In Lennerstrand, G., and Bachy-y-Rita, P., editors: Basic mechanisms of ocular motility and their clinical implications, Wenner-Gren Center International Symposium series, vol. 24, Elmsford, N.Y., 1975, Pergamon Press.

Künzle, H., and Akert, K.: Efferent connections of cortical area 8 (frontal eye field) in *Macaca fascicularis:* a reinvestigation using the autoradiographic technique, J. Comp. Neurol. **173:**147, 1977.

Kuypers, H.G.J.M.: Corticobulbar connexions to the pons and lower brain-stem in man, Brain **81:**364, 1958.

Lawrence, D.G., and Hopkins, D.A.: The development of motor control in the rhesus monkey: evidence concerning the role of corticomotoneuronal connections, Brain **99:**235, 1966.

Lawrence, D.G., and Kuypers, H.G.J.M.: The functional organization of the motor system in the monkey, I: the effects of bilateral pyramidal lesions; II: the effects of lesions of the descending brain-stem pathways, Brain **91:**1 and 15, 1968. *Two classic papers on the chronic effects of selective corticospinal lesions in primates, including information about which other descending pathways are able to compensate for loss of the corticospinal tract.*

Lynch, J.C., et al.: Parietal lobe mechanisms for directed visual attention, J. Neurophysiol. **40:**362, 1977.

Phillips, C.G., and Porter, R.: Corticospinal neurones: their role in movement, New York, 1977, Academic Press, Inc. *An interesting, well-written account of the development and current state of knowledge about the corticospinal tract.*

Polit, A., and Bizzi, E.: Processes controlling arm movements in monkeys, Science **201:**1235, 1978. *An article dealing with the motor abilities of a monkey receiving no afferent input from one arm.*

Raphan, T., and Cohen, B.: Brainstem mechanisms for rapid and slow eye movements, Ann. Rev. Physiol. **40:**527, 1978.

Russell, J.R., and DeMyer, W.: The quantitative cortical origin of pyramidal axons of *Macaca rhesus,* Neurol. **11:**96, 1961.

Schiller, P.H., True, S.D., and Conway, J.L.: Effects of frontal eye field and superior colliculus ablations on eye movements, Science **206:**590, 1979.

Stein, R.B.: Peripheral control of movement, Physiol. Rev. **54:**215, 1974.

Talbott, R.E., and Humphrey, D.R., editors: Posture and movement, New York, 1979, Raven Press.

Wiesendanger, M.: The pyramidal tract: recent investigations on its morphology and function, Ergeb. Physiol. **61:**72, 1969.

CHAPTER 13

BASAL GANGLIA

In 1817 James Parkinson, an English country physician, published a brief monograph entitled *An Essay on the Shaking Palsy*, in which he described the symptoms of several individuals who had the disease that now bears his name. Parkinsonian patients, as described in more detail later in this chapter, are characterized by tremor, generally increased muscle tone, and difficulty in initiating voluntary movements (which are unusually slow once begun). Disorders of this sort, whose signs typically include involuntary movements and generalized alterations in muscle tone, have come to be associated with damage to the basal ganglia. They are often referred to as *extrapyramidal disorders*, although as explained in the last chapter, such terminology can be somewhat misleading; for example, at least some of the involuntary movements are actually effected through the corticospinal tract.

TERMINOLOGY

The term "basal ganglia" originally referred to all the masses of gray matter buried within the cerebrum and thus included the *putamen, caudate nucleus, globus pallidus, amygdala, claustrum,* and occasionally even the *thalamus* (Figs. 13-1 and 13-2). However, it is now used to refer to those structures whose damage causes "extrapyramidal" syndromes. This list of structures includes at least one brainstem nucleus but excludes some nuclei buried within the cerebrum. Thus the amygdala, claustrum, and thalamus are usually no longer spoken of as basal ganglia, since the amygdala is part of the limbic system, the claustrum has an unknown function, and the thalamus is part of a multitude of different pathways. Use of the term "basal ganglia" still varies, but most people mean the combination of caudate nucleus, putamen, globus pallidus, *subthalamic nucleus,* and *substantia nigra;* some include the *red nucleus* and the brainstem reticular formation as well.

Various names are applied to different combinations of members of the basal ganglia (Fig. 13-3). The putamen

and globus pallidus together comprise the *lenticular* (Latin = lens-shaped) (or *lentiform*) *nucleus*. Bridges of gray matter growing across the internal capsule between the putamen and the caudate nucleus give this region a striped appearance in certain planes of section, so the combination of the caudate and lenticular nuclei is called the *corpus striatum*. The caudate nucleus and putamen have a common embryological origin, identical histological appearances, and similar connections, so both together are called the *neostriatum,** or simply the *striatum*. Thus the striatum is a major subdivision of the corpus striatum.

These assorted names give rise to prefixes and suffixes that are used to describe fibers coming from or going to different members of the basal ganglia. "Strio-" and "-striate" are used for the striatum; thus *striopallidal* fibers go from the caudate nucleus or putamen to the globus pallidus, while *corticostriate* fibers go from the cerebral cortex to the caudate nucleus or putamen. The globus pallidus is also called the *pallidum*, so *pallidothalamic* fibers go from the globus pallidus to the thalamus. *Nigroreticular* fibers go from the substantia nigra to the reticular formation.

TOPOGRAPHY

The lenticular nucleus is shaped somewhat like a wedge cut from a sphere (Figs. 13-1 and 13-2). The putamen (Latin = husk), which is approximately coextensive with the insula, forms the outermost portion of this wedge. It is separated from the more medial globus pallidus by a thin *lateral medullary lamina* of myelinated fibers. The globus pallidus is itself divided into medial and lateral portions by a *medial medullary lamina*. In unstained sections through the lenticular nucleus, the globus pallidus has a distinctively pale appearance as a

---

*"Neo-" refers to the fact that the neostriatum is generally considered to be a recent phylogenetic acquisition. Using similar terminology, the globus pallidus and the amygdala are occasionally referred to as the *paleostriatum* and the *archistriatum*, respectively.

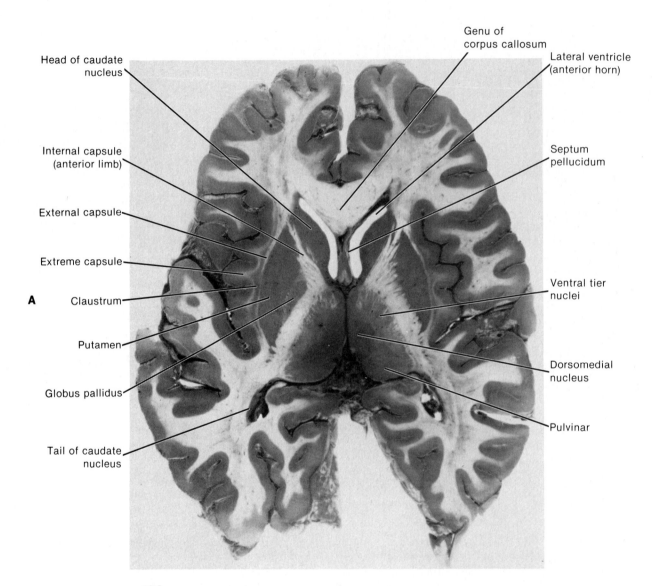

Head of caudate nucleus

Internal capsule (anterior limb)

External capsule

Extreme capsule

Claustrum

Putamen

Globus pallidus

Tail of caudate nucleus

Genu of corpus callosum

Lateral ventricle (anterior horn)

Septum pellucidum

Ventral tier nuclei

Dorsomedial nucleus

Pulvinar

A

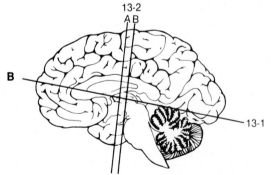

13-2
A B

B

13-1

Fig. 13-1. A, Basal ganglia and surrounding structures as seen in an approximately horizontal section. **B,** Planes of section for Figs. 13-1 and 13-2.

Fig. 13-2. Basal ganglia and surrounding structures as seen in coronal sections. (Shown on opposite page.)

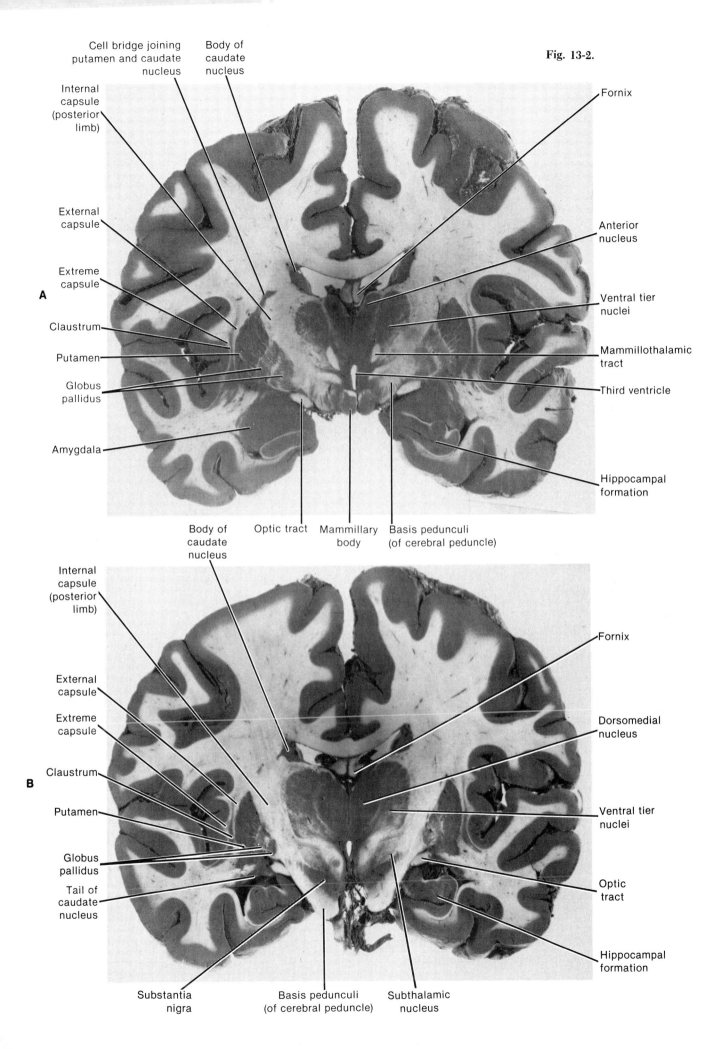

Cell bridge joining
putamen and caudate
nucleus

Body of
caudate
nucleus

Fig. 13-2.

Internal
capsule
(posterior
limb)

Fornix

External
capsule

Anterior
nucleus

Extreme
capsule

A

Ventral tier
nuclei

Claustrum

Mammillothalamic
tract

Putamen

Third ventricle

Globus
pallidus

Amygdala

Hippocampal
formation

Body of
caudate
nucleus

Optic tract

Mammillary
body

Basis pedunculi
(of cerebral peduncle)

Internal
capsule
(posterior
limb)

Fornix

External
capsule

Dorsomedial
nucleus

Extreme
capsule

B

Claustrum

Putamen

Ventral tier
nuclei

Globus
pallidus

Optic
tract

Tail of
caudate
nucleus

Hippocampal
formation

Substantia
nigra

Basis pedunculi
(of cerebral peduncle)

Subthalamic
nucleus

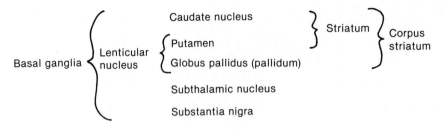

Fig. 13-3. Terminology associated with the basal ganglia.

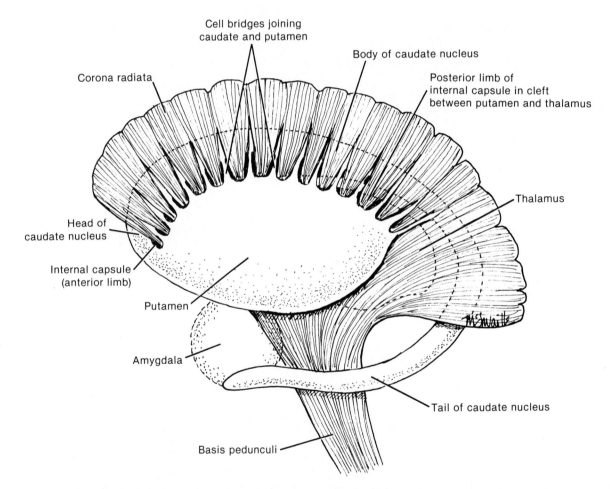

Fig. 13-4. Schematic drawing of what the corpus striatum, amygdala, thalamus, and internal capsule would look like if they were all isolated from the rest of the brain.

result of the large number of myelinated fibers that traverse it, terminate in it, and originate in it. (In myelin-stained sections like those shown in Figs. 13-8 and 13-11, it will therefore be relatively dark.)

The caudate nucleus starts out embryologically from the same mass of cells that gives rise to the putamen. In the course of development, the caudate nucleus remains in the wall of the lateral ventricle and grows around with it in a C-shaped course. The caudate nucleus of the adult

has an enlarged *head* that bulges into the anterior horn, a *body* that forms the lateral wall of the body of the ventricle, and a slender *tail* that borders on the inferior horn (Figs. 2-15 to 2-19, 13-1, 13-2, and 13-4). The caudate nucleus and putamen retain their embryological continuity just above the orbital surface of the frontal lobe, where the head of the caudate fuses with the anterior part of the putamen. In the temporal lobe, the tail of the caudate nucleus is continuous with the amygdala, which

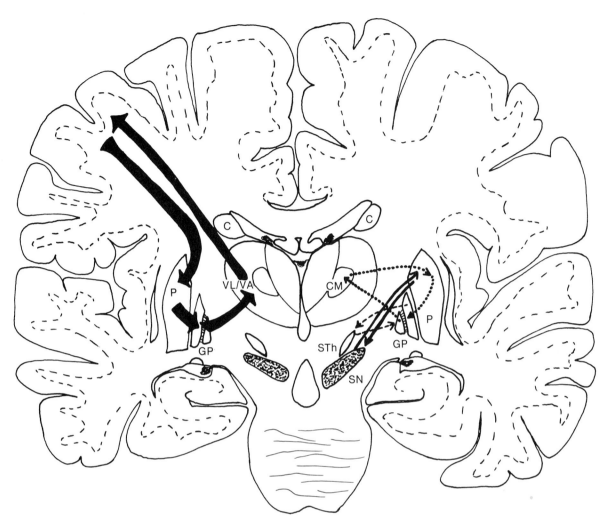

Fig. 13-5. Major neural circuits involving the basal ganglia; plane of section similar to Fig. 13-2, *B*. The major circuit is shown on the left: from widespread cortical areas, through the corpus striatum and the VL/VA complex of the thalamus, and back to motor and premotor cortex. Other circuits are shown on the right: (1) reciprocal connections between the striatum and substantia nigra (solid lines); (2) reciprocal connections between the globus pallidus and subthalamic nucleus (dashed lines); and (3) loop from the globus pallidus to the centromedian nucleus, the striatum, and back to the globus pallidus (dotted lines). For the sake of simplicity, no connections of the caudate nucleus are shown, but they are approximately the same as those of the putamen. Some artistic liberties were taken in putting the VL/VA complex and the centromedian nucleus in the same plane, since the VL/VA is actually slightly anterior to this section. *C*, Caudate nucleus; *CM*, centromedian nucleus of thalamus; *GP*, globus pallidus; *P*, putamen; *SN*, substantia nigra; *STh*, subthalamic nucleus; *VL/VA*, ventral lateral and ventral anterior nuclei of thalamus.

in turn is continuous with the putamen (Figs. 13-2 and 13-4), but these physical continuities are of no apparent functional significance.

CONNECTIONS OF THE BASAL GANGLIA

The corpus striatum forms by far the largest part of the basal ganglia, yet it has no way to directly affect motor neurons (Fig. 12-2). Thus the only way the corpus striatum can play a role in the control of movement is by somehow influencing one or more of the descending

pathways already mentioned. The principal way in which it does so is by way of the neural circuit shown in Fig. 13-5. The striatum (caudate nucleus and putamen) is the major "afferent" center of the basal ganglia, receiving inputs from widespread areas of the cerebral cortex. The striatum projects to the globus pallidus, which in turn projects to the VL/VA complex of the thalamus. Since the VL/VA projects to the motor and premotor cortex, this is a route by which the basal ganglia can influence the activity of the corticospinal tract.

The same route permits effects on the rubrospinal and reticulospinal tracts, since numerous corticorubral and corticoreticular fibers originate in motor and premotor cortex.

The remaining connections of the basal ganglia are, to a great extent, additional neural loops grafted onto or into the major circuit just described (Fig. 13-5). Reciprocal connections between the striatum and the substantia nigra form one such loop; reciprocal connections between the globus pallidus and the subthalamic nucleus form a second; and a pathway from the intralaminar nuclei through the striatum and globus pallidus and back to the intralaminar nuclei forms a third loop.

In the account that follows, only the best documented connections of the basal ganglia are described. Sad to say, the function of most of these connections is unknown. The best we can do at present is consider the consequences of disruption of some of them.

Striatum

The caudate nucleus and putamen receive inputs from the cerebral cortex, the substantia nigra, and the intralaminar nuclei of the thalamus (Fig. 13-6). The cortical input is by far the most massive of the three. These fibers originate in all areas of the cortex, pass through the internal and external capsules, and end in a roughly topographical pattern in the striatum; the projection from the motor and somatosensory cortex is particularly

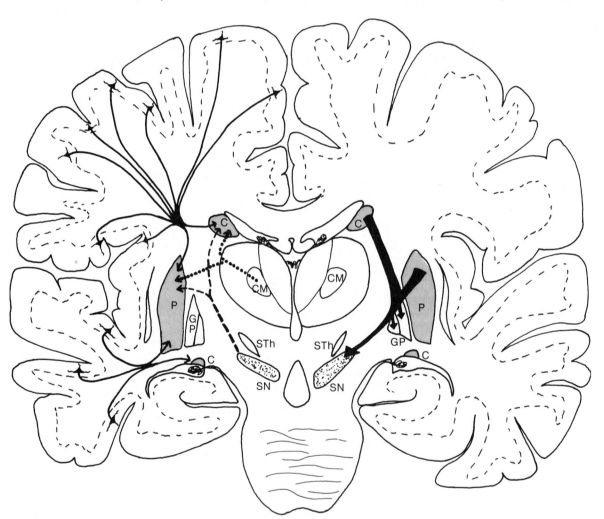

Fig. 13-6. Connections of the striatum (putamen and caudate nucleus); afferents to the striatum on the left, efferents from the striatum on the right. Plane of section and abbreviations as in Fig. 13-5. Major inputs to the striatum are from widespread cortical areas (solid lines), the substantia nigra (dashed lines), and the intralaminar nuclei of the thalamus, especially the centromedian nucleus (dotted lines). The striatal outputs go to both segments of the globus pallidus and to the substantia nigra. For the sake of simplicity, the connections of the tail of the caudate nucleus are mostly omitted, but they are like those of the rest of the caudate nucleus.

heavy. Thus the basal ganglia are constantly informed about most aspects of cortical function. The substantia nigra projects to all areas of the striatum in a point-to-point fashion by way of very fine axons that use dopamine as their neurotransmitter. Destruction of this *nigrostriatal* pathway is the major factor causing Parkinson's disease. Finally, the intralaminar nuclei, especially the centromedian nucleus, project to the striatum. Many of these same fibers, as mentioned in Chapter 10, have collateral branches that end in the cerebral cortex. This *thalamostriate* pathway is particularly well developed in primates, but virtually nothing is known of its function. As described later in this chapter, various clinical findings can be associated with damage to different parts of the basal ganglionic system; however, there are no particular symptoms that we can ascribe to malfunction of the thalamus–corpus striatum–thalamus loop.

Striatal efferents collect into numerous bundles of myelinated fibers that converge on the globus pallidus. These *striopallidal* fibers give off branches to both segments of the globus pallidus; then many of them con-

tinue caudally to end in the substantia nigra. Since the major output of the substantia nigra is back to the striatum (Fig. 13-5), the striatum must depend on the globus pallidus for most of the influence it exerts on the control of movement.

Globus pallidus

Afferents to both segments of the globus pallidus arise in the striatum and the subthalamic nucleus (Fig. 13-7). As Fig. 13-8 shows, the subthalamic nucleus is located right across the internal capsule from the globus pallidus. The small bundles of fibers that cross the internal capsule and interconnect these two nuclei are collectively called the *subthalamic fasciculus*.

Although the two segments of the globus pallidus have similar inputs, their efferents are separate and distinct (Fig. 13-7). The lateral segment projects through the subthalamic fasciculus to the subthalamic nucleus. The medial pallidal segment projects mainly to the thalamus through two collections of fibers (Fig. 13-9). One collection, the *lenticular fasciculus*, runs directly

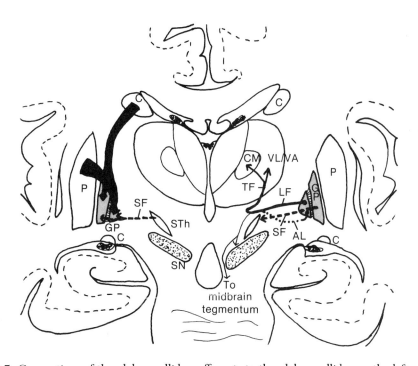

Fig. 13-7. Connections of the globus pallidus; afferents to the globus pallidus on the left, efferents from the globus pallidus on the right. Plane of section as in Fig. 13-5. Major inputs project to both segments of the globus pallidus from the striatum (solid line) and the subthalamic nucleus (dashed lines). Efferents from the lateral pallidal segment project back to the subthalamic nucleus (dashed line). Efferents from the medial pallidal segment go mainly to the VL/VA complex and the centromedian nucleus of the thalamus; a smaller number go to the substantia nigra, the midbrain tegmentum (and thence to the reticular formation) and to the habenula (not shown). *AL*, Ansa lenticularis; *C*, caudate nucleus; *CM*, centromedian nucleus of thalamus; *GP*, globus pallidus; *LF*, lenticular fasciculus; *P*, putamen; *SF*, subthalamic fasciculus; *SN*, substantia nigra; *STh*, subthalamic nucleus; *TF*, thalamic fasciculus; *VL/VA*, ventral lateral and ventral anterior nuclei of thalamus.

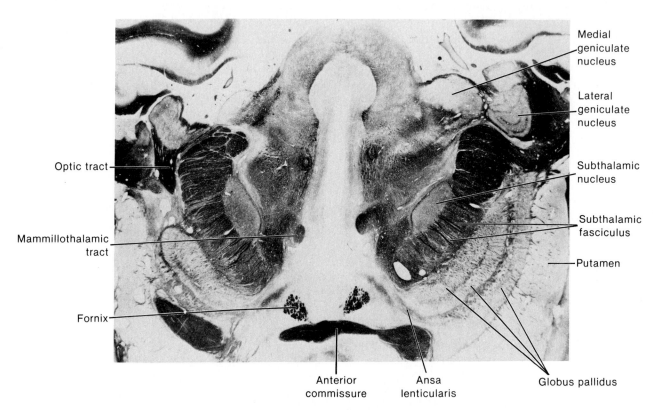

Fig. 13-8. The subthalamic fasciculus as seen in a horizontal section (same section as Fig. 11-10). Subthalamic fasciculus is a collective term for the small bundles of fibers that pass through the internal capsule interconnecting the subthalamic nucleus and the globus pallidus.

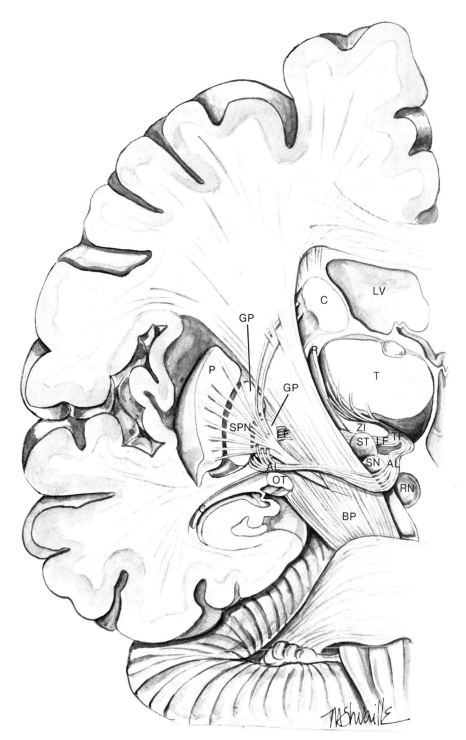

Fig. 13-9. Schematic drawing of the paths of the ansa lenticularis and the lenticular fasciculus as seen in an anterior view of a partially dissected brain. The ansa lenticularis loops around the medial edge of the internal capsule, while the lenticular fasciculus passes through the internal capsule. The two bundles join to form the thalamic fasciculus. The subthalamic fasciculus is not indicated in this drawing. *AL*, Ansa lenticularis; *BP*, basis pedunculi; *C*, caudate nucleus; *GP*, globus pallidus; *LF*, lenticular fasciculus; *LV*, lateral ventricle; *OT*, optic tract; *P*, putamen; *R*, thalamic reticular nucleus; *RN*, red nucleus; *SN*, substantia nigra; *SPN*, striopallidal and strionigral fibers; *ST*, subthalamic nucleus; *T*, thalamus; *TF*, thalamic fasciculus; *ZI*, zona incerta. (Modified from Nieuwenhuys, R., et al.: The human central nervous system, New York, 1978, Springer-Verlag, Inc.)

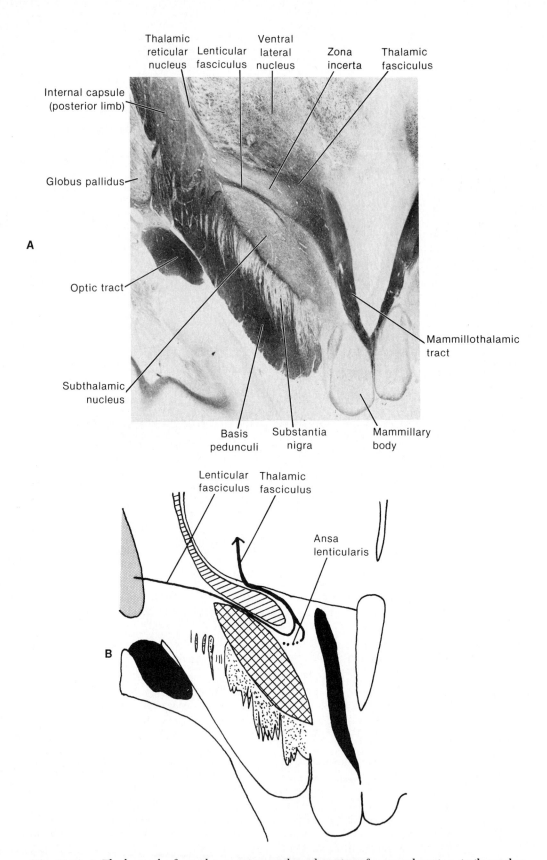

Fig. 13-10. A, The lenticular fasciculus seen in an enlarged portion of a coronal section similar to that shown in Fig. 10-9. The path of the fibers in the lenticular fasciculus is shown in **B,** as is part of the course of the ansa lenticularis, which loops around the medial edge of the internal capsule (out of the plane of section; dotted portion) and joins the lenticular fasciculus to form the thalamic fasciculus.

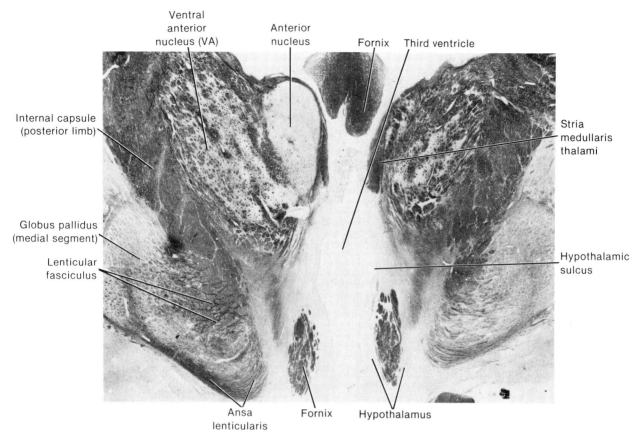

Fig. 13-11. The ansa lenticularis seen in an enlarged portion of a coronal section similar to that shown in Fig. 10-10.

through the internal capsule and then passes medially as a sheet of fibers between the subthalamic nucleus and the zona incerta (Fig. 13-10). At the medial edge of the zona incerta, the lenticular fasciculus makes a hairpin turn in a lateral and dorsal direction and enters the thalamus. The second collection loops around the medial edge of the internal capsule as the *ansa lenticularis* (Latin, ansa = loop) (Figs. 13-9 and 13-11); it joins the lenticular fasciculus to form the *thalamic fasciculus* and enters the thalamus. The thalamic fasciculus then terminates in the VL/VA complex and in the intralaminar nuclei, particularly the centromedian nucleus. The VL and VA project to the motor and premotor cortex, thus completing the principal circuit of the basal ganglia (Fig. 13-5).

A few fibers leave the ansa lenticularis and lenticular fasciculus to end in the habenula, in the substantia nigra, and in a portion of the midbrain tegmentum that in turn projects to the reticular formation. However, their numbers are meager compared to the major outputs to the thalamus and subthalamic nucleus.

Subthalamic nucleus

The contacts of the subthalamic nucleus are simple and straightforward, consisting for the most part of reciprocal connections with the globus pallidus (Fig. 13-12). Subthalamic efferents to the substantia nigra and to the VL/VA have also been described, but these are relatively few in number.

Substantia nigra

The major contacts of the substantia nigra are its reciprocal connections with the caudate nucleus and putamen (Fig. 13-12). However, recent work has shown that nigral connections are somewhat more extensive than had been realized previously. Additional inputs are received from the globus pallidus, subthalamic nucleus, and hypothalamus. Additional outputs go to the thalamus (the VL/VA), the superior colliculus, and the reticular formation. The latter two are of considerable interest, since they raise the possibility that the basal ganglia could influence motor neurons via tectospinal and reticulospinal pathways without going through the cere-

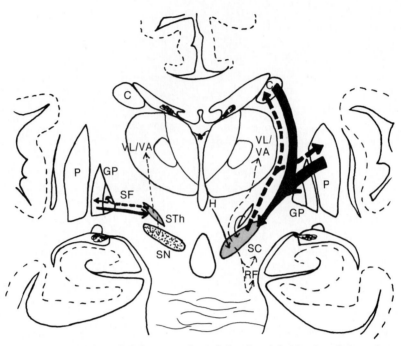

Fig. 13-12. Connections of the subthalamic nucleus (left side of diagram) and the substantia nigra (right side of diagram). Afferents to these structures are drawn in solid lines, efferents from them in dashed lines. Plane of section as in Fig. 13-5. Major contacts of the subthalamic nucleus are its reciprocal connections with the globus pallidus (via the subthalamic fasciculus); a few subthalamic efferents project to the substantia nigra and to the VL/VA. Major contacts of the substantia nigra are its reciprocal connections with the striatum. Additional nigral afferents arise in the globus pallidus, hypothalamus, and subthalamic nucleus. Additional nigral efferents project to the VL/VA, the superior colliculus, and the reticular formation. *C*, Caudate nucleus; *GP*, globus pallidus; *H*, hypothalamus; *P*, putamen; *RF*, reticular formation; *SC*, superior colliculus; *SF*, subthalamic fasciculus; *SN*, substantia nigra; *STh*, subthalamic nucleus; *VL/VA*, ventral lateral and ventral anterior nuclei of thalamus.

bral cortex first. Although little is known about the physiology of this alternative descending influence, it seems very likely that the route through the cerebral cortex is of considerably greater importance.

SOME FUNCTIONAL ASPECTS OF THE BASAL GANGLIA

Involuntary movements and disturbances of muscle tone figure prominently in most disorders involving the basal ganglia. The involuntary movements are customarily subdivided into tremors and states of *chorea*, *athetosis*, and *ballismus*. The disturbances of tone may be such that tone is increased in flexors and extensors generally (as in the rigidity of Parkinson's disease), or tone may be increased in only some muscles so that the patient's body is bent or twisted into an abnormal, relatively fixed posture. The latter condition is called *dystonia*. In still other cases, tone may be decreased.

Patients with chorea (Greek = dance) exhibit a series of nearly continuous rapid movements of the face,

tongue, or limbs (usually the distal portions of the limbs). The movements often resemble fragments of normal voluntary movements. *Huntington's chorea* is a hereditary disorder in which there is widespread degeneration of the cells of the striatum and the cerebral cortex. Typically symptoms first appear between the ages of 30 and 50 as involuntary choreiform movements. The movements slowly become more pronounced, and this symptom is followed by or accompanied by gradually developing dementia. The chorea is presumably caused by striatal degeneration and the dementia by cortical degeneration. This is a particularly nasty disease, since it is inherited in a dominant fashion but is usually not manifested until after individuals are old enough to have started families. There is at present no test that can determine if a potential victim is indeed a carrier, so there is no way to determine whether half of his or her children are likely to be affected.

Athetosis (Greek = without position) is characterized by slow, writhing movements, most pronounced in the hands and fingers, so that a patient may be unable to keep the affected limb in a fixed position (hence the name "athetosis"). The responsible lesion seems to be in the striatum. All intermediate forms between chorea and athetosis are seen, and questionable cases are often referred to as *choreoathetosis*. No one knows why a particular lesion in the striatum should induce one state rather than the other, although there is a tendency to associate chorea with damage to the caudate nucleus and athetosis with damage to the putamen.

Hemiballismus (Greek, ballismus = jumping about) is one of the most dramatic of the disorders of the basal ganglia. Its most prominent characteristic is wild flailing movements of one arm and leg. The responsible lesion is in the contralateral subthalamic nucleus. Hemiballismus is most often seen in older people, having been caused by a stroke involving a small ganglionic branch of the posterior cerebral artery. The reason movements are seen contralateral to the lesion is apparent from Fig. 13-12: each subthalamic nucleus is related by way of the globus pallidus and the VL/VA to the ipsilateral motor cortex; the motor cortex is concerned with movements of the contralateral side of the body.

Parkinsonism is the most common and probably the best-known disease involving the basal ganglia. The symptoms are quite variable in relative severity and onset, but they usually include tremor, rigidity, and difficulty in moving. The tremor is a *resting tremor*, characteristically involving the hands in a "pill-rolling" movement; it diminishes during voluntary movement and increases during emotional stress. The *rigidity* is caused by increased tone in all muscles although strength is nearly normal and reflexes are not particularly affected. The rigidity may be uniform throughout the range of movements imposed by an examiner (called *plastic* or *lead-pipe rigidity*), or it may be interrupted by a series of very brief relaxations (called *cog-wheel rigidity*). Thus Parkinsonian rigidity is quite distinct from spasticity, in which tone is increased selectively in the extensors of the leg and the flexors of the arm and can be overcome in the clasp-knife reaction, and in which stretch reflexes are hyperactive. Finally, the difficulty in moving (*bradykinesia*, or slow movements; *hypokinesia*, or few movements) is shown by such things as decreased blinking, an expressionless face, and the absence of the arm movements normally associated with walking. Bradykinesia and hypokinesia are fundamental deficits and are not simply the result of rigidity.

Treatment of disorders

Most disorders of the basal ganglia include striking positive signs (for example, tremor, rigidity, and ballistic movements), in which motor neurons are made to fire when they should not; they frequently include nega-tive signs as well (for example, hypokinesia), in which motor neurons cannot easily be made to fire by their owner. The positive signs led to the notion that the globus pallidus (through which most of the output of the basal ganglia funnels) is able to instigate excessive activity in the motor pathways but that this excitatory activity is normally held in check by the other members of the basal ganglia. Destruction of the striatum, subthalamic nucleus, or substantia nigra would then release the globus pallidus from some of its restraints. Since the principal effect of the globus pallidus is on motor and premotor cortex by way of the VL/VA complex, it was reasoned some time ago that destruction of this part of the thalamus would break the loop and thereby relieve the symptoms. Somewhat astoundingly, this turns out to be true. Stereotactic lesions in the VL/VA region (*thalamotomy*; the VL is the principal target) or in the medial segment of the globus pallidus are reasonably successful in relieving the tremor and rigidity of parkinsonism, the flailing movements of hemiballismus, and some (but not all) other involuntary movements and abnormalities of tone. In the case of hemiballismus, the excessive activity of the basal ganglia is apparently expressed solely through the corticospinal tract. This tract has been sectioned in the cerebral peduncle in a few humans (on the side contralateral to the ballistic movements) for the relief of hemiballismus. The involuntary movements were permanently abolished and a transient flaccid paralysis ensued on the side contralateral to the surgery; however, as explained in the last chapter, there were rather limited long-term deficits.

Unfortunately such surgery has no effect on negative signs such as hypokinesia, as though the basal ganglia normally play a role in the design or initiation of movement, so that once they are damaged this particular function is lost.

Considering the proximity of the VL/VA to the internal capsule and considering that thalamotomy does not relieve the negative signs, this surgery has always been a last resort, and other forms of treatment have long been sought. Postmortem examination of the brains of patients with parkinsonism indicated that damage is most consistently evident in the substantia nigra, reflecting degeneration of the pigmented nigral cells that normally manufacture dopamine and transport it to the striatum. It was therefore reasoned that if the dopamine could somehow be replaced, the symptoms might be ameliorated. Since dopamine does not cross the blood-brain barrier, it is necessary to administer *l*-dopa (levodopa), a precursor of dopamine that does cross the barrier. This form of therapy has proven to be highly successful for many but not all parkinsonian patients.

The many common features of the various syndromes caused by damage to diverse parts of the basal ganglia give rise to the concept of these neural structures as forming a finely tuned system in which malfunction of any part can throw the whole system out of balance. The study of the balancing mechanisms in neurochemical terms is currently a very active area of research. Thus a decrease in dopamine levels in the striatum causes parkinsonian symptoms. This can occur naturally (in Parkinson's disease) or as a side effect of drugs that act as dopamine antagonists (such as the phenothiazines used for psychiatric disorders). In contrast, increased levels of dopamine in the striatum, as in parkinsonian patients who receive too much *l*-dopa, can cause choreiform and athetoid movements as though the system were now tilted in the opposite direction. Great interest has been generated by the recent discovery that striatal synthesis of the transmitter γ-aminobutyric acid (GABA) is decreased in patients with Huntington's chorea. A number of other transmitters in the basal ganglia are known or suspected, but their study is at a very early stage.

ADDITIONAL READING

Brownstein, M.J.: Biochemical anatomy of the extrapyramidal system. In Fuxe, K., and Calne, D.B., editors: Dopaminergic ergot derivatives and motor function, Elmsford, N.Y., 1979, Pergamon Press.

Carpenter, M.B.: Athetosis and the basal ganglia: review of the literature and study of forty-two cases, Arch. Neurol. Psychiatr. 63:875, 1950.

DeLong, M.R., and Georgopoulos, A.P.: Physiology of the basal ganglia: a brief overview, Adv. Neurol. 23:137, 1979.

DeLong, M.R., and Strick, P.L.: Relation of basal ganglia, cerebellum, and motor cortex units to ramp and ballistic limb movements, Brain Res. 71:327, 1974. *One hypothesis about the basal ganglia is that they are responsible for the generation of slow movements, and the cerebellum is involved with rapid movements. Recordings from single cells in the basal ganglia indicate that while there may be some validity to this concept, things are not quite that simple.*

Denny-Brown, D.: The basal ganglia and their relation to disorders of movement, New York, 1962, Oxford University Press.

Dray, A.: The striatum and substantia nigra: a commentary on their relationships, Neurosci. 4:1407, 1979.

Flowers, K.: Some frequency response characteristics of Parkinsonism on pursuit tracking, Brain 101:19, 1978.

Flowers, K.: Lack of prediction in the motor behavior of Parkinsonism, Brain 101:35, 1978.

Goldman, P.S., and Nauta, W.J.H.: An intricately patterned prefrontocaudate projection in the rhesus monkey, J. Comp. Neurol. 171:369, 1977. *Recent results that indicate that the traditional view of the striatum as a uniformly organized structure is probably an oversimplification.*

Graybiel, A.M., and Ragsdale, C.W., Jr.: Histochemically distinct compartments in the striatum of human, monkey, and cat demonstrated by acetylthiocholinesterase staining, Proc. Nat. Acad. Science 75:5723, 1978. *Additional recent results, complementary to those of Goldman and Nauta, indicating that the striatum is a jigsaw puzzle in terms of both connections and neurotransmitters.*

Hallett, M., Shahani, B.T., and Young, R.R.: Analysis of stereotyped voluntary movements at the elbow in patients with Parkinson's disease, J. Neurol. Neurosurg. Psychiatry 40:1129, 1977.

Hopkins, D.A., and Niesser, L.W.: Substantia nigra projections to the reticular formation, superior colliculus and central gray in the rat, cat and monkey, Neurosci. Lett. 2:253, 1976.

Hore, J., Meyer-Lohmann, J., and Brooks, V.B.: Basal ganglia cooling disables learned arm movements of monkeys in the absence of visual guidance, Science 195:584, 1977. *Some exciting work bearing on the possible role of the basal ganglia in the formulation of voluntary movements.*

Kemp, J.M., and Powell, T.P.S.: The connexions of the striatum and globus pallidus: synthesis and speculation, Philos. Trans. R. Soc. Lond. B262:441, 1971.

Martin, J.P.: The basal ganglia and posture, Tunbridge Wells, U.K., 1967, Pitman Medical Publishing Co., Ltd.

Molina-Negro, P.: Surgery for abnormal movements. In Rasmussen, T., and Marino, R., editors: Functional neurosurgery, New York, 1979, Raven Press.

Nauta, H.J.W., and Cole, M.: Efferent projections of the subthalamic nucleus: an autoradiographic study in monkey and cat, J. Comp. Neurol. 180:1, 1978.

Nauta, W.J.H., and Domesick, V.B.: The anatomy of the extrapyramidal system. In Fuxe, K., and Calne, D.B., editors, Dopaminergic ergot derivatives and motor function, Elmsford, N.Y., 1979, Pergamon Press.

Poirier, L.J., Sourkes, T.L., and Bédard, P.J., editors: The extrapyramidal system and its disorders, Adv. Neurol., vol. 24, 1979.

Spokes, E.G.S.: Neurochemical alterations in Huntington's chorea: a study of post-mortem brain tissue, Brain 103:179, 1980.

Stern, G.: The effects of lesions in substantia nigra, Brain 89:449, 1966. *An example of one of the major obstacles in studying the function of the basal ganglia: experimental lesions generally do not reproduce the symptoms of human diseases.*

Teräv, H., and Calne, D.B.: Developments in understanding the physiology and pharmacology of Parkinsonism, Acta Neurol. Scand. 60:1, 1979.

Whittier, J.R.: Ballism and the subthalamic nucleus (nucleus hypothalamicus; corpus Luysi). Review of the literature and study of thirty cases, Arch. Neurol. Psychiatr. 58:672, 1947.

Yahr, M.D., editor: The basal ganglia, New York, 1976, Raven Press.

CHAPTER 14

CEREBELLUM

Cerebellum literally means "little brain," and in a real sense it is. This semidetached mass of neural tissue covers most of the posterior surface of the brainstem, anchored there by three pairs of fiber bundles called *cerebellar peduncles*. Sensory inputs of virtually every description find their way to the uniquely structured cortex of the cerebellum, which in turn projects (via a set of *deep cerebellar nuclei*) to various sites in the brainstem and thalamus. Although the cerebellum is extensively concerned with the processing of sensory information, and although it has no way to influence motor neurons directly, it is considered part of the motor system because cerebellar damage results in abnormalities of equilibrium, of muscle tone and postural control, and of coordination of voluntary movements.

GENERAL PLAN OF THE CEREBELLUM
Gross anatomy

The outside of the cerebellum has a banded appearance, as though its surface were folded like an accordion (Figs. 14-1 and 14-2). This folding is a successful device for increasing the cerebellar surface area: if the cortex could be drawn out into a flat sheet, it would be over 1 m long. Deep fissures, most easily seen in sagittal sections (Fig. 14-4), indent the cerebellar surface. Smaller fissures indent the walls of these deep fissures, with the result that the entire cerebellar surface is made up of cortical ridges called *folia*, most of which are transversely oriented. Beneath the cortex is a mass of white matter, the *medullary center* of the cerebellum, which is composed of fibers going to or coming from the cerebellar cortex.

The first fissure to appear during development is the *posterolateral fissure*, which separates the *flocculonodular lobe* from the *corpus cerebelli*. In humans, the corpus cerebelli is by far the larger of the two, and the posterolateral fissure is so deep that the *flocculus* of each side is almost pinched off from the rest of the

cerebellum (Figs. 14-3 and 14-5). The *primary fissure*, a prominent landmark in midsagittal sections of the cerebellum, subdivides the corpus cerebelli into *anterior* and *posterior lobes* (Figs. 14-4 and 14-5).

The cerebellum may also be subdivided into longitudinal zones, perpendicular to the fissures, which cut across the anterior, posterior, and flocculonodular lobes (Fig. 14-5). The most medial zone, straddling the midline, is the *vermis* (Latin = worm). On either side of the vermis is the *intermediate* (or *paravermal*) *zone*. The most lateral portions, which comprise most of the cerebellum, are the *cerebellar hemispheres*. The vermis is fairly clearly set off from more lateral portions on the inferior surface of the cerebellum (Fig. 14-2), but other longitudinal lines of separation are not very obvious from the outside (for example, Fig. 14-1). The demarcation into longitudinal zones is based on function and on patterns of connections, as will be described shortly. Cerebellar cortex has the same structure everywhere and is smoothly continuous from one hemisphere across the midline to the other. The fissures that carve the cerebellum into *lobules* and folia are also continuous across the midline, so that each transverse wedge of cerebellum has a vermal portion and a more lateral portion. Thus the *nodulus* is the vermal portion of the flocculonodular lobe and continues laterally into the flocculus. An assortment of exotic names is applied to the lobules and the vermal areas of the corpus cerebelli (Fig. 14-5), and a Roman numeral system is used as well for the vermis, but for the most part these names and numbers are of limited utility in clinical settings. The *tonsils* are the hemispheral portion just across the posterolateral fissure from the flocculi; appropriately enough, their vermal continuation is the *uvula*.

The cerebellum is attached to the brainstem by three substantial peduncles on each side. The *inferior cerebel-*

Text continued on p. 242.

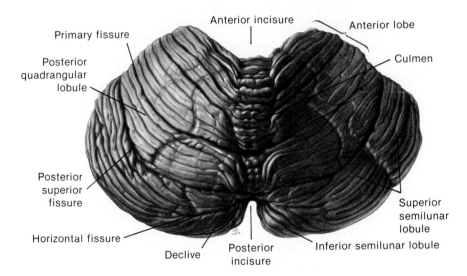

Fig. 14-1. Superior surface of the cerebellum (the surface normally covered by the tentorium cerebelli). (From Mettler, F.A.: Neuroanatomy, ed. 2, St. Louis, 1948, The C.V. Mosby Co.)

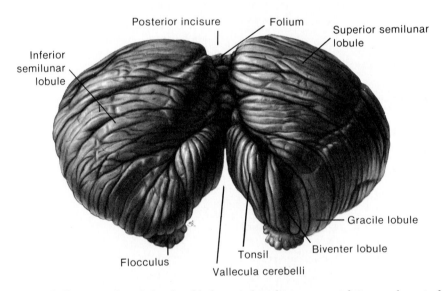

Fig. 14-2. Cerebellum seen from behind and below, as though one were sighting up the spinal cord. (From Mettler, F.A.: Neuroanatomy, ed. 2, St. Louis, 1948, The C.V. Mosby Co.)

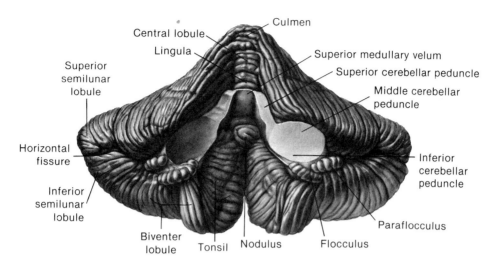

Fig. 14-3. Ventral surface of a cerebellum that had been removed from the brainstem by severing the cerebellar peduncles. The view is as if one were looking up from the floor of the fourth ventricle toward its roof. (From Mettler, F.A.: Neuroanatomy, ed. 2, St. Louis, 1948, The C.V. Mosby Co.)

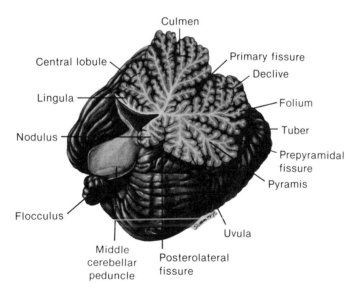

Fig. 14-4. Medial surface of a hemisected cerebellum, demonstrating the depth of many of the cerebellar fissures and the way in which the fissures divide the vermis into a number of lobules. The same fissures continue laterally and divide up the cerebellar hemispheres. (From Mettler, F.A.: Neuroanatomy, ed. 2, St. Louis, 1948, The C.V. Mosby Co.)

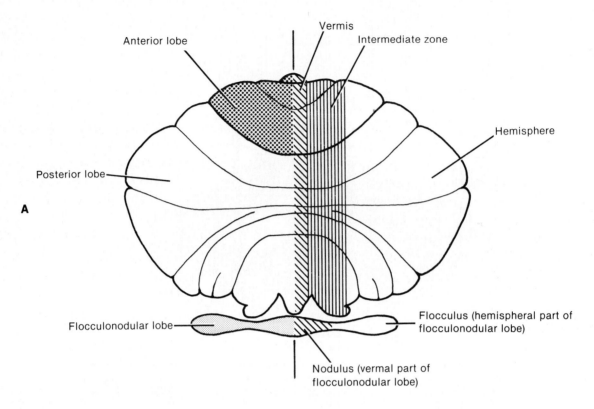

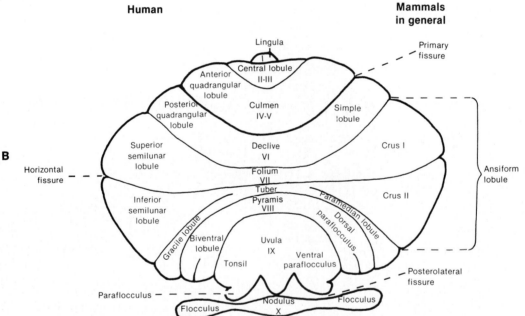

Fig. 14-5. Cerebellar terminology on a schematic cerebellum projected as though the cerebellum were flattened out with its vermis now in one plane (compare with Figs. 14-1 to 14-4). **A**, General division into transversely oriented lobes (on the left side of the diagram) and into longitudinal zones (on the right). **B**, Terminology for the various subdivisions of the vermis (including Roman numerals) and lobules of the hemispheres. On the left side of the diagram are terms classically used for the human cerebellum. On the right side are terms from comparative anatomy used more frequently in describing the cerebella of experimental animals. (Modified from Larsell, O.: Anatomy of the nervous system, ed. 2, New York, 1951, Appleton-Century-Crofts.)

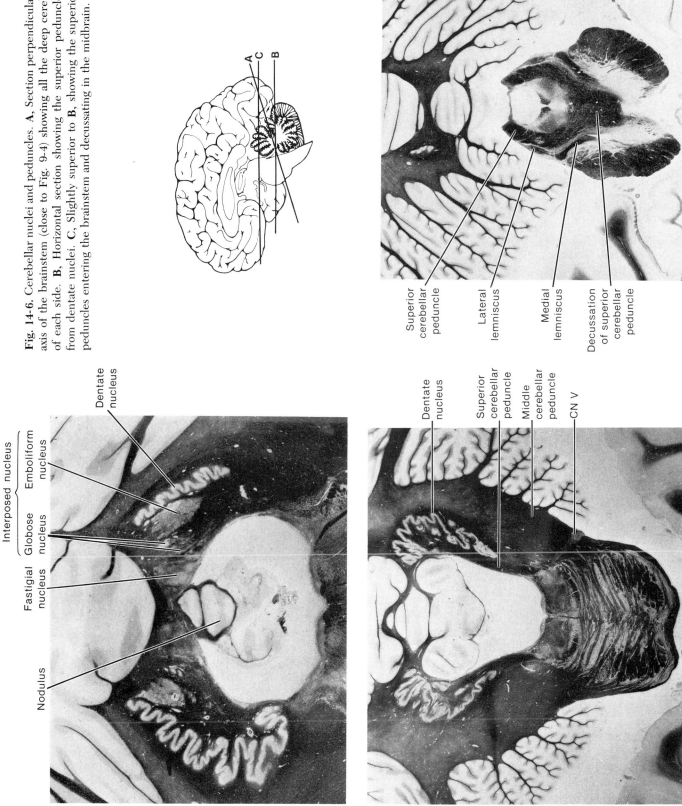

Fig. 14-6. Cerebellar nuclei and peduncles. **A,** Section perpendicular to the long axis of the brainstem (close to Fig. 9-4) showing all the deep cerebellar nuclei of each side. **B,** Horizontal section showing the superior peduncles emerging from dentate nuclei. **C,** Slightly superior to **B,** showing the superior cerebellar peduncles entering the brainstem and decussating in the midbrain.

A

Nodulus

Fastigial nucleus

Interposed nucleus
Globose nucleus
Emboliform nucleus

Dentate nucleus

B

Dentate nucleus

Superior cerebellar peduncle

Middle cerebellar peduncle

CN V

C

Superior cerebellar peduncle

Lateral lemniscus

Medial lemniscus

Decussation of superior cerebellar peduncle

lar peduncle (or *restiform body**) (Figs. 8-8 and 8-9) is composed mainly of afferents to the cerebellum from the spinal cord and brainstem. The *middle cerebellar peduncle* (or *brachium pontis*) (Fig. 8-10) is the largest of the three. It is composed virtually exclusively of afferents to the cerebellum from the *pontine nuclei*, principally of the contralateral side. The *superior cerebellar peduncle* (or *brachium conjunctivum†*) (Figs. 8-11 to 8-15 and 14-6) contains the major efferent pathways from the cerebellum.

A series of *deep cerebellar nuclei* is buried in the medullary center of each side of the cerebellum (Fig. 14-6). The most lateral is the *dentate nucleus*, a crumpled sheet of cells that looks strikingly like the inferior olivary nucleus. Most of the fibers in the superior cerebellar peduncle originate from the dentate nucleus and emerge from its medially facing mouth, or *hilus*. Medial to the dentate nucleus are the *emboliform nucleus* and the *globose nucleus*. In most nonhuman cerebella, the equivalent cells form a single nuclear mass called the *interposed nucleus* (or *nucleus interpositus*), and so

---

*There is a bit of a logical inconsistency in using the terms "inferior cerebellar peduncle" and "restiform body" interchangeably. The *juxtarestiform body*, carrying vestibular traffic to and from the cerebellum, is also part of the inferior cerebellar peduncle. In common usage, the logical inconsistency is often ignored.

†A similar logical inconsistency exists in using the terms "superior cerebellar peduncle" and "brachium conjunctivum" synonymously. "Brachium conjunctivum" refers specifically to the large mass of cerebellar efferents bound mostly for the red nucleus and thalamus, whereas the total superior cerebellar peduncle also includes a few cerebellar afferents such as those of the anterior spinocerebellar tract.

even in human neuroanatomy the term "interposed nucleus" is often used for the combination of the emboliform and globose nuclei. Finally, the most medial of the deep cerebellar nuclei is the *fastigial nucleus*.

Cerebellar cortex

The cortex of the cerebellum has a uniform and fairly simple three-layered structure (Fig. 14-7). The most superficial layer is the *molecular layer*, consisting mainly of the axons and dendrites of various cerebellar neurons. Deep to the molecular layer is a single layer of large neurons called *Purkinje cells*. Finally, adjacent to the medullary center is the *granular layer*, composed mainly of small *granule cells* arranged in a stratum many cells thick. The molecular and granular layers also contain characteristic types of interneurons (Fig. 14-8), but the fundamental circuitry of the cerebellar cortex can be described in terms of Purkinje cells, granule cells, and the afferents to the cortex (Fig. 14-9).

Purkinje cells are the only neurons whose axons leave the cortex. They are, in addition, among the most anatomically distinctive neurons to be found in the nervous system. Each Purkinje cell has an intricate, extensive dendritic tree that is flattened out in a plane perpendicular to the long axis of the folium in which it resides (Fig. 14-9). Each granule cell sends its axon into the molecular layer, where it bifurcates to form a fine, unmyelinated *parallel fiber* running along the long axis of the folium. In its course, therefore, each parallel fiber passes through and synapses on the dendritic trees of a succession of Purkinje cells (as many as 500 of them). Each of us is estimated to have an incredible 10^{10} granule

Purkinje cell layer   Molecular layer   Granular layer

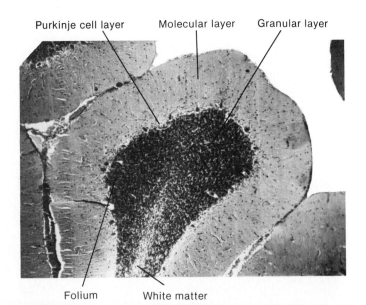

Folium   White matter

Purkinje cell layer   Molecular layer   Granular layer

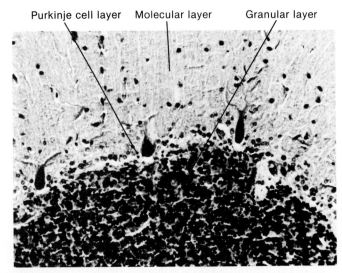

Fig. 14-7. Low-power and high-power micrographs of the cerebellar cortex showing its three layers. (From Willis, W.D., Jr., and Grossman, R.G.: Medical neurobiology, ed. 2, St. Louis, 1977, The C.V. Mosby Co.)

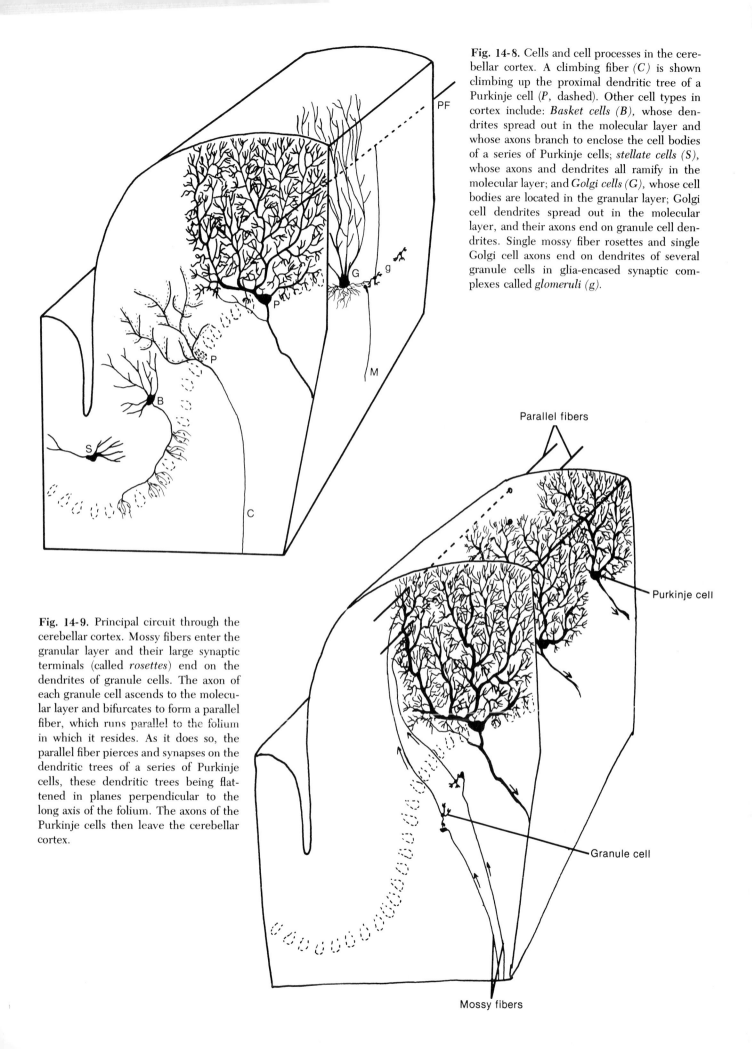

Fig. 14-8. Cells and cell processes in the cerebellar cortex. A climbing fiber (*C*) is shown climbing up the proximal dendritic tree of a Purkinje cell (*P*, dashed). Other cell types in cortex include: *Basket cells (B)*, whose dendrites spread out in the molecular layer and whose axons branch to enclose the cell bodies of a series of Purkinje cells; *stellate cells (S)*, whose axons and dendrites all ramify in the molecular layer; and *Golgi cells (G)*, whose cell bodies are located in the granular layer; Golgi cell dendrites spread out in the molecular layer, and their axons end on granule cell dendrites. Single mossy fiber rosettes and single Golgi cell axons end on dendrites of several granule cells in glia-encased synaptic complexes called *glomeruli (g)*.

Fig. 14-9. Principal circuit through the cerebellar cortex. Mossy fibers enter the granular layer and their large synaptic terminals (called *rosettes*) end on the dendrites of granule cells. The axon of each granule cell ascends to the molecular layer and bifurcates to form a parallel fiber, which runs parallel to the folium in which it resides. As it does so, the parallel fiber pierces and synapses on the dendritic trees of a series of Purkinje cells, these dendritic trees being flattened in planes perpendicular to the long axis of the folium. The axons of the Purkinje cells then leave the cerebellar cortex.

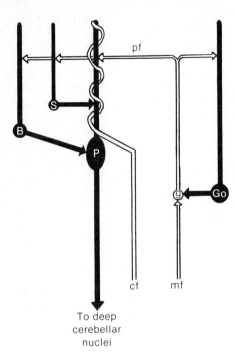

To deep
cerebellar
nuclei

Fig. 14-10. Major interconnections in cerebellar cortex; inhibitory connections shown in black, excitatory in white. One striking thing about the cerebellar cortex is the large amount of inhibition used in processing there: The mossy fiber (mf)–granule cell (g) inputs and the climbing fiber (cf) inputs are excitatory, but everything else is inhibitory. Golgi cells (Go) make inhibitory feedback connections onto granule cells. Basket cells (B) and stellate cells (S) make inhibitory synapses on the cell bodies and dendrites, respectively, of Purkinje cells (P). Finally, all synapses of Purkinje cells, as far as we know, are inhibitory. (Modified from Thach, W.T.: Cerebellar output: properties, synthesis and uses, Brain Res. 40:89, 1972.)

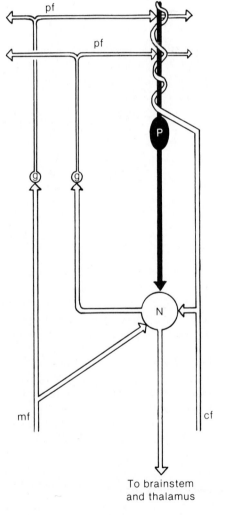

To brainstem
and thalamus

Fig. 14-11. Schematic diagram of general interconnections of cerebellar cortex and deep cerebellar nuclei. Mossy fibers (mf) and climbing fibers (cf) both send collaterals to cells of deep nuclei (N) before continuing to cerebellar cortex, where climbing fibers end directly on Purkinje cells (P), and mossy fibers influence Purkinje cells indirectly through granule cell (g)–parallel fiber (pf) pathway. Purkinje cells in turn end on cells of deep nuclei, and deep nuclei send mossy fibers to cortex as well as massive numbers of fibers to extracerebellar sites in brainstem and thalamus. (Modified from Thach, W.T.: Cerebellar output: properties, synthesis and uses, Brain Res. 40:89, 1972.)

cells, and individual Purkinje cells receive synapses from perhaps 10^5 of them.

There are two sets of afferent fibers to the cerebellar cortex: *climbing fibers* and *mossy fibers*. A climbing fiber ends directly on each Purkinje cell, winding around the proximal portions of its dendrites like ivy climbing a trellis. The origin of climbing fibers has been a matter of dispute for years, but it is currently thought that most or all of them arise in the contralateral inferior olivary nucleus. By elimination, then, all the rest of the afferents to the cerebellar cortex are mossy fibers. Mossy fibers end on the dendrites of granule cells, so this is an indirect route to the Purkinje cells (mossy fiber → granule cell → parallel fiber → Purkinje cell).

Deep nuclei

Although Purkinje cell axons are the only route out of the cerebellar cortex, few of them leave the cerebellum itself. Rather, they project to the deep nuclei, which in turn give rise to the cerebellar output. However, it has become clear in recent years that the deep nuclei are not just simple relay stations; they have a more intricate relationship with the cerebellar cortex than had been realized previously (Fig. 14-11). For example, climbing fibers and many mossy fibers send collateral branches to the deep nuclei. Nuclear cells are thus in a position to sample the same inputs the cortex receives and to compare the original inputs to the results of cortical computations on them. Furthermore, in addition to giving rise to axons that leave the cerebellum, the deep nuclei project back to the same areas of cerebellar cortex from which they receive Purkinje axons. The functional implications of these recently discovered connections are unknown, but they make it less surprising that the consequences of cerebellar damage are much more severe and long-lasting when the deep nuclei are included in the lesion.

Functional divisions

The cerebellum is involved in equilibrium, in muscle tone and postural control, and in the coordination of voluntary movements; thus it would seem reasonable for it to receive vestibular, spinal, and cerebral cortical inputs. This is indeed the case, and even though the cerebellar cortex has the same anatomical appearance everywhere, different areas are concerned with particular functions. The flocculonodular lobe and part of the uvula receive vestibular inputs, and so this area is referred to as the *vestibulocerebellum*. Most of the vermal and paravermal regions (except for the nodulus and uvula) receive spinal inputs and so are called the *spinocerebellum*. Projections from the cerebral cortex (via relays in the pontine nuclei) form the major input to the cerebellar hemispheres, so the hemispheres are some-

times referred to as the *pontocerebellum* or, more often the *neocerebellum*.* There is a certain amount of overlap of these functional divisions in terms of connections. For example, the spinocerebellum receives afferents from pontine nuclei, and parts of it receive vestibular afferents as well.

Different areas of the cerebellar cortex are preferentially related not only to particular inputs but also to particular deep nuclei. The dentate nucleus receives projections mainly from the cerebellar hemispheres, the interposed nucleus from the paravermal cortex, and the fastigial nucleus from the vermis.

CEREBELLAR INPUTS

The cerebellar cortex receives some of its complement of mossy fibers from the deep cerebellar nuclei; the remaining mossy fibers carry information from three principal extracerebellar sources (Fig. 14-12): (1) the vestibular nerve and nuclei, (2) the spinal cord, and (3) the cerebral cortex (via pontine nuclei). The climbing fiber input to the cerebellar cortex, as mentioned previously, arises in the inferior olivary nucleus.

Vestibular system

Some primary vestibular afferents enter the cerebellum through the juxtarestiform body and end as mossy fibers in the flocculonodular lobe, the uvula, and the fastigial nucleus. A larger number of secondary fibers, arising in the vestibular nuclei, follow the same course to the flocculus and most of the vermis, bilaterally.

Spinal cord

A great deal of somatosensory information (principally from various mechanoreceptors of the skin, muscles and joints) reaches the vermal and paravermal cortex. Some of it reaches the cerebellum directly via the spinocerebellar tracts and the cuneocerebellar tract (Fig. 7-15). Some arrives indirectly by way of the reticular formation (remember that the lateral and paramedian reticular nuclei of the medulla project to the cerebellum). Not surprisingly, similar information from the head also reaches the cerebellum from the trigeminal system. All the trigeminal nuclei participate in this projection to some extent, but the bulk of it arises in the rostral two thirds of the spinal nucleus (nucleus interpolaris and nucleus oralis). The anterior spinocerebellar

---

*Many authors use the terms "archicerebellum," "paleocerebellum," and "neocerebellum" synonymously with "vestibulocerebellum," "spinocerebellum," and "pontocerebellum" in reference to what is thought to be the phylogenetic sequence of development of these different cerebellar areas. Unfortunately, different authors use these terms in slightly different ways. "Vestibulocerebellum," "spinocerebellum," and "neocerebellum," as defined here, seem to be the most common usage of the terminology at present.

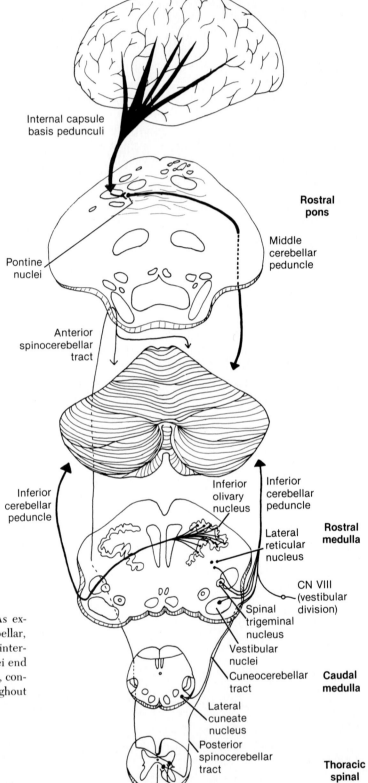

Fig. 14-12. Principal inputs to the cerebellar cortex. As explained further in the text, spinocerebellar, cuneocerebellar, and trigeminocerebellar fibers end in the vermis and intermediate zone; fibers from the vestibular nerve and nuclei end mainly in the flocculonodular lobe; pontocerebellar fibers, conveying information from the cerebral cortex, end throughout the cerebellar cortex, as do olivocerebellar fibers.

TABLE 7

Inputs to cerebellar cortex*

Tract	Origin	Termination	Peduncle
Anterior spino-cerebellar	Contralateral spinal cord	Vermis and intermediate zone, mostly ipsilateral to origin† (recrosses in cerebellum)	Superior
Posterior spino-cerebellar	Clarke's nucleus	Vermis and intermediate zone, mostly ipsilateral†	Inferior
Cuneocerebellar	Lateral cuneate nucleus	Vermis and intermediate zone, mostly ipsilateral†	Inferior
Vestibulo-cerebellar‡	Vestibular ganglion	Ipsilateral flocculus, nodulus, and uvula	Inferior (juxtaresti-form body)
Vestibulo-cerebellar§	Vestibular nuclei	Flocculus and vermis, bilaterally	Inferior (juxtaresti-form body)
Reticulo-cerebellar	Lateral and paramedian reticular nuclei	Mainly vermis and intermediate zone, mostly ipsilateral	Inferior
Trigeminocere-bellar	Spinal and main sensory nuclei of trigeminal nerve	Vermis and intermediate zone, mostly ipsilateral†	Inferior
Olivocerebellar	Inferior olivary and accessory olivary nuclei	All contralateral areas	Inferior
Pontocerebellar	Pontine nuclei	All contralateral areas except nodulus; some to ipsilateral vermis	Middle
Tectocerebellar	Superior and inferior colliculi	Vermis and intermediate zone	Superior

*Inputs from deep cerebellar nuclei not included.
†Bilateral in posterior lobe (compare Fig. 14-13).
‡Primary afferents.
§Second order fibers.

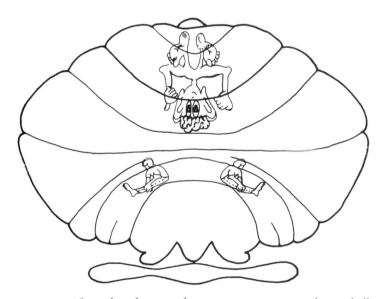

Fig. 14-13. Arrangement of visual, auditory, and somatosensory inputs to the cerebellar cortex. Such maps have never actually been determined physiologically for the human cerebellum. Rather, they are inferred from data such as that of Snider (1950) for monkeys. The mapping is not nearly as precise as in the sensory and motor areas of the cerebral cortex. The large eyes and ears of the upper homunculus are meant to indicate that this is the region that receives auditory and visual inputs.

tract and a reported projection from the mesencephalic trigeminal nucleus travel in the superior cerebellar peduncle, but all the rest of the somatosensory input from both body and head traverses the inferior cerebellar peduncle (Table 7).

Electrophysiological studies have shown that this projection ends somatotopically in a peculiar and interesting way. Each part of the body is mapped three times onto the cerebellar cortex, once ipsilaterally in a pattern mostly contained in the anterior lobe and again bilaterally in the posterior lobe (Fig. 14-13). In each of the three somatotopic maps, the head is nearest the primary fissure and the trunk is adjacent to the midline.

Cerebral cortex

You may recall that the basis pedunculi of the cerebral peduncle is considerably larger than the medullary pyramid. One basis pedunculi contains about 21 million fibers, of which only about 1 million continue on into the ipsilateral pyramid. Some of the remaining 20 million fibers are bound for the reticular formation or for the motor nuclei of cranial nerves, but the vast majority end in ipsilateral pontine nuclei. The pontine nuclei of one side contain about 12 million cells that project through the middle cerebellar peduncle to virtually all parts of the cerebellar cortex.* Almost all of these fibers cross the midline in the basis pontis and end on the contralateral side of the cerebellum; indeed the pathway is usually treated as entirely crossed. However, a few fibers (particularly some of those destined for the vermis) end ipsilaterally.

The corticopontocerebellar pathway is therefore a mammoth one, dwarfing the corticospinal tract by comparison. All areas of the cerebral cortex project to the pontine nuclei, but contributions from the vicinity of the central sulcus predominate (that is, from the motor and premotor cortex and from somatosensory cortex and adjacent parts of the parietal lobe). There are projections from other parts of the cortex, such as auditory and visual areas, but these are not as heavy as the others just mentioned. The vermis preferentially receives its cortical input from the motor cortex of the precentral gyrus, and the pathway is somatotopically organized so that the pontocerebellar fibers end in the same pattern as do those carrying information from the spinal cord (Fig. 14-13). The cerebellar hemispheres, in contrast, receive most of their cortical input from premotor, somatosensory, and association areas of the cerebral cortex.

Inferior olivary nucleus

The inferior olivary nucleus (actually a complex of a *principal* and two *accessory* olivary nuclei) is unique

among structures providing afferents to the cerebellum. All olivary efferents emerge medially, enter the contralateral inferior cerebellar peduncle, and blanket the entire contralateral cerebellar cortex with climbing fibers.

The information these climbing fibers convey comes from diverse sources, including the spinal cord, the red nucleus, the cerebral cortex, and the cerebellum itself. Fibers from the ipsilateral red nucleus, forming the bulk of the central tegmental tract, are the numerically most important olivary input. Spinal inputs, all crossed, reach the inferior olivary complex both directly (via *spino-olivary fibers*) and indirectly (through relays in the posterior column nuclei). Some fibers from the cerebral cortex of both sides, mostly from motor cortex, also reach the olive. Finally, there is a topographically highly organized projection from the contralateral dentate and interposed nuclei to the inferior olivary complex (Fig. 14-15).

A structure with these sorts of connections would be expected to play an important role in cerebellar function. This appears to be the case, since selective destruction of the inferior olive in experimental animals has acute effects similar to those of destruction of the entire contralateral half of the cerebellum (described shortly). However, selective olivary destruction is exceedingly rare in human pathology. Damage in this part of the brainstem is likely to affect the nearby pyramid and/or inferior cerebellar peduncle as well, and it becomes difficult to sort out those symptoms for which olivary damage is responsible.

Other inputs

Electrophysiological studies have also shown that responses to visual and auditory stimuli can be recorded from the vermis, approximately midway along its length (Fig. 14-13). The anatomical routes by which this information reaches the cerebellum are not known with certainty, but there are likely to be at least two routes. The auditory and visual areas of the cerebral cortex can influence the cerebellum by way of the standard corticopontocerebellar pathway. In addition, fibers from the superior and inferior colliculi convey visual and auditory information, respectively, to the cerebellum. They may do so by way of relays in pontine nuclei, although some authors have described a direct *tectocerebellar* projection through the superior cerebellar peduncle. Visual information also reaches the flocculus, where it is used in the control of eye movements.

CEREBELLAR OUTPUTS

The output of the cerebellar cortex is entirely in the form of the axons of Purkinje cells. Some of these, arising in the flocculonodular lobe and in parts of the vermis of both anterior and posterior lobes as well, leave the

---

*The nodulus receives no pontocerebellar fibers. The flocculus probably receives some, although not all authors agree on this point.

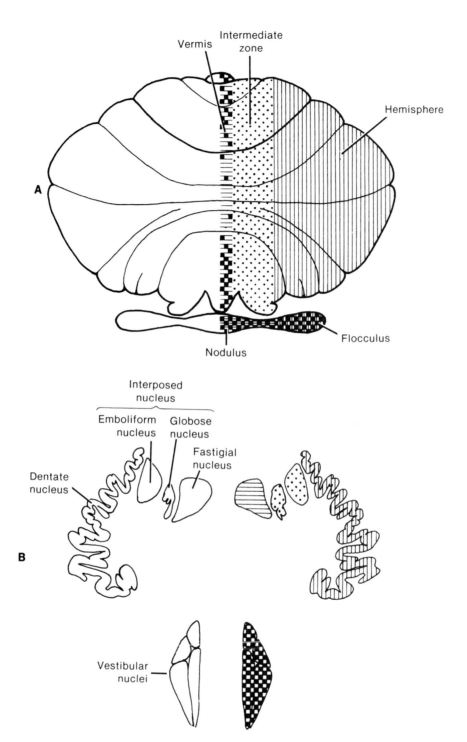

Fig. 14-14. Projections from cerebellar cortex to deep cerebellar nuclei and vestibular nuclei. The cortex is generally divided into three longitudinal zones that project in a medial-to-lateral sequence to the fastigial, interposed, and dentate nuclei. Superimposed on this is a projection from the vermis and flocculonodular lobe directly to the vestibular nuclei. (Modified from Jansen, J., and Brodal, A.: Das Kleinhirn. In Möllendorff's Handbuch der mikroskopischen Anatomie des Menschen IV/8, Heidelberg, 1958, Springer-Verlag, Inc.)

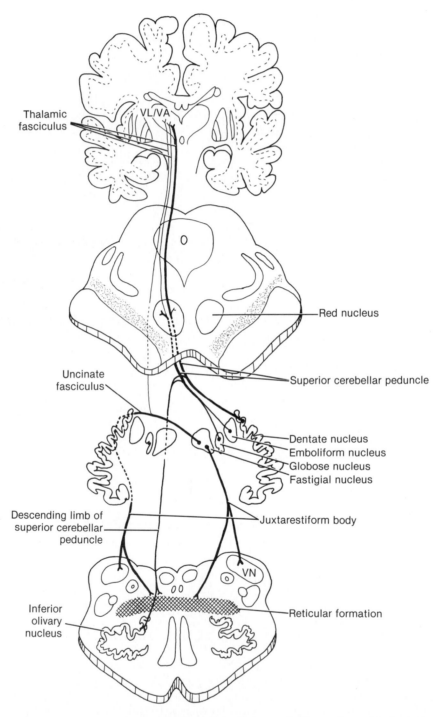

Fig. 14-15. Principal efferent connections of the deep cerebellar nuclei. The fastigial nucleus projects bilaterally to the vestibular nuclei and the reticular formation; a few fibers reach the contralateral VL/VA complex. The interposed nucleus (globose + emboliform) projects heavily to the red nucleus and less heavily to the VL/VA complex; the dentate nucleus does just the opposite. Both the interposed and dentate nuclei also send fibers to the contralateral inferior olivary complex and reticular formation.

cerebellum via the juxtarestiform body and end in the vestibular nuclei. This then provides the only reasonably direct access the cerebellar cortex has to motor neurons of the spinal cord (via the vestibulospinal tracts); all other Purkinje axons end in the deep cerebellar nuclei. They do so in an orderly medial-to-lateral way: the vermis projects to the fastigial nucleus, the paravermal or intermediate zone projects to the interposed nucleus, and the lateral hemisphere projects to the dentate nucleus (Fig. 14-14). The flocculonodular lobe sends some fibers to both the dentate and the fastigial nuclei, in addition to its outputs to the vestibular nuclei.

The output connections of the fastigial nucleus are distinctive, whereas those of the dentate and interposed nuclei are similar to each other. In addition to the connections described in the next three sections, all the deep nuclei project back to the cerebellar cortex.

Fastigial nucleus

The fastigial output is primarily directed to the brainstem, ending in the vestibular nuclei of both sides and in the reticular formation, mainly contralaterally (Fig. 14-15). Fibers that will end ipsilaterally go right out through the juxtarestiform body. Those bound for contralateral targets cross the midline within the cerebellum, loop over the superior cerebellar peduncle as the *uncinate fasciculus* (or *hook bundle*), and descend through the contralateral juxtarestiform body. A few fibers also project to the contralateral VL/VA complex of the thalamus.

Dentate and interposed nuclei

The major output from the cerebellum is the brachium conjunctivum, which arises in the dentate and interposed nuclei and leaves the cerebellum as the bulk of the superior cerebellar peduncle. This peduncle joins the brainstem in the rostral pons (Figs. 8-11 and 14-6); at this level some fibers turn caudally as the *descending limb of the superior cerebellar peduncle* and end in the reticular formation and the inferior olivary nucleus. Most of the fibers, however, continue rostrally, decussate in the midbrain (Figs. 8-13 to 8-15 and 14-6), and reach the red nucleus, where most of the fibers from the interposed nucleus and a minority of the dentate fibers terminate. The remaining fibers pass through or around the red nucleus, join the thalamic fasciculus, and end in the VL/VA complex of the thalamus. The projections of these two cerebellar nuclei therefore differ mainly in emphasis. The interposed nucleus preferentially influences the red nucleus, whereas the dentate nucleus preferentially influences the thalamus.

SOME FUNCTIONAL ASPECTS OF THE CEREBELLUM

The cerebellum is a great delight for anatomists and physiologists because of its uniform, precisely organized cortex and its well worked out connections. It is also something of an embarrassment, because in the final analysis we do not understand too much about how it works. However, characteristic motor disorders and no sensory deficit whatever follow cerebellar damage. Based on the nature of these motor disabilities (detailed in the next section), and on the anatomy and physiology of different parts of the cerebellum, a few general comments about function can be made.

The lateral hemispheres form the largest part of the human cerebellum. The major neural circuit in which they are involved is the great loop from widespread areas of the cerebral cortex to the cerebellum and back to the motor cortex (Fig. 14-16). This circuitry suggests that the cerebellar hemispheres could be involved somehow in the planning of movements, acting by influencing the output of motor cortex. Consistent with this notion, it has been found that most neurons in the dentate nucleus change their firing rates before voluntary movements occur, and indeed many of them change firing rates even before activity in motor cortex changes. (This is not to say that voluntary movements are initiated in the cerebellum, since in anticipation of a movement, various areas of cerebral association cortex become active long before the dentate nucleus does.) Thus the currently most prevalent hypothesis about the function of the hemisphere–dentate nucleus portion of the cerebellum is that it participates in the programming of voluntary movements, particularly learned, skillful movements that become more rapid, precise, and automatic with practice. This is consistent with the clinical observation that although a great deal of compensation may take place after cerebellar injury, deficits in skilled learned movements (for example, piano playing) may be permanent. Note that the connections between cerebral and cerebellar hemispheres are almost entirely crossed (Fig. 14-16). This means that, for example, the left side of the cerebellum is related to motor cortex on the right. Since the right motor cortex controls the left side of the body, it would be expected (and is observed) that the symptoms of unilateral cerebellar damage are found on the ipsilateral side of the body.

The major inputs to the intermediate or paravermal cortex are superimposed, somatotopically arranged projections from motor cortex and spinal cord (Figs. 14-13 and 14-17). The major output of this part of the cerebellum is via the interposed nucleus to the red nucleus and also back to the motor cortex (through the VL/VA) (Fig. 14-17). Thus the intermediate cerebellum can influence spinal cord motor neurons through the corticospinal tract and also through the rubrospinal (or rubroreticulospinal) pathway. This has led to the hypothesis that the intermediate cerebellar cortex somehow compares motor commands from the cerebral cortex to the actual position and velocity of the moving part, and

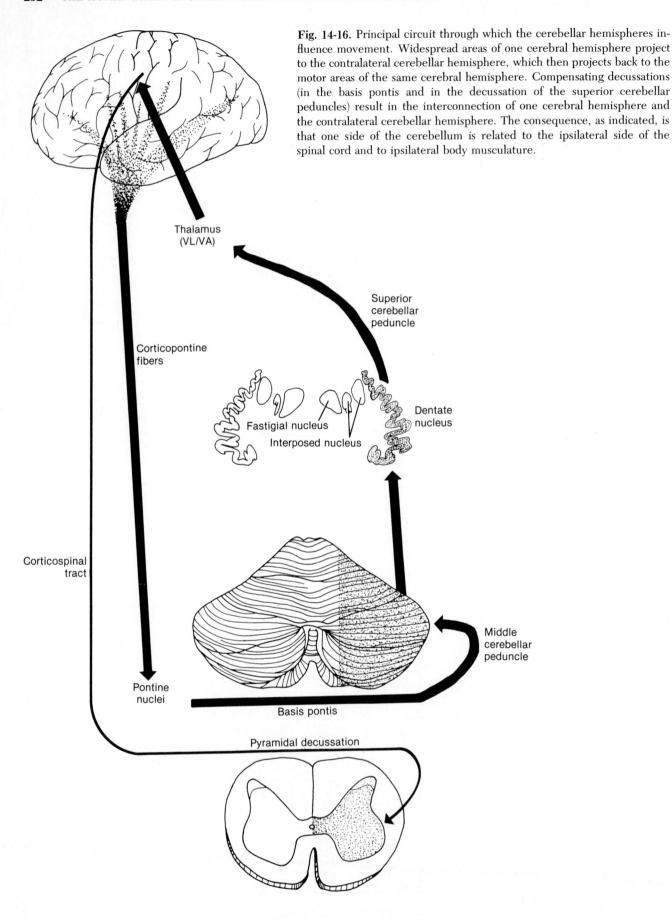

Fig. 14-16. Principal circuit through which the cerebellar hemispheres influence movement. Widespread areas of one cerebral hemisphere project to the contralateral cerebellar hemisphere, which then projects back to the motor areas of the same cerebral hemisphere. Compensating decussations (in the basis pontis and in the decussation of the superior cerebellar peduncles) result in the interconnection of one cerebral hemisphere and the contralateral cerebellar hemisphere. The consequence, as indicated, is that one side of the cerebellum is related to the ipsilateral side of the spinal cord and to ipsilateral body musculature.

Thalamus
(VL/VA)

Superior
cerebellar
peduncle

Corticopontine
fibers

Fastigial nucleus

Dentate
nucleus

Interposed nucleus

Corticospinal
tract

Middle
cerebellar
peduncle

Pontine
nuclei

Basis pontis

Pyramidal decussation

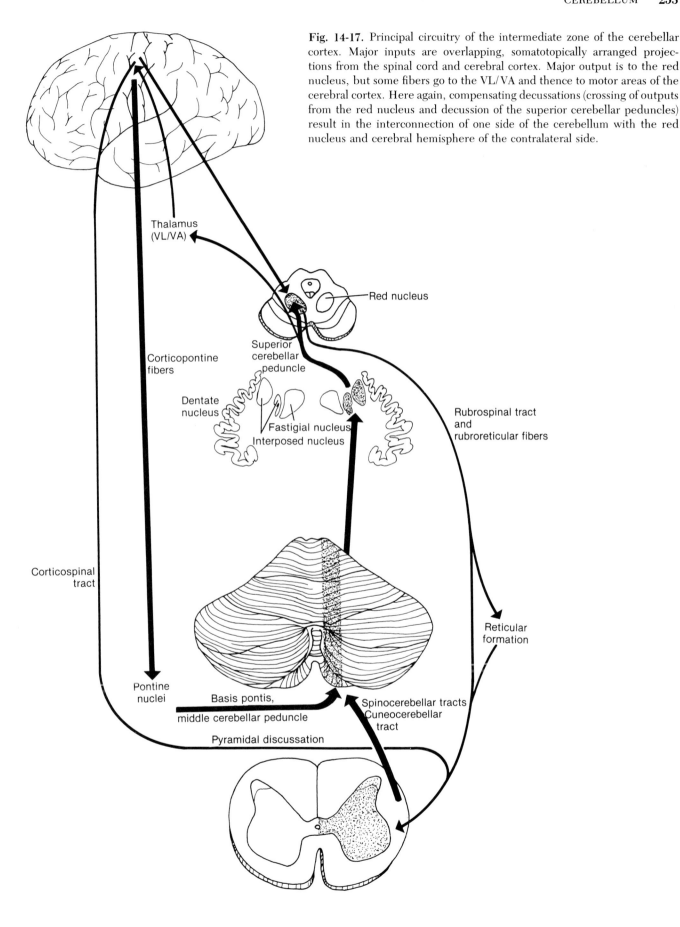

Fig. 14-17. Principal circuitry of the intermediate zone of the cerebellar cortex. Major inputs are overlapping, somatotopically arranged projections from the spinal cord and cerebral cortex. Major output is to the red nucleus, but some fibers go to the VL/VA and thence to motor areas of the cerebral cortex. Here again, compensating decussations (crossing of outputs from the red nucleus and decussion of the superior cerebellar peduncles) result in the interconnection of one side of the cerebellum with the red nucleus and cerebral hemisphere of the contralateral side.

Thalamus
(VL/VA)

Red nucleus

Superior
cerebellar
peduncle

Corticopontine
fibers

Dentate
nucleus

Fastigial nucleus
Interposed nucleus

Rubrospinal tract
and
rubroreticular fibers

Corticospinal
tract

Reticular
formation

Pontine
nuclei

Basis pontis,
middle cerebellar peduncle

Spinocerebellar tracts
Cuneocerebellar
tract

Pyramidal discussation

then, by way of the interposed nucleus, issues correcting signals. This is consistent with the observation that most neurons of the interposed nucleus have firing rates related to voluntary movements, but unlike those of dentate neurons, their rates tend to change *during* movement rather than prior to it. Note that here again a given side of the cerebellum winds up affecting ipsilateral motor neurons (for example, left side of cerebellum → right red nucleus → left side of spinal cord).

The vermis includes the representation of the trunk conveyed by the spinocerebellar tracts. Its major outputs reach the vestibular nuclei and the reticular formation both through the fastigial nucleus and through direct projections to the vestibular nuclei. The vestibulospinal and reticulospinal tracts then influence spinal motor neurons. Since this part of the cerebellum has so little effect on more rostral levels of the CNS, it seems reasonable that it should be most concerned with the regulation of posture and of stereotyped movements that are programmed in the brainstem and spinal cord. For example, the cerebellum-vestibulospinal pathway has been shown to be partly responsible for rhythmic modulation of the basic pattern of walking movements generated in the spinal cord.

The principal connections of the flocculonodular lobe are with the vestibular nerve and nuclei, implying that they should have something to do with the maintenance of equilibrium. As discussed in the next section, this is indeed the case, and damage to this part of the cerebellum causes a general dysequilibrium, as though some controls had been removed from the vestibular nuclei. In addition, the flocculus seems to have a special role in the coordination of slow eye movements, which is not surprising in view of the involvement of the vestibular nuclei in eye movements. Deciding how to visually track a moving target is not as easy as it sounds, since a target's image will move across the retina if the target moves, if the eyes move, or if the head moves. Some Purkinje cells in the flocculus receive all three kinds of information, make the appropriate computations, and reflect true target velocity in their output.

Clinical observations

In spite of the fact that the cerebellum is clearly divided into longitudinal vermal-intermediate-hemispheric zones, syndromes referrable to individual zones are rarely seen clinically. In order to destroy only the intermediate zone on one side, for example, a lesion would need to extend from the superior surface of the cerebellum near the midbrain to the inferior surface of the cerebellum overlying the medulla. The lesion would also need to extend into the depths of the cerebellar fissures. It is extremely unlikely that this could happen without damaging other parts of the cerebellum and possibly parts of the brainstem as well. As a result, what

is typically seen clinically are problems referrable to the flocculonodular lobe or to one or both sides of the corpus cerebelli as a whole.

Flocculonodular lobe. The nodulus sits on the roof of the caudal part of the fourth ventricle. Tumors, called *medulloblastomas*, occasionally arise in the roof of the ventricle, usually in young children, and are the most common cause of damage to the flocculonodular lobe. Affected individuals have a general loss of equilibrium — they sway from side to side when standing, walk with a staggering, wide-based gait, and tend to fall over. The basic mechanisms used in moving the limbs are unaffected, since when the trunk is supported (for example, when lying in bed), movements of the arms and legs are normal. In contrast to the findings after damage to the cerebellar hemispheres, there is no tremor, and both reflexes and muscle tone remain normal. Nystagmus frequently accompanies cerebellar damage (particularly damage to its inferior portions), but it is often difficult to rule out involvement of the eighth nerve or the vestibular nuclei. As a further consequence of these tumors, the lateral and median apertures of the fourth ventricle may be squeezed shut, with ensuing noncommunicating hydrocephalus.

Corpus cerebelli. The malnutrition often accompanying chronic alcoholism causes a degeneration of the cerebellar cortex that tends to start at the anterior end of the anterior lobe and march backwards. A great deal of the anterior lobe is occupied by vermis and paravermis (Fig. 14-5), and the legs are represented most anteriorly (Fig. 14-13). The result is a syndrome (called the *anterior lobe syndrome*) in which the legs are primarily affected, and the most prominent symptom is a broad-based, staggering gait, similar in many ways to that seen after damage to the flocculonodular lobe. In the anterior lobe syndrome, however, there is a general incoordination or *ataxia* (Greek = lack of order) of leg movements, even when the trunk is supported.

Most of the cerebellum is made up of the lateral hemisphere, and with a few exceptions like the one just mentioned, this is the region most heavily damaged in lesions of the corpus cerebelli. The result is called the *neocerebellar syndrome*, which is characterized by a variable combination of changes in muscle tone, reflexes, and the coordination of voluntary movements, all ipsilateral to the side of the lesion.

Widespread decreases in muscle tone (*hypotonia*) may follow small lesions, so that the limbs offer little resistance to passive movement and muscles feel abnormally soft and flaccid. Stretch reflexes are often reduced (*hyporeflexia*), and as a result of the hypotonia a limb may swing back and forth after a reflex contraction (*pendular reflexes*).

Most prominent, however, is a lack of coordination of voluntary movements. This is caused by a fundamental deficit in the timing of movements and the regulation of their rates. As shown in Fig. 14-18, voluntary movements take longer than usual to initiate, and there are problems in stopping them or changing their direction. This is manifest in a number of different ways: patients are likely to overshoot or undershoot targets *(dysmetria);* corrective movements when the patient nears a target have the appearance of a tremor *(intention tremor);* and rapid alternating movements, such as repeatedly pronating and supinating the forearm, may be especially difficult *(adiadochokinesia).* Note that the intention tremor of cerebellar disease is quite different from the resting tremor seen in disorders of the basal ganglia, partly because it is seen during voluntary movements and partly

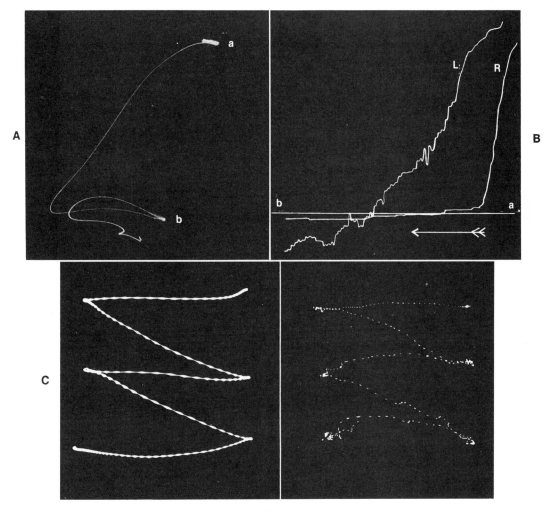

Fig. 14-18. Movements made by patients with cerebellar lesions (all involving one or both hemispheres), recorded by the simple but ingenious technique of photographing a light bulb attached to the patient's finger (A and C) or by recording the movement on a revolving drum. **A,** A patient attempts to touch his nose (at *b*) with the tip of his finger, starting from point *a* above his head; the movement has two distinct parts to it instead of being a smooth, continuous sweep (decomposition of movement), and the patient misjudges the range (dysmetria), striking his nose and then making irregular corrective movements. **B,** A patient with left-sided cerebellar damage attempts to stretch two similar springs and then keep them stretched to the level of the line *ab;* time progresses from right to left in this record. The normal right arm *(r)* moves promptly and appropriately, but the left arm *(l)* starts slowly, moves slowly, makes many small corrective movements, overshoots the line *ab,* and is then unable to maintain a constant stretch. **C,** A patient with right-sided cerebellar damage moves each hand back and forth between a series of small targets; the light attached to his fingertip was flashing at a constant rate, so the separation between bright spots is a measure of finger velocity. The left hand (on left) performs smoothly and accurately, but the right hand (on right) moves at varying speeds and has particular difficulty stopping and changing direction. (From Holmes, G.: The cerebellum of man, Brain **62:**1, 1939.)

because it is not so rhythmic or regular. When complex movements involving more than one joint are performed, the timing of different parts may be defective in different ways, leading to *decomposition of movement* (Fig. 14-18, *A*). The complex movements used in speaking may be affected in this way, in which case the normal flow and rhythm of speech is disrupted; successive syllables may emerge slowly and separated from each other (*scanning speech*).

In view of current notions of the function of the cerebellar hemispheres in the preprogramming of skilled voluntary movements, it is interesting to note that the neocerebellar syndrome is not accompanied by any sensory deficits. The British neurologist Gordon Holmes described a patient who had incurred damage to his right cerebellar hemisphere and who said, "The movements of my left arm are done subconsciously, but I have to think out each movement of the right arm. I come to a dead stop in turning and have to think before I start again."

ADDITIONAL READING

Allen, G.I., and Tsukahara, N.: Cerebrocerebellar communication systems, Physiol. Rev. **54**:957, 1974.

Amici, R., Avanzini, G., and Pacini, L.: Cerebellar tumors, clinical analysis and physiopathologic correlations, Munich, 1976, S. Karger.

Angevine, J.B., Jr., Mancall, E.L., and Yakovlev, P.I.: The human cerebellum: an atlas of gross topography in serial sections, Boston, 1961, Little, Brown and Co. *A review of various systems of cerebellar nomenclature and terminology together with a collection of beautiful sections cut in several different planes.*

Armstrong, D.M.: The mammalian cerebellum and its contribution to movement control, Int. Rev. Physiol. **17**:239, 1978. *An extensive, up-to-date physiologically oriented review.*

Batton, R.R., III, et al.: Fastigial efferent projections in the monkey: an autoradiographic study, J. Comp. Neurol. **174**:281, 1977.

Brecha, N., and Karten, H.J.: Accessory optic projections upon oculomotor nuclei and vestibulocerebellum, Science **203**:913, 1979. *A recently unravelled route by which visual information used in guiding eye movements reaches the cerebellum.*

Chan-Palay, V.: Cerebellar dentate nucleus: organization, cytology and transmitters, New York, 1977, Springer-Verlag, Inc.

Courville, J., de Montigny, C., and Lamarre, Y.: The inferior olivary nucleus, New York, 1980, Raven Press.

Desclin, J.C.: Histological evidence supporting the inferior olive as the major source of climbing fibers in the rat, Brain Res. **77**:365, 1974.

Dow, R.S., and Moruzzi, G.: The physiology and pathology of the cerebellum, Minneapolis, 1958, University of Minnesota Press.

Eccles, J.: Cerebellar function in the control of movement. In Rose, F.C., editor: Physiological aspects of clinical neurology, Oxford, 1977, Blackwell Scientific Publications, Ltd.

Flumerfelt, B.A., Otabe, S., and Courville, J.: Distinct projections to the red nucleus from the dentate and interposed nuclei in the monkey, Brain Res. **50**:408, 1973.

Gould, B.B., and Graybiel, A.M.: Afferents to the cerebellar cortex in the cat: evidence for an intrinsic pathway leading from the deep nuclei to the cortex, Brain Res. **110**:601, 1976.

Hendry, S.H.C., Jones, E.G., and Graham, J.: Thalamic relay nuclei for cerebellar and certain related fiber systems in the cat, J. Comp. Neurol. **185**:679, 1979.

Hoddevik, G.H.: The pontine projection to the flocculo-nodular lobe and the paraflocculus studied by means of retrograde transport of horseradish peroxidase in the rabbit, Exp. Brain Res. **30**:511, 1977.

Holmes, G.: The cerebellum of man, Brain **62**:1, 1939. *Still the all-time great description of the neocerebellar syndrome in man and the source of the striking illustrations used in Fig. 14-18.*

Ikeda, M.: Projections from the spinal and the principal sensory nuclei of the trigeminal nerve to the cerebellar cortex in the cat, as studied by retrograde transport of horseradish peroxidase, J. Comp. Neurol. **184**:57, 1979.

Ito, M.: Recent advances in cerebellar physiology and pathology, Adv. Neurol. **21**:59, 1978.

Kalil, K.: Projections of the cerebellar and dorsal column nuclei upon the inferior olive in the rhesus monkey: an autoradiographic study, J. Comp. Neurol. **188**:43, 1979.

Larsell, O., and Jansen, J.: The comparative anatomy and histology of the cerebellum: the human cerebellum, cerebellar connections, and the cerebellar cortex, Minneapolis, 1972, University of Minnesota Press.

Lechtenberg, R., and Gilman, S.: Speech disorders in cerebellar disease, Ann. Neurol. **3**:285, 1978. *Cerebellar speech disorders are generally considered to be caused by damage to the vermis, but this report presents an alternative view.*

Massion, J., and Rispal-Padel, L.: Spatial organization of the cerebello-thalamo-cortical pathway, Brain Res. **40**:61, 1972.

Meyer-Lohmann, J., Hore, J., and Brooks, V.B.: Cerebellar participation in generation of prompt arm movements, J. Neurophysiol **40**:1038, 1977. *What happens to voluntary movements when one dentate nucleus is temporarily disabled.*

Miles, F.A., and Fuller, J.H.: Visual tracking and the primate flocculus, Science **189**:1000, 1975.

Mower, G., et al.: Visual pontocerebellar projections in the cat, J. Neurophysiol. **43**:355, 1980.

Murphy, M.G., and O'Leary, J.L.: Neurological deficit in cats with lesions of the olivocerebellar system, Arch. Neurol. **24**:145, 1971.

Orlovsky, G.N.: Activity of vestibulospinal neurons during locomotion, Brain Res. **46**:85, 1972. *The activity is rhythmically modulated, and the modulation disappears after cerebellar lesions.*

Palay, S.L., and Chan-Palay, V.: Cerebellar cortex: cytology and organization, New York, 1974, Springer-Verlag, Inc. *A beautiful book, full of Golgi-stained cells and electron micrographs.*

Ritchie, L.: Effects of cerebellar lesions on saccadic eye movements, J. Neurophysiol. **39**:1246, 1976.

Shepherd, G.M.: The synaptic organization of the brain, ed. 2, New York, 1979, Oxford University Press. *A nice, readable book about a number of areas of the CNS; Chapter 10 covers the cerebellum.*

Snider, R.S.: Recent contributions to the anatomy and physiology of the cerebellum, Arch. Neurol. Psychiatr. **64**:196, 1950. *A summary of the electrophysiologically determined mapping of the cerebral cortex and the body surface onto the cerebellar cortex.*

Soechting, J.F., et al.: Changes in a motor pattern following cerebellar and olivary lesions in the squirrel monkey, Brain Res. **105**:21, 1976.

Tolbert, D.L., Bantli, H., and Bloedel, J.R.: Organizational features of the cat and monkey cerebellar nucleocortical projection, J. Comp. Neurol. **182**:39, 1978.

Thach, W.T.: Timing of activity in cerebellar dentate nucleus and cerebral motor cortex during prompt volitional movement, Brain Res. **88**:233, 1976.

Victor, M., Adams, R.D., and Mancall, E.L.: A restricted form of cerebellar cortical degeneration occurring in alcoholic patients, Arch Neurol. **1**:578, 1959.

Westheimer, G., and Blair, S.M.: Oculomotor defects in cerebellectomized monkeys, Invest. Ophthalmol. **12**:618, 1973.

CHAPTER 15

CEREBRAL CORTEX

The cerebral cortex is a sheet of neurons and their interconnections, about 2.5 sq ft in area, that plates the corrugated surface of the cerebral hemispheres in a layer just a few millimeters thick. Fig. 15-1, 15-2, and 15-3 show the gross topography of this cortical covering.

One of the more striking changes that has occurred in the course of evolution of brains in vertebrate animals is the tremendous increase in the relative size of the cerebral hemispheres and the even greater increase in the area of cerebral cortex on their surfaces. One inference drawn from this fact (and one abundantly supported by clinical evidence) is that the cerebral cortex has a great deal to do with the abilities and activities we think of as reaching their highest level of development in humans (or in some cases as existing uniquely in humans). Obvious examples are language and abstract thinking. This is, of course, not the only function of the cerebral cortex; basic aspects of perception, movement, and adaptive response to the outside world also depend on it.

HISTOLOGY
Terminology

The cerebral cortex does not have the same structure everywhere. Almost all the cortex that can be seen from the outside of the brain is of a type called *neocortex*, "neo-" referring to the common notion that it first appeared fairly late in vertebrate evolution (some neocortex, or its functional equivalent, actually may be present in all vertebrates, but mammals have much more than other vertebrates do). Neocortex accounts for more than 90% of the total cortical area. The remainder is made up of *paleocortex* and *archicortex*, named in reference to their supposedly more ancient origins.* Paleocortex covers some restricted parts of the base of the telencephalon (Fig. 15-4), and archicortex comprises the hippocampal formation.

All neocortical areas go through a period during development in which they have a six-layered structure. As discussed shortly, this layered appearance persists in only some areas of the adult brain, but in view of its uniform early development, the neocortex is also referred to as *homogenetic cortex* or *isocortex*. In contrast, paleocortex and archicortex never go through such a six-layered stage and are referred to collectively as *heterogenetic cortex* or *allocortex* (Greek, allo = other). The hippocampal formation is a component of the limbic system, and the paleocortex, which develops in conjunction with the olfactory system, is closely interconnected with limbic structures. Both, therefore, are considered in Chapter 16, and the remainder of this chapter deals with the neocortex.

Cell types

The two principal neuronal cell types in the neocortex are *stellate* (or *granule*) *cells* and *pyramidal cells*. Stellate cells come in a wide assortment of shapes, but they are basically small (in the range of less than 10 μm) multipolar neurons with short axons that do not leave the cortex. Pyramidal cells are named for their shape (Fig. 15-5): a long *apical dendrite* leaves the top of each pyramidal cell and ascends vertically toward the cortical surface, and a series of *basal dendrites* emerge from nearer the base of the cell and spread out horizontally. Pyramidal cells range in size from 10 μm in diameter all the way up to the 70 to 100 μm giant pyramidal cells (*Betz cells*) of the motor cortex, which are among the largest neurons in the CNS. Most pyramidal cells have long axons that leave the cortex to reach either other cortical areas or various subcortical sites. Therefore stellate cells are the principal interneurons of the neocortex, while pyramidal cells are the principal output neurons.

The apical dendrites of pyramidal cells are studded with numerous small projections called *dendritic spines*. These spines are the preferential site of synaptic contacts onto pyramidal cell dendrites and have been the

---

Pallium is Latin for mantle or cloak, and the neocortex, paleocortex, and archicortex are sometimes called, respectively, the *neopallium*, *paleopallium*, and *archipallium*.

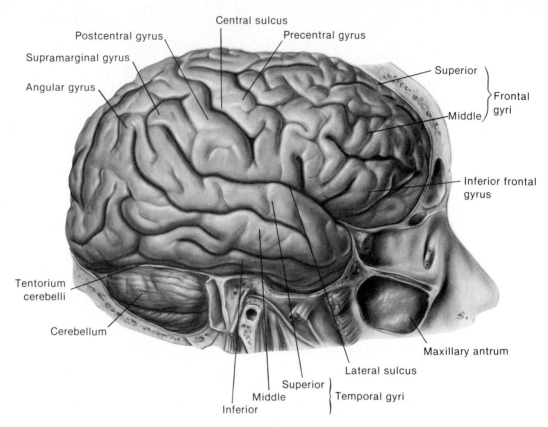

Fig. 15-1. Lateral surface of the cerebral hemisphere with the major gyri indicated. (From Mettler, F.A.: Neuroanatomy, ed. 2, St. Louis, 1948, The C.V. Mosby Co.)

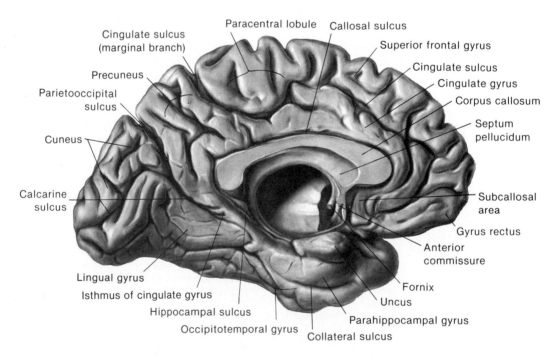

Fig. 15-2. Medial surface of the cerebral hemisphere after the brainstem, cerebellum, and diencephalon have been removed; major gyri and other features are indicated. (From Mettler, F.A.: Neuroanatomy, ed. 2, St. Louis, 1948, The C.V. Mosby Co.)

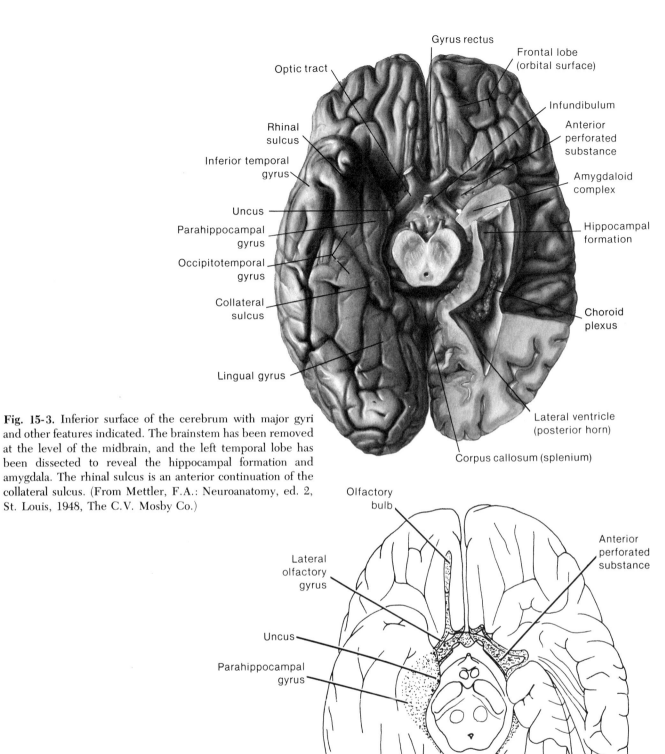

Fig. 15-3. Inferior surface of the cerebrum with major gyri and other features indicated. The brainstem has been removed at the level of the midbrain, and the left temporal lobe has been dissected to reveal the hippocampal formation and amygdala. The rhinal sulcus is an anterior continuation of the collateral sulcus. (From Mettler, F.A.: Neuroanatomy, ed. 2, St. Louis, 1948, The C.V. Mosby Co.)

Fig. 15-4. Inferior surface of the brain, with non-neocortical areas of the telencephalon stippled. Note that the vast majority of the cortical surface is neocortex. (Modified from Von Economo, C., and Koskinas, G.N.: Die Cytoarchitektonik der Hirnrinde des erwachsenen Menschen, Heidelberg, 1925, Julius Springer.)

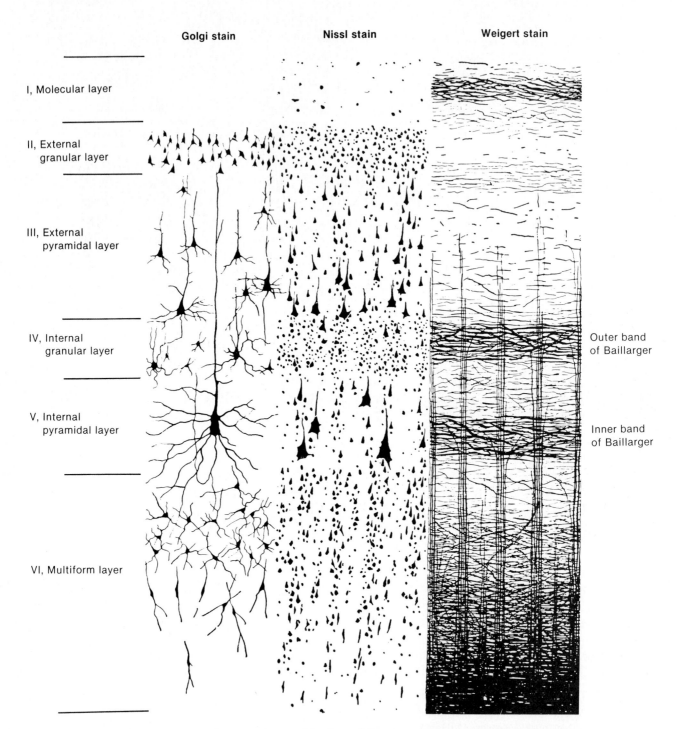

Fig. 15-5. Cross section of neocortex stained by three different methods; the six cortical layers are indicated. The Golgi stain reveals the shapes of the arborizations of cortical neurons by completely staining a small percentage of them. The Nissl method stains the cell bodies of all neurons, showing their shapes and packing densities. The Weigert method stains myelin, revealing the horizontally oriented bands of Baillarger as well as vertically oriented collections of cortical afferents and efferents. (From Ranson, S.W., and Clark, S.L.: The anatomy of the nervous system, ed. 10, Philadelphia, 1959, W.B. Saunders Company.)

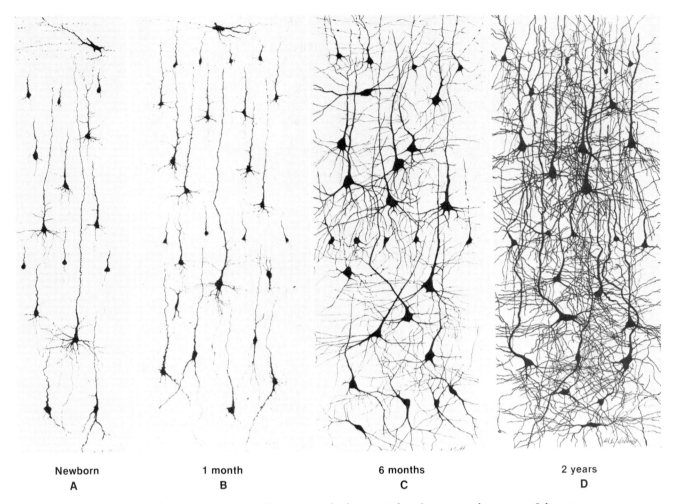

Newborn	1 month	6 months	2 years
A	B	C	D

Fig. 15-6. Golgi-stained sections of human cerebral cortex taken from equivalent areas of the anterior portion of the middle frontal gyrus at different ages. Note that although the packing density of cortical neurons does not appear to change, there is a tremendous increase in the complexity of dendritic arborizations with increasing age. (From Conel, J.L.: The postnatal development of the human cerebral cortex, Cambridge, Mass., Harvard University Press. **A,** Vol. I, 1939; **B,** vol. II, 1941; **C,** vol. IV, 1951; **D,** vol. VI, 1959. Reprinted by permission.)

source of considerable interest and some mystery as well. They are not merely a device for increasing dendritic surface area, since the portions of a dendrite located between spines are sparsely populated with synaptic contacts. It has been suggested that dendritic spines may be the sites of synapses that are selectively modified as a result of learning, since small changes in the geometry of a spine could cause relatively large changes in its electrical properties and therefore in the efficacy of that synapse. Certain cases of mental retardation are accompanied by faulty development of dendritic spines, but which is cause and which is effect (if either) is not known. Certainly, however, the most remarkable change that occurs in the cortex after birth is the tremendous expansion of the dendritic trees of its neurons (Fig. 15-6) and a parallel increase in the numbers of

dendritic spines. It should be noted that spines are not unique to cortical pyramidal cells; they are also found on the dendrites of some other neurons, such as Purkinje cells and many striatal interneurons.

Other neocortical cell types (in addition to the stellate and pyramidal cells) include *horizontal cells* (or *cells of Cajal*), *fusiform cells,* and *cells of Martinotti.* Horizontal cells ramify within the most superficial cortical layer; they are prominent during development, but most disappear after birth. Fusiform cells are found in the deepest cortical layer; they are spindle shaped, with a tuft of dendrites emerging from each end of the spindle (Fig. 15-5) and an axon that leaves the cortex. Cells of Martinotti are found in all cortical layers and are unusual in having axons that ascend toward the surface.

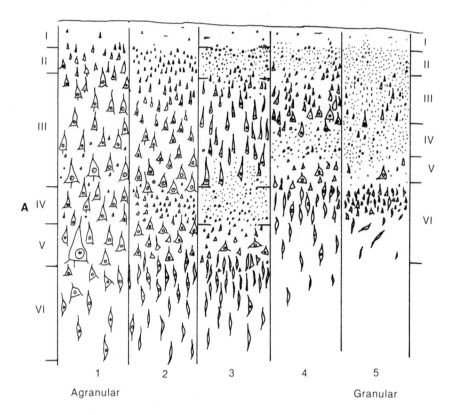

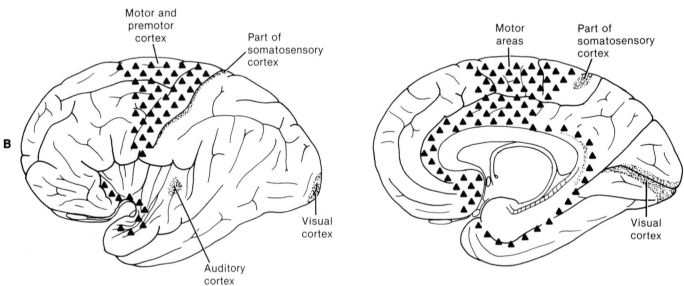

Fig. 15-7. **A,** Different types of neocortex. At the two extremes are the heterotypical cortices: agranular cortex dominated by pyramidal cells and granular cortex (koniocortex) dominated by stellate cells. Areas with intermediate structures in which six layers can be discerned are homotypical and were divided into three types by von Economo: *2*, frontal type; *3*, parietal type; *4*, polar type. **B,** Distribution of heterotypical cortex. The lateral view, on the left, is drawn as though the lateral sulcus had been pried open, exposing the insula. Agranular cortex is found primarily in motor areas, granular cortex primarily in sensory areas (compare to Fig. 15-14). (Modified from Von Economo, C.: The cytoarchitectonics of the human cerebral cortex, Oxford, 1929, Oxford University Press.)

Cortical layers

The cells of the neocortex are arranged in a series of six layers, more apparent in some areas than in others. Most superficial is a cell-poor *molecular layer*, and deepest is the *polymorphic* (or *multiform*) *layer*, which is populated largely by fusiform cells. In between these two are four layers alternately populated mostly by stellate cells or mostly by pyramidal cells. The layers are commonly designated by Roman numerals and by names, as indicated in Fig. 15-5.

Myelin staining reveals vertically oriented bundles of cortical afferents and efferents as well as horizontal bands through which these fibers and intracortical axons spread (Fig. 15-5). Two particularly prominent horizontal bands are contained in layers IV and V and are called, respectively, the *outer* and *inner bands of Baillarger.*

The six neocortical cell layers are not equally prominent everywhere. Areas that give rise to many long axons (for example, the motor cortex) would be expected to have numerous large pyramidal cells, and this is indeed the case (Fig. 15-7). In these areas, stellate cells are relatively scarce, and layers II through V are dominated by pyramidal cells to the extent that individual layers are no longer obvious. Because of the lack of stellate (granule) cells, such cortex is called *agranular*. In contrast, primary sensory areas project mainly to adjacent cortical areas and do not give rise to many long axons. They have a corresponding dearth of large pyramidal cells; here too, layers II through V look like one continuous layer, but in this case they are dominated by stellate cells (Fig. 15-7). Such cortex is therefore called *granular cortex* or *koniocortex* (Greek, konio = dust, referring to the numerous tiny cells). There is a continuum of structural types ranging between thick (4.5 mm) agranular cortex and thin (1.5 mm) granular cortex (Fig. 15-7). The intermediate kinds, in which the six neocortical layers can be seen, are called *homotypical* cortices (as opposed to granular and agranular cortices, which are collectively called *heterotypical*).

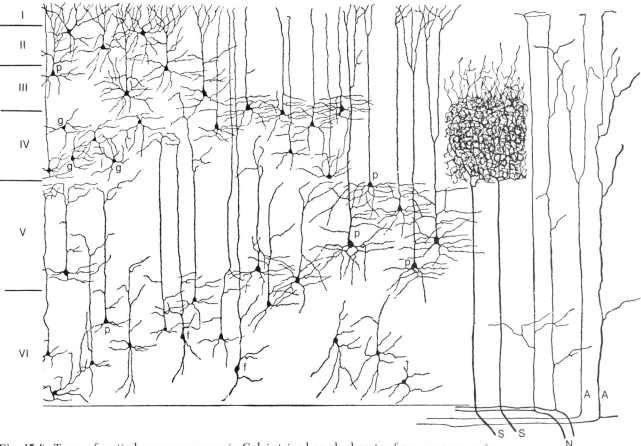

Fig. 15-8. Types of cortical neurons as seen in Golgi-stained cerebral cortex from a mouse; main types of cortical afferents shown on the right. Cells: *f*, fusiform cells; *g*, granule (stellate) cells; *p*, pyramidal cells. Afferents: *A*, association fibers from other cortical areas; *N*, fibers from nonspecific thalamic nuclei; *S*, fibers from specific thalamic nuclei. Note the strongly vertical orientation of many cortical elements. (From Lorente de Nó, R.: Cerebral cortex: architecture, intracortical connections, motor projections. In Fulton, J.F.: Physiology of the nervous system, ed. 3, Oxford, 1949, Oxford University Press.)

Cortical connections

Afferents to the cortex can come from only two general places: other cortical areas or subcortical sites. Afferents from other cortical sites, which are discussed at various points in this chapter, may arise in the same hemisphere *(association fibers)* or in the contralateral hemisphere *(commissural fibers)*. The single major subcortical source of afferents is the thalamus, and its pattern of projections was described in Chapter 10. Other subcortical sites, such as the locus ceruleus, also provide some afferents to the cortex.

These various types of incoming fibers ramify within the cortex in different patterns (Fig. 15-8). For example, specific thalamic afferents end in a dense arborization located in the lower part of layer III and in layer IV*; fibers from other thalamic nuclei and from other cortical

---

*Since the line of Gennari in the striate cortex represents a particularly large outer band of Baillarger and is located in layer IV, it is often assumed that it represents the massive projection from the lateral geniculate nucleus to the striate cortex. However, cutting all the afferents to the striate cortex does not cause the line of Gennari to disappear, and the true nature of this structure is unknown.

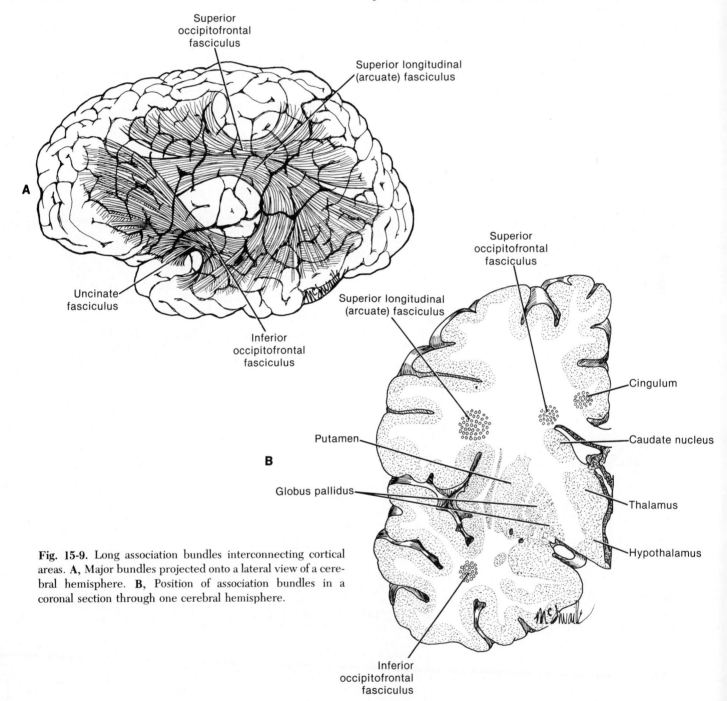

Fig. 15-9. Long association bundles interconnecting cortical areas. **A,** Major bundles projected onto a lateral view of a cerebral hemisphere. **B,** Position of association bundles in a coronal section through one cerebral hemisphere.

areas ascend vertically and terminate diffusely along their course in distinctive patterns (for example, those from association nuclei end mostly in layer I, those from intralaminar nuclei in layer VI, and those from other cortical areas in layers II and III).

Efferents from the cortex, like afferents to it, must be connected either with other cortical areas or with subcortical sites. Efferents to subcortical sites have been mentioned in various places throughout this book. Most of them descend through the internal capsule along a pathway that (for some) continues through the cerebral peduncle, the basal part of the pons, and the medullary pyramids, finally reaching the spinal cord. Along this pathway many other structures are contacted, including (but by no means limited to) the caudate nucleus and putamen, the thalamus, the superior colliculus (from visual areas), the red nucleus, the reticular formation, motor neurons of cranial and spinal nerves, and various

sensory nuclei of the brainstem and spinal cord. Some corticostriate fibers travel through the external capsule.

Most efferents to the cortex of the contralateral hemisphere pass through the corpus callosum, as described later in this chapter (Fig. 15-18). Those interconnecting parts of the temporal lobes (particularly the middle and inferior temporal gyri) traverse the anterior commissure. Efferents to ipsilateral cortical areas come in all lengths, from very short ones that never leave the cortex to U-shaped fibers that dip under one sulcus to reach the next gyrus and longer association fibers that travel to a different lobe. The longer fibers collect into reasonably well-defined bundles (Fig. 15-9) that can be found by gross dissection (Fig. 15-10). The most prominent of these association bundles are the *superior longitudinal fasciculus*, the *superior* and *inferior occipitofrontal fasciculi*, and the *cingulum*. The superior longitudinal fasciculus (also called the *arcuate fasciculus*) sweeps along

Superior longitudinal
(arcuate) fasciculus

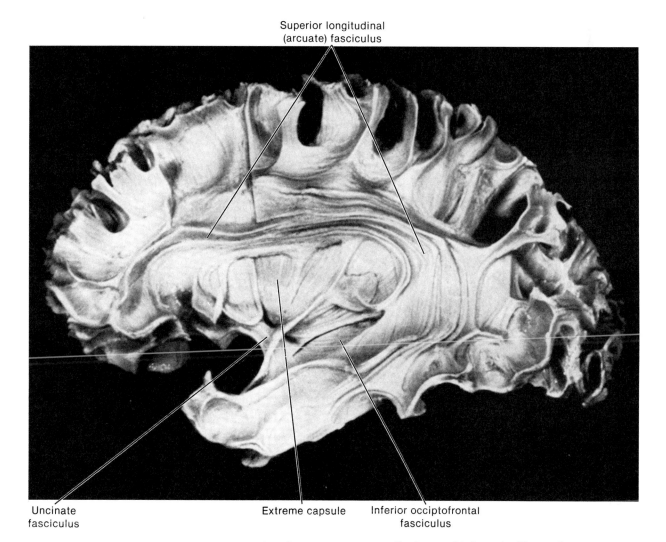

Uncinate
fasciculus

Extreme capsule

Inferior occiptofrontal
fasciculus

Fig. 15-10. Some long association bundles as seen in a partially dissected left cerebral hemisphere. (From Ludwig, E., and Klingler, J.: Atlas cerebri humani, Boston, 1956, Little, Brown and Co.)

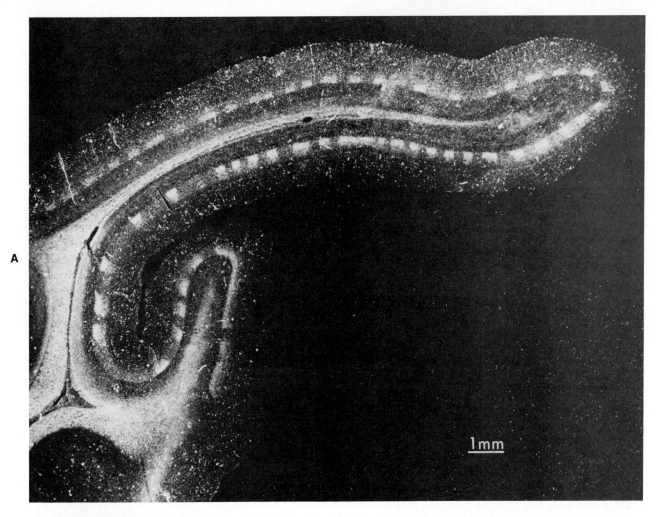

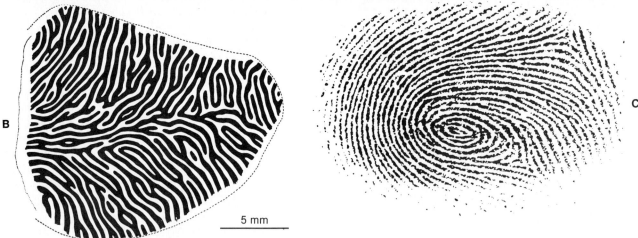

Fig. 15-11. Cortical columns in the visual cortex of rhesus monkeys. **A**, Autoradiograph of a section through the visual cortex of a monkey whose ipsilateral eye had been injected with a radioactive amino acid 2 weeks prior to sectioning. The amino acid was taken up by the ganglion cells of that eye, transported to the lateral geniculate nucleus (presumably after being packaged into proteins), taken up by geniculate cells, and then transported to the visual cortex. Ocular dominance columns for the injected eye show up as light areas in layer IV (where the optic radiation terminates) in this autoradiograph seen with dark-field optics; the interspersed dark areas are ocular dominance columns for the contralateral eye. **B**, Reconstruction of the ocular dominance columns (seen as though you were looking down on the cortical surface) showing that the columns are really more or less parallel slabs. **C**, Fingerprint of human index finger to the same scale as **B**. (From Hubel, D.H., and Wiesel, T.N.: Functional architecture of macaque monkey visual cortex, Proc. R. Soc. Lond. **B198**:1, 1977. Courtesy of Dr. David Hubel. By permission of the Controller of Her Britannic Majesty's Stationery Office.)

in a great arc above the insula from the frontal lobe to posterior portions of the hemisphere, where it fans out among the parietal, occipital, and temporal lobes. The superior occipitofrontal fasciculus, as its name implies, runs between the frontal and occipital lobes parallel to the corpus callosum for much of its course. Within the hemisphere, the superior occipitofrontal fasciculus is located between the corpus callosum and the caudate nucleus, and so it is also called the *subcallosal bundle*. The inferior occipitofrontal fasciculus passes below the insula from the frontal lobe through the temporal lobe and back to the occipital lobe. Its fibers fan out at both ends of the fasciculus, and those that hook around the margin of the lateral sulcus to interconnect the orbital cortex and anterior temporal cortex are often considered separately as the *uncinate fasciculus* (Latin, uncus = hook). Finally, the cingulum courses beneath the cingulate gyrus and continues around beneath the parahippocampal gyrus to nearly complete a circle. None of these association bundles should be thought of as discrete, point-to-point pathways from one place to another; rather, fibers enter and leave them all along their courses.

Cortical columns

In spite of the fact that the cortex is horizontally laminated, one gets the strong impression that there is also a vertical organization ("vertical" meaning perpendicular to the surface). Apical dendrites of pyramidal cells have vertical courses, as do afferents to the cortex and the axons of some intracortical cells (Fig. 15-8); even the cell bodies of cortical neurons often look as though they are arranged in vertical columns (Fig. 15-5). Physiological studies and newer types of anatomical studies have now shown that this is not just an illusion. If an electrode is slowly advanced through the somatosensory cortex along a path perpendicular to the cortical surface, all the cells encountered are found to respond to the same type of stimulus delivered to about the same region of the body with about the same latency. Similarly all the cells along a vertical path through the visual cortex respond best to bars or edges with the same orientation in about the same part of the visual field; if the electrode is moved over 50 μm or so, cells with a different preferred stimulus orientation are encountered. Furthermore each cell along such a vertical path responds better to stimulation of one eye than to stimulation of the other eye; cells in a nearby vertical region may have not only a different preferred stimulus orientation but also a different preferred eye. The picture that is now emerging is of the organization of the cortex into vertical slabs or columns, each 50 to 500 μm wide, in which some parameter (for example, stimulus orientation) is constant for all cells. Vertical slabs of different types (for example, stimulus orientation or ocular dominance) may intersect one another in patterns that are still largely unknown.

We do not yet know the extent to which columnar organization is used in the cortex generally. For most areas this is presently impossible to determine physiologically, because we cannot define the "best" stimulus for the cells in most parts of the cortex. However, some of the new anatomical tracing techniques make it possible to visualize the columns (Fig. 15-11), and there are indications that columnar organization is widespread. For example, it has now been shown that in at least some cortical areas, afferents from the thalamus, from other ipsilateral cortical areas, and from contralateral cortical areas each end in vertical slabs separated by slabs that do not receive that particular kind of input.

LOCALIZATION OF FUNCTION

Just as there has been a long controversy about whether the nature of a stimulus is signalled by the type of peripheral receptor that is activated or by the pattern of activity in many receptors, so too there has been a controversy about localization of function in the cerebral cortex. At one extreme have been those who maintain (in a kind of phrenology moved inwards) that particular patches of cortex are the unique sites of particular functions. At the other extreme have been those who maintain that very large areas of cortex form uniform fields in which functions are not localized and that complex activities depend on the amount of such cortex that is intact, not on the particular areas. As is often the case, the truth appears to lie somewhere in between. Consider the "simple" visual examination of an object, for example. This involves analysis of its size, shape, color, movement, and position in space; correlation of that object with objects seen in the past; cross-correlation of the appearance of the object with its sound, smell, and other properties; and decision making about whether to run away, to grab it, etc. Not surprisingly, large expanses of cortex are involved in even simple activities like this, and performance of complex tasks can be impaired by damage to widely separated cortical areas. Nevertheless many years of clinical experience have shown that reasonably predictable deficits are found after damage at various cerebral sites. This could mean that a given function is actually localized in a particular area, that the area performs one crucial step in the function, or that the area facilitates the activity of one or more other structures. Whichever is the case, the consistent association of some deficits with certain areas of damage provides a useful diagnostic tool, and we often speak as though functions are localized to specific cortical areas.

Anatomical maps

Seeing that various cortical areas are structurally distinct from one another in fairly obvious ways (for example, granular versus agranular cortex), a number of anatomists have sought to map the cortex in terms of

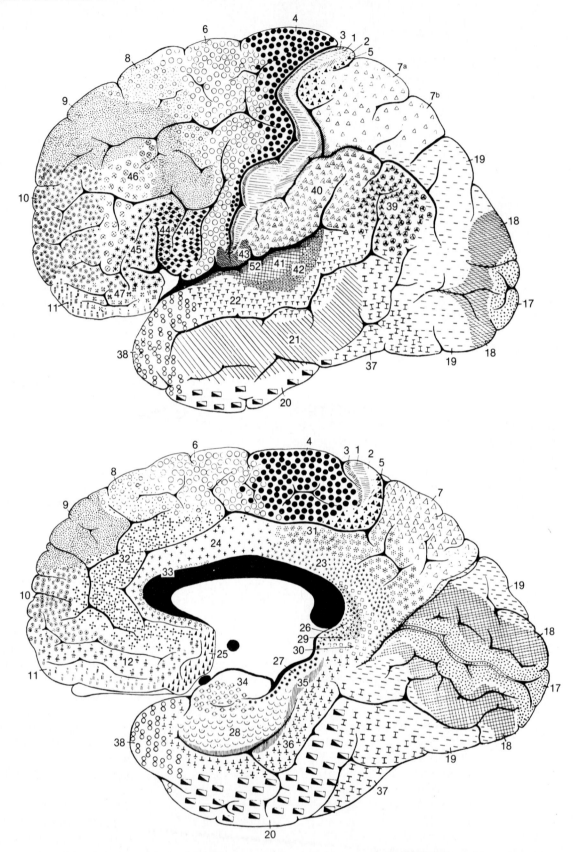

Fig. 15-12. Brodmann's anatomically defined areas of the human cerebral cortex. (From Von Economo, G., and Koskinas, G.N.: Die cytoarchitektonik der Hirnrinde des erwachsenen Menschen, Heidelberg, 1925, Julius Springer.)

TABLE 8

Selected Brodmann's areas

Lobe	Number	Location	Other names
Frontal	4	Precentral gyrus, paracentral lobule	Primary motor area
	6	Superior and middle frontal gyri, precentral gyrus	Premotor area
	8	Superior and middle frontal gyri	Inferior portion = frontal eye field
	44,45	Opercular and triangular parts of inferior frontal gyrus	Broca's area
Parietal	3,1,2	Postcentral gyrus, paracentral lobule	Primary somatosensory area; SI
	5,7	Superior parietal lobule	Somatosensory association area
	39	Inferior parietal lobule	Angular gyrus*
	40	Inferior parietal lobule	Supramarginal gyrus*
Occipital	17	Banks of calcarine fissure	Primary visual area; VI
	18,19	Surrounding 17	Visual association area; VII, VIII
Temporal	41	Superior temporal gyrus	Primary auditory area; AI
	42	Superior temporal gyrus	Auditory association area; AII
	22	Superior temporal gyrus	Auditory association area; posterior portion = Wernicke's area

*Included in Wernicke's area by many authors.

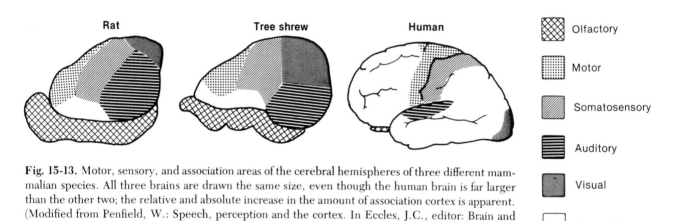

Fig. 15-13. Motor, sensory, and association areas of the cerebral hemispheres of three different mammalian species. All three brains are drawn the same size, even though the human brain is far larger than the other two; the relative and absolute increase in the amount of association cortex is apparent. (Modified from Penfield, W.: Speech, perception and the cortex. In Eccles, J.C., editor: Brain and conscious experience, New York, 1966, Springer-Verlag, Inc.)

these differences and often of considerably more subtle differences. One mapping system whose terminology has come into widespread use is that devised by Brodmann (Fig. 15-12), who divided the cortex of each hemisphere into 52 areas. The boundaries between many of these areas are not precise, as they often grade into each other by degrees. In addition, as noted previously, the correlation of functions with specific anatomical areas is not nearly as precise as was once hoped. Nevertheless many of the numbers proposed by Brodmann are commonly used for reference purposes (Table 8).

Cortical areas

The neocortex of each cerebral hemisphere is traditionally considered as made up of *primary sensory areas* (receiving inputs from thalamic relay nuclei), a *primary motor area* (giving rise to the pyramidal tract), and *association areas*. In this view, the somatosensory cortex occupies the postcentral gyrus, the visual cortex the banks of the calcarine sulcus, the auditory cortex a small part of the superior temporal gyrus, and the motor cortex the precentral gyrus. These areas are characterized by a topographical organization in which the body surface, the outside world, or the range of audible frequencies is mapped onto the cortical surface (Figs. 11-12 and 12-4). The maps are distorted in such a way that highly discriminating or finely controlled items have a disproportionately large representation (for example, the fovea in the visual cortex or the fingers in the motor and somatosensory cortex).

These primary areas come to occupy relatively less and less of the cortical surface over the course of mammalian evolution (Fig. 15-13), and most of the human neocortex is of the association variety. Association cortex in turn is commonly divided into two broad types. The area adjacent to a primary area is generally considered to be devoted to an elaboration of the business of that primary area. Thus areas 18 and 19, which surround the primary visual cortex, are referred to as the *visual association cortex*. Similarly the superior parietal lobule, much of the superior temporal gyrus, and the premotor cortex are involved in somatosensory, auditory, and motor functions, respectively. This still leaves the inferior parietal lobule and large portions of the frontal and temporal lobes, which would then be concerned somehow with high-level intellectual functions.

While there is a great deal of validity to this broad view of cortical organization, it is also clear that it is a considerable oversimplification in some respects. For one thing, the distinction between primary areas and association areas is not nearly so clear as the traditional formulation implies. One example given in an earlier chapter is the finding that the pyramidal tract originates not just from the classical primary motor cortex but also from other areas, including the somatosensory cortex. As another example, we now know there are *several* separate, distinct, and topographically arranged representations of motor and sensory functions in the cortex. In addition, the concepts that primary sensory areas receive all the input (which is then acted on in some more complex fashion by the association cortex) and that motor activity is formulated in association areas and then funnels down to the primary motor area for expression are certainly not completely correct. Monkeys (and humans as well) with extensive damage to the precentral or postcentral gyrus are not rendered unable to move or to perceive tactile stimuli. They are impaired in these capacities, but the fact that they suffer only a partial disability indicates that other cortical areas play a role as well and that these other areas can function independently of the primary areas, at least to some extent. The details of the ways in which different areas of the cortex and other parts of the CNS cooperate to produce something like a simple voluntary movement or a simple visual perception are still largely mysterious. The best we can do at present is specify some known cortical connections and the consequences of damage to some cortical areas.

Sensory areas

Somatosensory cortex. Somatosensory information traveling rostrally in the medial lemniscus and in the spinothalamic and trigeminothalamic tracts relays in the VPL/VPM of the thalamus and projects through the posterior limb of the internal capsule mainly to areas 3, 1, and 2. These are three long, parallel strips of cortex that together occupy almost the entire postcentral gyrus; most of area 3 is in the posterior wall of the central sul-

cus. These areas are not only structurally distinct from one another, but they also differ slightly in their connections; in fact, the body surface is mapped separately in each area in terms of different types of sensory input. Cells in area 3 mostly reflect activity of slowly adapting cutaneous receptors, those of area 1 rapidly adapting cutaneous receptors, and those of area 2 deep receptors such as those of joints. The result is a map in which the progression from tongue to contralateral toe is spread out along an inferior-superior line (Fig. 12-4) and in which the progression from skin to interior is spread out along a much shorter anterior-posterior line. Since this is the most prominent (but not the only) area concerned with somatic sensation, it is often referred to as the *first somatosensory area*, or *SI*. Another parallel strip of cortex (area 3a), located in the depths of the central sulcus between areas 3 and 4, should probably be included in SI, since it receives information from muscle receptors. The fact that none of area 3a is exposed at the surface of the brain has contributed to the long-held (but apparently erroneous) notion that muscle receptors have no cortical representation and do not contribute to conscious experience.

A *second somatosensory area* (SII) has also been described; it receives its inputs both from the VPL/VPM and from the SI. It occupies part of the parietal operculum, and much of it is buried in the lateral sulcus, possibly extending onto the insula (Fig. 15-14). SII is also somatotopically organized but in an order that is the reverse of that in SI; that is, the face areas of both maps are adjacent to one another, and the rest of the SII map extends into the lateral sulcus. The cells in SII tend to have bilateral receptive fields so that touching either of two symmetrically placed sites will activate them.

Stimulation of the postcentral gyrus in conscious humans produces sensations usually described as a tingling or numbness in a contralateral part of the body whose location is related in an orderly way to the site stimulated (Fig. 12-4). The sensations generally do not resemble those caused by natural stimuli like bending a hair or touching the skin, presumably because electrical stimulation of the cortex is a poor imitation of the pattern of activity set up by natural stimuli. Interestingly, sensations of pain can rarely be elicited from the postcentral gyrus. Destruction of the postcentral cortex causes a considerable impairment of the finer aspects of somatic sensation (such as judging the exact location or intensity of a stimulus) and a serious deficit in the sense of position and movement of the affected parts, but such damage does not abolish tactile sensation or sensation of pain. Indeed on the few occasions when removal of the postcentral cortex was tried as a treatment for intractable pain, the patient's pain was usually relieved only partially and briefly, and this was often followed by a hy-

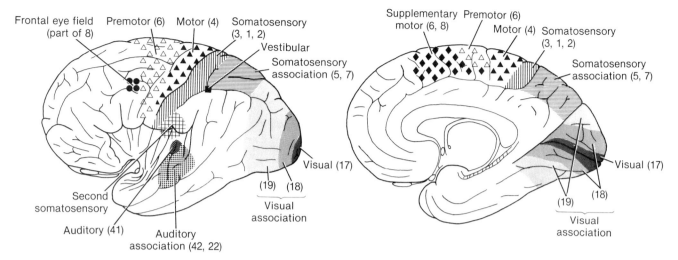

Fig. 15-14. Summary diagram of some functional areas of the cerebral cortex. The lateral view, on the left, is drawn as though the lateral sulcus had been pried open, exposing the insula. These functional areas are generally associated with one of Brodmann's anatomically defined areas, and the Brodmann number is indicated in parentheses when appropriate; the correspondence, however, is often only approximate. The probable location of the primary vestibular cortex is indicated by a black square.

perpathic state reminiscent of thalamic pain. In contrast, many SII cells in experimental animals respond to noxious stimuli, and stimulation of SII in humans is often painful. There are a few scattered reports indicating that destruction of SII in humans causes abolition or reduction of pain with little tactile deficit. These clinical observations taken together suggest that SI has a special role in discriminative tactile sensation and that SII has a special role in the perception of pain. These are not, however, the exclusive provinces of each. The fact that hyperpathia can follow damage to SI indicates that this cortical area is involved in perception of pain; conversely, some tactile deficits have been described after SII damage in monkeys.

Visual cortex. The retinotopic projection from the lateral geniculate nucleus to the banks of the calcarine sulcus, conveying information about the contralateral visual field, was described in Chapter 11. This primary visual cortex (called the *striate cortex*) corresponds to area 17 of Brodmann's map. Lateral parts of the visual field are represented anteriorly, the fovea has a disproportionately large representation located posteriorly, and the vertical meridian is represented along the upper and lower borders of area 17 (Fig. 11-12). Although area 17 looks fairly small on maps such as that in Fig. 15-12, it really occupies a substantial amount of the cortical surface and only appears small because most of it forms the walls of the deep calcarine sulcus.

A two-part visual association cortex occupies the rest of the occipital lobe. Area 18 (the *parastriate cortex*) surrounds area 17 and is itself surrounded by area 19 (the

peristriate cortex). This association cortex receives its visual information both from area 17 and via the superior colliculus–pulvinar pathway. Areas 18 and 19 are themselves complex mosaics of smaller, retinotopically organized areas, one interested in the movements of objects, another in the colors of objects, and still others in other properties.

The relative roles of primary visual cortex and visual association cortex in human vision are poorly understood. It seems safe to say that the primary area is extremely important, since its destruction results in a total or near-total loss of conscious awareness of visual stimuli. A simplified view of its function, then, would be that the primary visual cortex does some initial processing on inputs from the lateral geniculate nucleus (for example, combining inputs from the two eyes and beginning to analyze depth), then distributes this information to the various subareas of the visual association cortex where motion, color, and other parameters are analyzed more elaborately. If this is true, then bilateral lesions of the visual association cortex could conceivably disrupt single aspects of visual function. (Such cases would also be extremely rare, because they would need to involve symmetrically placed areas and would need to spare the optic radiations). A few cases have in fact been reported in which bilateral damage to the inferior surfaces of the occipital lobes caused color blindness but left vision otherwise more or less normal.

Auditory cortex. The superior surface of the temporal lobe forms one wall of the lateral sulcus. Two *transverse temporal gyri* cross the posterior part of this surface and form Brodmann's areas 41 and 42. Area 41 is granular cortex (like areas 3 and 17) and receives most of the auditory radiation from the medial geniculate nucleus via the sublenticular part of the internal capsule; thus it serves as the *primary auditory cortex*, or *AI*. Just as the body is mapped onto the postcentral gyrus *(somatotopy)* and the retina is mapped onto striate cortex *(retinotopy)*, so the spectrum of audible frequencies is mapped onto area 41 *(tonotopy)*. Area 42 is adjacent to area 41 and receives auditory information both from area 41 and from the medial geniculate nucleus. This is analogous to the arrangement found in the second somatosensory area (SII), so area 42 is often referred to as AII.* The cortex surrounding area 41 in monkeys includes at least four different subareas, each with its own tonotopic map. The same is assumed to be true for humans, but the exact details of the arrangement of these multiple maps with respect to area 42 are not known. Area 42 is itself flanked by area 22, which forms much of the superior temporal gyrus and is called the *auditory association cortex.*

At levels rostral to the cochlear nuclei, both ears are represented in the auditory pathway of each side of the brain, although the contralateral ear predominates (Chapter 9). As a result, even total destruction of the auditory cortex has relatively little effect. An individual with such damage may have some difficulty localizing sounds on the contralateral side and may have some subtle hearing loss that is greater for the contralateral ear, but the deficits are not nearly comparable in magnitude to those that follow damage to the somatosensory or visual cortex. On the other hand, if the auditory association cortex of area 22 is damaged in the dominant hemisphere, severe language problems may ensue, as discussed later in this chapter.

Other sensory areas. Gustatory information, relayed from the VPM through the posterior limb of the internal capsule, apparently reaches the parietal operculum and part of the insula. This seems like a logical place for gustatory cortex, since it is adjacent to the representation of the tongue in the somatosensory cortex; however, this probable gustatory area is rarely exposed during surgical procedures, so little direct information is available about it for humans. A few cases have been reported in which stimulation of the parietal operculum or underlying insula caused sensations of taste or in which seizures originating in this vicinity were preceded by an aura that included sensations of taste.

The vestibular area was long thought to be located in the superior temporal gyrus near the auditory cortex,

since stimulation of this region sometimes produces a sensation of movement or dizziness. However, more recent work on monkeys has shown that the most direct cortical projection from the vestibular nerve is to the parietal lobe adjacent to the representation of the head in the primary somatosensory cortex. The most likely location in humans (determined by extrapolation from monkeys and not by direct observation) is in the walls of the intraparietal sulcus near its junction with the postcentral sulcus (Fig. 15-14). The feelings of dizziness elicited by stimulation of the superior temporal gyrus may indicate that there is a secondary vestibular area in the temporal lobe.

The olfactory system is unique in that it does not relay in the thalamus and that the primary olfactory cortex is paleocortical rather than neocortical. Since it is closely connected with elements of the limbic system, the olfactory cortex is discussed separately in the next chapter.

Motor areas

Just as the somatosensory, visual, and auditory systems have multiple representations in the cortex, so too there are several areas from which movements can be elicited. The *primary motor cortex* corresponds to Brodmann's area 4, occupying a tapering strip in the precentral gyrus. Area 4 is agranular, the thickest cortex in the brain, containing a preponderance of pyramidal cells including the giant pyramidal cells (Betz cells). In the midnineteenth century, before the motor cortex had been explored electrically, the British neurologist Hughlings Jackson predicted the pattern in which movements are mapped on the precentral gyrus, based on his careful observation of patients with epileptic foci in this area. He noted that such patients typically had seizures that started as a twitching in one part of the body and then spread to other regions on the same side in a sequence that was similar from one patient to another. This sequence corresponds to the now-familiar homunculus for the motor cortex, which is generally parallel to the homunculus found in the somatosensory cortex (Fig. 12-4). As might be expected from the distortions of the motor homunculus, Jackson also observed that these seizures were more likely to begin as twitchings of the fingers or lips. Such attacks are still referred to as *jacksonian seizures* and the spread of motor activity as a *jacksonian march.* Stimulation of area 4 in conscious humans causes discrete movements involving one muscle or a small group of muscles (such as flexion of a single finger joint), which the patient is unable to prevent.* The movements are always contralateral to the side stimulated except in movements of the palate, the pharynx, the masseter, and often the tongue (but not the face),

---

*Terminology for area 42 varies among authors. Since it receives direct projections from the medial geniculate nucleus, some include it in the primary auditory cortex. Since it receives projections from area 41, others refer to it as part of the auditory association cortex.

---

*However, the patient has no sensation of *willing* the movement.

where the movements are bilateral; this corresponds nicely to the partly crossed–partly uncrossed corticobulbar projection (Fig. 12-6).

Several cortical areas in addition to area 4 give rise to corticospinal fibers and to other cortical efferents that participate in motor control (Fig. 12-5). Among them is area 6, which is also agranular cortex similar to area 4 except that it lacks Betz cells. Movements can be elicited by stimulating area 6 (the *premotor area*), but the threshold is slightly higher than in the case of area 4, the movements are slower, and they are more likely to involve larger groups of muscles. Corticospinal fibers also arise in the somatosensory cortex of the postcentral gyrus, and movements can be elicited from this region too, according to a pattern identical to the somatosensory homunculus. Finally, there is a *supplementary motor area* on the medial surface of the hemisphere; it is located anterior to the representation of the foot in the primary motor cortex, in the medial extensions of areas 6 and 8 (Fig. 15-14). Stimulation of the supplementary motor area causes movements that are usually described as the assumption of postures and may involve muscles on both sides of the body. The patient may, for example, turn his head and trunk to the contralateral side while raising his contralateral arm.

The multiple representation of movements in the cerebral cortex, with a primary area and several other nearby areas, is strikingly similar to the situation with sensory systems. In this case too, the primary motor area seems to be the most important in terms of the deficits that follow its destruction. Lesions of area 4 cause an initial contralateral flaccid paralysis, which resolves fairly quickly into hemiparesis accompanied by mild spasticity. The paresis is worse for more distal muscles, and its effects are seen most when fine, skilled movements (such as individual finger movements) are attempted. There is disagreement as to the degree of spasticity (or whether there is any at all) following damage that is entirely restricted to area 4, but the spasticity is certainly slight compared to that seen in cases of more widespread cortical damage or of lesions of the internal capsule. Selective damage to area 6 or to the supplementary motor cortex has no significant lasting effect, but if such damage accompanies destruction of the primary motor area, then fullblown spastic hemiparesis results.

Higher functions

Humans use language, create visual art and music, and otherwise behave in ways totally or nearly totally beyond the capacities of nonhuman species. Such behavior therefore can be studied only in humans, in contrast to our ability to obtain useful information about basic aspects of motor and sensory systems from experimental animals. This obviously constrains us to examin-

ing the effects of naturally occurring lesions of the brain or the effects of neurosurgical procedures, neither of which is likely to affect single anatomical areas in isolation. Our knowledge of higher mental functions is therefore based on clinical case studies, often on small numbers of patients with very rare lesions; as a result, it is not very satisfactory from a strictly scientific point of view. Nevertheless, as in the case of motor and sensory cortex, damage to certain cortical areas results in predictable deficits.

Cerebral dominance. All the functions discussed thus far have been related equally to both cerebral hemispheres, so that the hemisphere in which a lesion occurs makes a difference only insofar as determining the side of the body on which a deficit is found. In contrast, it has long been known that language deficits are far more likely to occur after damage to the left hemisphere than after damage to the right. Thus it appears that language tends to be lateralized in the human brain, and the hemisphere that is more important for the comprehension and production of language is now commonly called the *dominant hemisphere*. Its mate is of course called the *nondominant hemisphere*, although this is rather chauvinistic terminology, since (as will be seen) the so-called nondominant hemisphere is quite superior in some things.

Nearly all right-handed people (more than 95%) have dominant left hemispheres. Left-handed people are more likely than right-handers to have dominant right hemispheres or to have some language representation in each hemisphere, but still the majority of left-handers are left-dominant. Thus the side that is dominant is correlated to some extent with handedness, but regardless of whether an individual is left-handed or right-handed, the left hemisphere is more likely to be dominant.

Brains, on casual inspection, look bilaterally symmetrical, but searches for an anatomical basis for the lateralization of language have revealed that a variety of asymmetries actually exist. As discussed in the next section, certain cortical areas abutting the lateral sulcus are very important for linguistic functions, and so the consistent asymmetries found in the vicinity of the lateral sulcus are of great interest in this regard. The part of the superior surface of the superior temporal gyrus located posterior to the primary auditory cortex is called the *planum temporale* and is, on the average, considerably larger on the left than on the right. Since the lateral border of the planum temporale forms part of the lower bank of the lateral sulcus, it stands to reason that the lateral sulcus should extend farther posteriorly on the left than on the right. This too has been found to be the case (Fig. 15-15). These asymmetries are present before birth, which seems to indicate that left-hemisphere

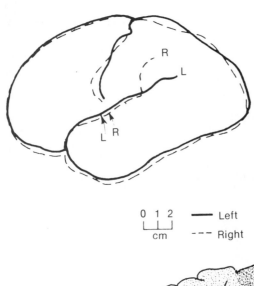

Fig. 15-15. Typical asymmetry of the two lateral sulci of a single human brain. Both hemispheres were photographed, then one of the photographs was reversed and superimposed on the other. Notice that the left lateral sulcus *(L)* extends farther posteriorly than does the right *(R)*, corresponding to the fact that the planum temporale is usually larger on the left. (From Rubens, A.B., Mahowald, M.W., and Hutton, J.T.: Asymmetry of the lateral (sylvian) fissures in man, Neurology **26**:620, 1976.)

0 1 2 —— Left
cm   --- Right

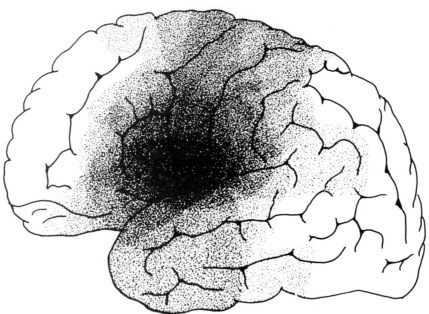

Fig. 15-16. Site of damage causing Broca's aphasia. The areas infarcted in 14 patients, all diagnosed as suffering from Broca's aphasia, were determined by radioisotope brain scan. All 14 lesions were then superimposed, indicating a focus of damage in the posterior part of the left inferior frontal gyrus. (From Kertesz, A., Lesk, D., and McCabe, P.: Isotope localization of infarcts in aphasia, Arch. Neurol. **34**:590, © 1977, American Medical Association.)

dominance for language is, at least in part, genetically determined. (This assumes, of course, that the connections of the planum temporale are as predetermined as its size.)

Language areas. Stimulation of the part of motor cortex where the mouth is represented causes an inability to speak and at the same time produces involuntary grunts, cries, or other forms of vocalization. This is similar to what happens when any other part of the motor cortex is stimulated: there is a discrete movement during which the patient is powerless to use those muscles for anything else. However, there are two areas whose stimulation on the dominant side cause the pa-

tient to cease speaking but not to do something else with the vocal muscles; more strikingly, stimulation of these areas can cause the patient to make linguistic errors or be unable to find appropriate words. The first of these two areas occupies the opercular and triangular parts of the inferior frontal gyrus and is called *Broca's area*. The second area occupies the posterior part of the superior temporal gyrus and much of the inferior parietal lobule. This posterior part of the superior temporal gyrus is called *Wernicke's area;* many extend the meaning of the term to include the inferior parietal lobule as well.

Inability to use language is called *aphasia* and can be divided into two broad types. The first type is asso-

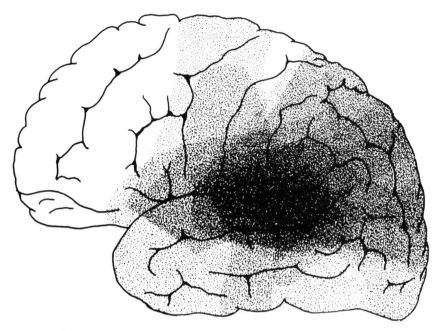

Fig. 15-17. Site of damage causing Wernicke's aphasia. The areas infarcted in 13 patients, all diagnosed as suffering from Wernicke's aphasia, were determined by radioisotope brain scan. All 13 lesions were then superimposed, indicating a focus of damage in the posterior part of the left superior temporal gyrus. (From Kertesz, A., Lesk, D., and McCabe, P.: Isotope localization of infarcts in aphasia, Arch. Neurol. 34:590, © 1977, American Medical Association.)

ciated with damage to Broca's area (Fig. 15-16). Broca's aphasics produce few words, either written or spoken, and have great difficulty producing them. They tend to leave out all but the most meaningful words in a sentence and to speak or write in a telegraphic manner. In marked contrast to their difficulties in producing language, Broca's aphasics have relatively little difficulty comprehending it. Broca's aphasia is also called *nonfluent, motor,* or *expressive aphasia.* The second type of aphasia is associated with damage to Wernicke's area (Fig. 15-17). Wernicke's aphasics are able to produce written and spoken words, but the words or the sequences in which they are used are defective in their linguistic content. There may be substitutions of one word for another *(paraphasia),* insertion of new and meaningless words *(neologisms),* or stringing together of words and phrases in an order that conveys little or no meaning *(jargon aphasia).* All of this suggests that the patient has difficulty comprehending whether his own speech makes sense, and indeed Wernicke's aphasics (in contrast to Broca's aphasics) are deficient in the comprehension of language generally. Because in this condition language can be produced but not understood, Wernicke's aphasia is also called *fluent, sensory,* or *receptive aphasia.*

These two broad types of aphasia are consistent with the notions that Broca's area contains the motor programs for the generation of language and Wernicke's area contains the mechanisms for the formulation of language. Destruction of Broca's area would then deprive the motor cortex of the instructions needed to generate language, but the muscles involved would be normal in other activities; comprehension of language would be relatively unaffected. Destruction of Wernicke's area would leave Broca's area unchecked so that words could be produced without regard for their meaning. This implies that there must be neural projections from Wernicke's area to Broca's area that would most likely travel in the superior longitudinal fasciculus (Fig. 15-9). It could be predicted that selective destruction of these fibers would also leave Broca's area unchecked and would result in fluent aphasia. Such cases have been reported (with lesions at the predicted site), in which the patient speaks like a Wernicke's aphasic but has intact comprehension, since Wernicke's area itself is undamaged. This syndrome is called *conduction aphasia.* Destruction of the angular gyrus in the dominant hemisphere causes a type of fluent aphasia in which the major deficit is an inability to name objects *(anomic aphasia).* This has been used to argue that the angular gyrus performs associations between objects and the symbols (such as words) for objects. According to this model then, the sequence of cerebral events that occurs during the verbal description of a seen object is as follows: visual information reaches the occipital lobe, is processed in various ways in areas 17, 18, and 19, and is projected to the dominant angular gyrus, which associates words with the object and its attributes; the words (or their cerebral representations) are transferred to Wernicke's area, which assembles them into sentences and activates the appropriate motor programs in Broca's area; these programs in turn activate the motor cortex.

As appealingly simple as such a model is (and as successful as it is in explaining a variety of aphasic disorders), it is certainly an oversimplification, and many investigators would violently disagree with it. For one thing, it requires an extraordinary degree of localization of very complex functions to specific small areas. For another, the types of aphasia just described are really abstractions, since they are never seen in pure form. This is partly because naturally occurring lesions are not neatly restricted to one of these areas and partly because aphasias may not exist in pure form. For example, Broca's aphasics typically have a comprehension deficit for grammatically complex statements; comprehension is only spared relative to the severe deficit in production of language. Nevertheless it is consistently found that within the cortical areas important for language, more anterior lesions result in greater deficits in production of language, and more posterior lesions result in greater deficits in comprehension.

Parietal lobe syndromes. Neurons in the primary somatosensory or visual cortices respond to easily defined and fairly simple stimuli like the onset of a light touch at a particular site on the back of the contralateral hand or a bar of light oriented at a specific angle and located in a particular part of the contralateral visual field. However, many of the neurons in the parietal association cortex (areas 5 and 7) of a monkey respond to considerably more complicated stimuli. Some respond to movement of the monkey's hand toward some desirable object (for example, a piece of food) but not at all to stretch of the muscles or rotation of the joints involved in the movement. Others respond only when the monkey visually fixates an object of interest and then continue to respond as the monkey tracks the object (if it moves). Removal of areas 5 and 7 causes a neglect of the contralateral half of the body: the limbs on that side are used little, and reaching with them is inaccurate.

The consequences of large lesions of the right parietal lobe in humans are similar to those seen in monkeys but more complex.* Such a patient has difficulty with spatial orientation to everything on the left and may completely ignore the halves of objects to the left as well as the left half of his own body. Such a lesion is rarely

confined to the parietal lobe and is often accompanied by hemiplegia and a hemisensory loss. The patient may deny that anything is wrong with the affected limbs and may even deny that they belong to him! In some cases, there is a general deficit in spatial orientation that shows up as a difficulty in following maps or in finding locations even in familiar surroundings. Contralateral neglect sometimes, but much less frequently, follows left parietal damage. This may be partly (but not entirely) a result of the fact that left parietal lesions are likely to encroach on Wernicke's area and cause much more prominent aphasic disturbances.

Other deficits likely to accompany parietal damage include very peculiar disabilities called *agnosias* and *apraxias*. Agnosia (Greek = lack of knowledge) means the inability to recognize objects when using a given sense, even though that sense is basically intact. A person with visual agnosia, for example, would be unable to recognize common objects by sight, even though the visual fields were perfectly intact and even though the ability to recognize the same objects using other senses (such as hearing or touch) might be intact. Apraxia (Greek = lack of action) means an inability to perform an action, even though the muscles required are perfectly sound and able to perform the same action in a different context. An apraxic patient might be unable to touch his nose with his index finger on request but would be quite capable of doing so spontaneously if his nose itched. There are a multitude of subcategories of agnosias and apraxias and numerous theories about whether some types are based on language deficits, spatial disorientation, or other more basic problems. Some (but not all) agnosias tend to be associated with bilateral parietal damage. Apraxias can result from a lesion on either side, although the exact nature of the apraxia depends on the side damaged.

Prefrontal cortex. The parts of each frontal lobe anterior to areas 4, 6, and 8 do not cause movements when stimulated and are called *prefrontal cortex.* This part of the brain expanded dramatically during mammalian evolution (Fig. 15-13) and now occupies the inside of the distinctive high forehead of humans. An early clue to the role of the prefrontal cortex in human behavior was provided by an unfortunate accident in the nineteenth century. In 1848, Phineas T. Gage, the foreman of a railroad construction crew, was setting a charge of explosives with a 13-pound, 3½-foot iron tamping rod. The charge exploded and blew the tamping iron through the front of his head, destroying a good deal of his prefrontal cortex. Remarkably, he survived the accident and regained his physical health in a few weeks. However, his personality changed dramatically. Before the accident, he was hard-working, responsible, clever, and thoroughly respectable. After the accident, he seemed to have lost most of his industriousness and

*In this discussion of parietal lobe syndromes, some types of symptoms are related to right-sided damage and others to left-sided damage. It is assumed (but in general not proven) that these sides correspond in a given patient to the sides non-dominant and dominant for language, respectively. Certainly this is true in the large majority of patients.

his awareness of social responsibilities.* He wandered aimlessly from job to job, exhibiting himself and his tamping iron in various carnivals, and was tactless and impulsive in his behavior, not particularly concerned about his future or the consequences of his actions.

Various means of separating the prefrontal cortex from the rest of the brain (procedures called *prefrontal lobotomy* or *prefrontal leukotomy*) were used in the first half of the twentieth century as a treatment for certain severe psychoses and other conditions, but these operations have been largely abandoned in favor of therapy with drugs. The procedures were done bilaterally, but similar (though less pronounced) effects were seen after unilateral operations. There was considerable variation from one patient to another, but individuals so treated typically became carefree and often apparently euphoric, which was the beneficial effect sought; someone suffering from intractable pain, for example, would admit that there was no decrease in the pain after a prefrontal leukotomy but would no longer be bothered by it. Unfortunately many of these individuals also lost some of their capacity to do things for a delayed reward and were inclined not to observe social norms in their behavior; powers of concentration, attention span, initiative and spontaneity, and abstract reasoning all suffered.

These effects are obviously difficult to quantify or to discuss in terms of anatomical bases. Equivalent lesions in nonhuman primates produce much less complex syndromes, at least as far as can be determined by objective measurements. All we can do at this juncture is point out that the prefrontal cortex has direct access to the activity of all the other cerebral lobes (via the long association bundles mentioned earlier) (Fig. 15-9) and so has abundant data at hand with which to work. The extensive interconnections between the prefrontal cortex and the dorsomedial nucleus of the thalamus also play an important role, as shown by the observation that lesions of the dorsomedial nucleus have effects similar to those of prefrontal leukotomy. Knowledge is scanty concerning the relationship of different aspects of the prefrontal syndrome to damage in different cortical areas, but it is clear that such localization exists, at least to some extent. For example, emotional changes seem to

be more related to damage to the orbital cortex and the intellectual deficits related more to damage to the lateral surface of the frontal lobe.

CORPUS CALLOSUM

The *corpus callosum*, interconnecting the two cerebral hemispheres, is by far the largest fiber bundle in the human brain. It contains more than 300 million axons. Most of these fibers interconnect mirror-image sites, but a substantial number end in areas different from those in which they arise (for example, area 17 of one hemisphere projects to areas 18 and 19 of the contralateral hemisphere). Nearly all cortical areas receive commissural fibers (Fig. 15-18), with a few notable exceptions like the hand area of the somatosensory cortex and all of area 17 not representing areas adjacent to the vertical midline. The commissural fibers to and from much of the temporal lobe, particularly the middle and inferior temporal gyri, pass through the *anterior commissure*.

We all know from common experience that something initially seen in one visual field can be identified if presented later in the contralateral visual field (for example, we can recognize a picture after it has been reversed left-to-right). The same is true for other sensory modalities such as touch*; similar transfers from one hemisphere to the other can be demonstrated easily in ex-

---

*Even though parts of the somatosensory and visual cortices receive no commissural fibers, all areas of the parietal and occipital association cortices do, so each hemisphere has access to data from the contralateral half of the body and the outside world.

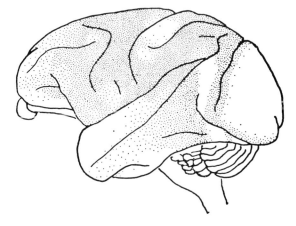

Fig. 15-18. Distribution of degenerating axon terminals after section of the corpus callosum and anterior commissure in a rhesus monkey. Note that with a few exceptions (for example, most of the primary visual cortex—exposed here on the lateral surface of the occipital lobe—and the hand area of somatosensory cortex), the cerebral cortex is blanketed with commissural connections. (From Myers, R.E.: Phylogenetic studies of commissural connexions. In Ettlinger, E.G., deReuck, A.V.S., and Porter, R., editors: Functions of the corpus callosum, Edinburgh, 1965, J. and A. Churchill, Ltd.)

---

*"The equilibrium or balance, so to speak, between his intellectual faculties and animal propensities, seems to have been destroyed. He is fitful, irreverent, indulging at times in the grossest profanity (which was not previously his custom), manifesting but little deference for his fellows, impatient of restraint or advice when it conflicts with his desires, at times pertinaciously obstinate, yet capricious and vacillating, devising many plans of future operation, which are no sooner arranged than they are abandoned . . . In this regard his mind was radically changed, so decidedly that his friends and acquaintances said that he was 'no longer Gage.' " (Harlow, H.M.: Recovery from the passage of an iron bar through the head, Mass. Med. Soc. Publ. 2:327, 1868.)

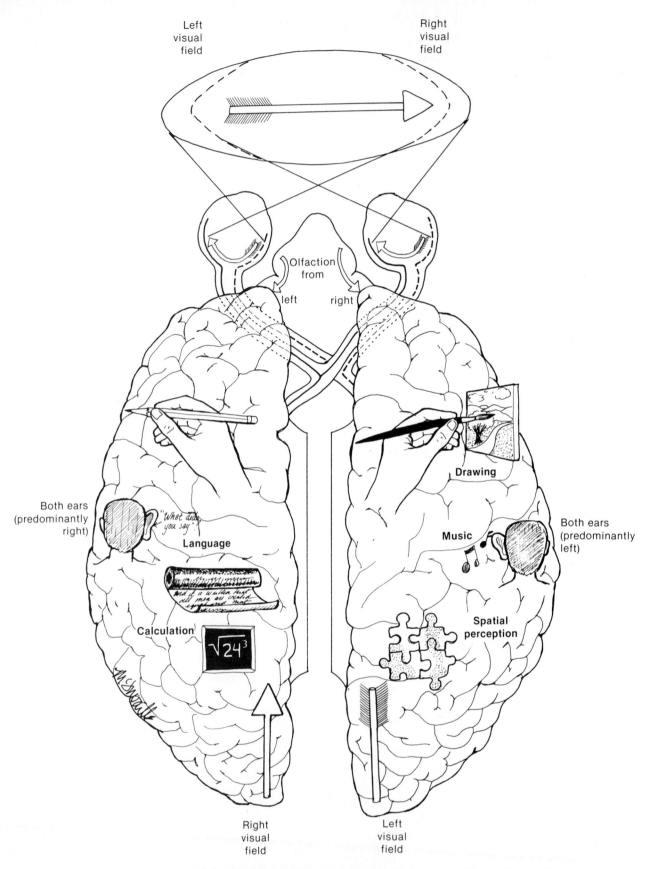

Fig. 15-19. Schematic illustration of the different functional specializations of the two hemispheres as determined from studies of patients after callosal section. (Modified from Sperry, R.W.: Lateral specialization in the surgically separated hemispheres. In Schmitt, F.O., and Worden, F.G., editors: The neurosciences: third study program, Cambridge, Mass., 1974, The MIT Press.)

perimental animals. The importance of the corpus callosum for these transfers can be shown dramatically in experiments involving bisection of the optic chiasm of experimental animals. This destroys all fibers crossing from each eye to the contralateral lateral geniculate nucleus, so anything presented to one eye only reaches the ipsilateral cerebral hemisphere. Such animals, despite having bitemporal visual field deficits, continue to show normal transfer of learning from one side to the other. However, if the corpus callosum is also sectioned, the animals no longer show this transfer. It is even possible to train them to give two completely different responses to the same stimulus, depending on which eye sees the stimulus.

Section of the corpus callosum has been used as a treatment of last resort for a few human patients suffering from intractable epilepsy, to prevent seizures from spreading from one hemisphere to the other. The procedure generally ameliorates the epilepsy, and the patients seem otherwise more or less unchanged, but careful testing reveals some remarkable alterations. Words flashed in the right visual field can be read normally, but words flashed in the left field cannot be read, and the patient denies having seen them. As far as spoken or written responses to visual stimuli are concerned, these "split-brain" patients behave as though they have a left homonymous hemianopsia. This is thoroughly consistent with the notion of dominance of the left hemisphere for language: visual stimuli in the right field reach the left hemisphere, which can organize and execute a spoken or written response; visual stimuli in the left field reach the right hemisphere, which no longer has access to the language areas. However, it is easy to show that the right hemisphere is still quite functional. For example, a picture of some object can be flashed in the left visual field and the patient asked to pick out that object manually from an assortment on a table; this can be done (usually with the left hand), even though the patient denies having seen anything. This is a clear indication that the right hemisphere has some capacity for the comprehension of language and the organization of nonverbal responses.

Continued testing of such patients has yielded some general concepts of hemisphere function that, by and large, confirm and extend the conclusions drawn from studies of patients with unilateral brain damage (Fig. 15-19). The left hemisphere in most people appears to be dominant not only for language but also for mathematical ability and the ability to solve problems in a sequential, logical fashion. The right hemisphere seems to be superior in musical skills, in recognition of faces, and in tasks requiring comprehension of spatial relationships; after callosal section a patient is likely to be able to draw and copy better with the left hand than with the right

hand. Problems are solved in a more comprehensive, holistic fashion by the right hemisphere. As noted previously, the right hemisphere also has some capacity for comprehension of language. The corpus callosum ordinarily welds the two hemispheres together into a unitary consciousness. After section of the corpus callosum, individuals develop close cooperation between their two hemispheres and subtle methods of cross-cuing, but nevertheless each hemisphere appears to have separate conscious experiences, creating a knotty philosophical problem.*

These same studies of split-brain patients also indicate that there is probably somewhat more bilaterality in the connections of somatic sensory and motor pathways than is commonly acknowledged. With time and practice, each hemisphere acquires not only a great deal of control over ipsilateral muscles but also considerable awareness of stimuli applied to the ipsilateral side of the body.

Disconnection syndromes

It stands to reason that we could not reach out for a seen object unless visual information could somehow influence the activity of the motor cortex. This has been corroborated experimentally in monkeys: cuts in the parietal lobe that destroy the long association bundles connecting the frontal and occipital lobes interfere with the ability to carry out movements guided by vision in the contralateral visual field. *Disconnection syndromes* similar in principle have been proposed (and in some cases have been shown fairly convincingly) to account for some of the complex disorders that follow cerebral damage in humans.

The classic example of a disconnection syndrome is *pure word blindness*, or *alexia without agraphia*. Patients with this rare condition are able to write (thus no agraphia) but are unable to read anything (alexia)—even words they have just finished writing; they almost always have a right homonymous hemianopsia as well. Alexia without agraphia occasionally follows a stroke that involves the left posterior cerebral artery and causes destruction of the left visual cortex (hence the hemianopsia) and of the splenium of the corpus callosum (Fig.

*"Everything we have seen so far indicates that the surgery has left these people with two separate minds, that is, two separate spheres of consciousness. What is experienced in the right hemisphere seems to be entirely outside the realm of awareness of the left hemisphere. This mental division has been demonstrated in regard to perception, cognition, volition, learning, and memory. One of the hemispheres, the left, dominant or major hemisphere, has speech and is normally talkative and conversant. The other, the minor hemisphere, however, is mute or dumb, being able to express itself only through nonverbal reactions." (Sperry, R.W. In Eccles, J.C., editor: Brain and conscious experience, New York, 1966, Springer-Verlag, Inc.) Not everyone agrees with Sperry's conclusion.

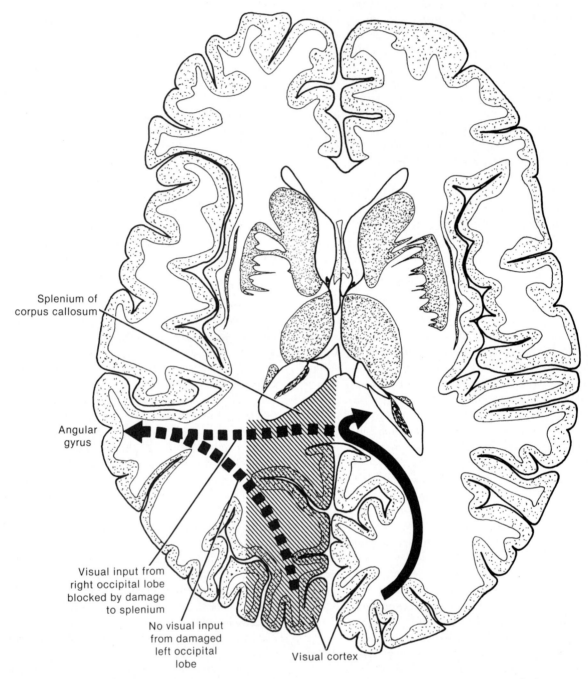

Splenium of
corpus callosum

Angular
gyrus

Visual input from
right occipital lobe
blocked by damage
to splenium

No visual input
from damaged
left occipital
lobe

Visual cortex

Fig. 15-20. Diagram of a lesion that would cause pure word blindness (alexia without agraphia). Destruction of the left visual cortex prevents information from the right visual field from reaching language areas of the left hemisphere, particularly the left angular gyrus. Destruction of the splenium of the corpus callosum prevents information from the left visual fields from reaching the language areas, since the route from the right visual cortex to the left hemisphere is blocked. The language areas themselves are undamaged, so the production of language and the comprehension of speech are intact.

15-20). As a result, the language areas (in particular the left angular gyrus) are cut off from all visual input: the destroyed left visual cortex can supply none, and the intact right visual cortex can supply none, since the route through the corpus callosum is blocked. Since the language areas are undamaged and still connected to the motor cortex, verbal and written language can still be produced.

Several other disconnection syndromes have been proposed or demonstrated, and the concept is valuable in terms of understanding some disorders of higher cerebral function. Callosal section represents an ultimate example. Conduction aphasia (discussed earlier), in which Broca's and Wernicke's areas are disconnected from each other, provides another example. Disconnections of language areas from different sensory areas or from motor cortex have been invoked to explain some cases of agnosia or apraxia.

CONSCIOUSNESS AND SLEEP

We all have an intuitive understanding of what consciousness means, but no satisfactory definition for it has yet been devised. Instead we usually settle for a listing of things that are present when consciousness is present; this list usually includes self-awareness, access to memories, and the ability to manipulate abstract ideas and to direct one's attention. Discussing the anatomical basis of consciousness is also difficult and ultimately probably impossible, since a complete description would require a solution to the age-old problem of the physical relationship between mind and brain. However, we can discuss anatomical structures whose well-being is important for the maintenance of consciousness. The first and most important point is that as far as we can tell, consciousness does not "reside" as a single entity in any particular part of the brain but rather arises somehow from interactions among many neural structures. Although the cerebral cortex is undoubtedly essential for many of the attributes associated with consciousness, remarkably large cortical areas can be destroyed without abolishing consciousness, and no single cortical area appears to be crucial for maintaining it. This is not to say that a fully intact cerebral cortex, all by itself, is conscious. As described in Chapter 8, the ascending reticular activating system (ARAS), part of the brainstem reticular formation, is essential for maintaining normal cortical function. The ARAS receives collaterals from virtually all sensory pathways and projects to the midline and intralaminar nuclei of the thalamus, which in turn project diffusely to widespread cortical areas. Bilateral destruction of the midbrain reticular formation or of the midline and intralaminar nuclei causes coma. (This does not imply that consciousness resides in the reticular formation: your car won't run without a battery, but when

it is running, the battery is not the source of power.) Finally, there is good reason to think that other structures such as the basal ganglia and the hypothalamus participate in the neural interactions whose result is consciousness.

Sleep is a reversible state of unconsciousness that is of great interest, not only because we spend so much time doing it but also because an understanding of the mechanisms of sleep might be expected to have a bearing on the mechanisms of consciousness in general. It was thought for a time that sleep was a passive process reflecting a decreased level of excitation of the ARAS and a consequent "shutting down" of the cerebral cortex. However, it is now apparent that active mechanisms play a major role and that specific neural structures can induce sleep by inhibiting the ARAS.

Our sleep is of two different kinds. The first, which includes several stages, is called *slow-wave* (or *synchronized*) *sleep*, because during it the electroencephalogram (EEG) is dominated by synchronous waves at various low frequencies, principally less than 4 Hz (*delta waves*). During slow-wave sleep, muscle tone is somewhat reduced, heart rate and breathing are slowed but steady, and subjects awakened from this state seldom report that they were dreaming. Roughly every 90 to 120 minutes we shift into the second type of sleep, called *desynchronized sleep*, in which the EEG is dominated by low-voltage, high-frequency activity that is not organized into obvious waves and is remarkably similar to the activity seen in the waking state. In spite of the fact that the EEG looks like that of wakefulness, an individual is harder to awaken from this stage than from slow-wave sleep; as a result, desynchronized sleep is also called *paradoxical sleep*. Desynchronized sleep has several other distinctive properties: there is a nearly complete abolition of muscle tone, and the transmission of impulses over at least some sensory pathways is greatly decreased; blood pressure falls, and heart rate and breathing become erratic. Superimposed on this background are coincident phasic events. There are bursts of inhibition of motor mechanisms, so that the last vestige of muscle tone is eliminated. Some twitching movements manage to break through the inhibition, most prominently bursts of rapid eye movements (REMs). The latter phenomenon gives rise to the most commonly used name for desynchronized sleep, which is *REM sleep*. Subjects awakened from REM sleep are likely to report that they were dreaming.

Many aspects of the anatomical substrate of sleep have been worked out in experimental animals, and the reticular formation figures prominently in these mechanisms (Fig. 15-21). Confirmation for humans is difficult to come by, since processes that damage the brainstem reticular formation to any great extent are usually fatal.

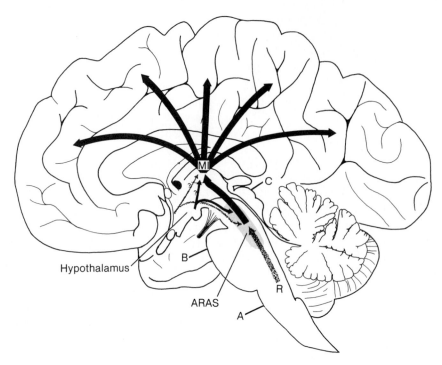

Fig. 15-21. Summary diagram of neural structures and connections important for maintenance of the sleep-waking cycle; sleep-inducing connections are stippled. The ascending reticular activating system (ARAS) maintains wakefulness by acting on the cerebral cortex in a generalized manner through the midline and intralaminar nuclei of the thalamus (*MI*). The ARAS is periodically turned off by projections from the medullary and pontine reticular formation (*R*), inducing sleep. Diencephalic centers are also capable of inducing sleep and wakefulness via connections that are not completely understood. Separate collections of neurons in the pons are responsible for triggering periods of REM sleep. Damage caudal to point *A* causes no changes in the sleep-wakefulness cycle. Damage at point *B* disconnects sleep-inducing portions of the reticular formation from the ARAS, causing nearly constant wakefulness of the forebrain. (However, such a lesion is extremely unlikely.) Damage at point *C* disconnects the ARAS from the forebrain, causing coma.

The following account is therefore based mainly on animal studies, but the clinical data available about humans are generally consistent with these results.

Stimulation of the midline and intralaminar nuclei at low frequencies produces sleep and synchronization of the EEG, so this part of the thalamus is considered to be a sort of final switching mechanism into which other sleep-inducing mechanisms funnel. The EEG of an animal whose brainstem has been transected in the rostral midbrain shows constant synchronized activity indicative of slow-wave sleep, at least in the acute stages after the operation. This reflects the fact that the ARAS has been disconnected from the forebrain. As long as the reticular formation is still connected to the forebrain (as, for example, after a transection of the upper cervical spinal cord), an animal shows all the standard EEG signs of cycling through wakefulness and the various stages of sleep. Some insight into what turns the ARAS off and on is provided by transecting the brainstem at a midpontine level. It might be expected that in such a case the animal would show either normal sleep and wakefulness

(if this lesion leaves enough of the reticular formation attached to the forebrain) or constant sleep (if too much of the reticular formation is removed by such a lesion). Instead the animal shows signs of constant wakefulness rostral to the lesion, at least during the acute stages after the operation. This indicates not only that the parts of the ARAS crucial for wakefulness are contained in the midbrain reticular formation but also that parts of the medullary and caudal pontine reticular formation are responsible for periodically turning the ARAS off and on. No one knows where the clockwork for this mechanism in the caudal brainstem is located, but there are indications that some cells of the *raphe nuclei* of the reticular formation, which use serotonin as their neurotransmitter, are important components. One piece of evidence supporting this concept is the observation that depletion of the brain's serotonin, either by pharmacological techniques or by destruction of the raphe nuclei, causes an insomnia that can be reversed promptly by administration of serotonin.

In addition to the brainstem mechanisms that regulate

sleep and wakefulness, there is a second system located more rostrally. Encephalitic damage to the posterior hypothalamus of humans causes the hypersomnia of sleeping sickness, and stimulation of this area in sleeping animals causes awakening. Conversely, damage to the general region of the preoptic area and orbital frontal cortex has been shown to cause insomnia, and stimulation of this area causes sleep. How this anterior "sleep center" and posterior "wakefulness center" interact with the brainstem mechanisms is not fully known. There are indications that in an intact animal the forebrain centers act in part directly on the ARAS to achieve a unified sleep-waking cycle. On the other hand, it is also known that 10 to 15 days after a mesencephalic transection the forebrain once again begins to cycle through the synchronized and desynchronized EEGs of apparent sleep and wakefulness, even though it is now independent of the ARAS.

The basic anatomical control mechanisms for REM sleep are more localized than are those for slow-wave sleep and are entirely contained in the caudal brainstem. This is shown perhaps most dramatically in the case of a cat with only those parts of its CNS up to the midpons left intact. Such an animal obviously is unable to show EEG signs of sleep and wakefulness, but at periodic intervals throughout the day and night, it does have episodes that include all the parts of REM sleep of which the spinal cord and caudal brainstem are capable. That is, there are periodic spells of decreased muscle tone and twitches of the lateral recti (the only way for REMs to be expressed in this condition).* The timing mechanism for the initiation of REM sleep is thought to be in the caudal pontine reticular formation. This timing mechanism somehow triggers neurons in the locus ceruleus or its immediate vicinity to mediate the tonic events of REM sleep such as the characteristic decrease of muscle tone; it also triggers the vestibular nuclei to cause the phasic events of REM sleep such as the REMs themselves and the transient abolition of the last little bit of muscle tone.

REM sleep normally occurs only in the midst of periods of slow-wave sleep, so it is assumed that the REM sleep mechanisms must ordinarily be primed or triggered by the centers for slow-wave sleep.

---

*These REMs in the absence of cerebral hemispheres are one bit of evidence for the generally accepted conclusion that, whatever the eye movements of REM sleep are, they do not represent "looking-at-a-dream" movements.

ADDITIONAL READING

Bremer, F.: Cerebral hypnogenic centers, Ann. Neurol. 2:1, 1977. "Hypnogenic" = sleep-inducing.

Brinkman, J., and Kuypers, H.G.J.M.: Cerebral control of contralateral and ipsilateral arm, hand and finger movements in the split-brain rhesus monkey, Brain 96:653, 1973.

Buser, P.A., and Rougeul-Buser, A., editors: Cerebral correlates of conscious experience, New York, 1978, Elsevier North-Holland, Inc.

Celesia, G.G.: Organization of auditory cortical areas in man, Brain 99:403, 1976.

Critchley, M.: The parietal lobes, London, 1953, Edward Arnold (Publishers), Ltd. The classic clinical work on the various syndromes resulting from parietal lesions.

Eccles, J.C., editor: Brain and conscious experience, New York, 1966, Springer-Verlag, Inc.

Galaburda, A.M., et al.: Right-left asymmetries in the brain, Science 199:852, 1978.

Geschwind, N.: Disconnexion syndromes in animals and man: part I, Brain 88:237, 1965. Part II, Brain 88:585, 1965. A scholarly and very influential paper arguing forcefully for the concept of complex syndromes caused by disconnections of various cerebral areas from one another.

Geschwind, N.: The organization of language and the brain, Science 170:940, 1970.

Goldman, P.S., and Nauta, W.J.H.: Columnar distribution of corticocortical fibers in the frontal association, limbic, and motor cortex of the developing rhesus monkey, Brain Res. 122:393, 1977. Pretty pictures.

Gordon, H.W., and Bogen, J.E.: Hemispheric lateralization of singing after intracarotid sodium amylobarbitone, J. Neurol. Neurosurg. Psychiatr. 37:727, 1974.

Gücer, G.: The effect of sleep upon the transmission of afferent activity in the somatic afferent system, Exp. Brain Res. 34:287, 1979.

Haaxma, R., and Kuypers, H.G.J.M.: Intrahemispheric cortical connexions and visual guidance of hand and finger movements in the rhesus monkey, Brain 98:239, 1975. Direct experimental demonstration of a type of disconnection syndrome.

Hecaen, H., and Albert, M.L.: Human neuropsychology, New York, 1978, John Wiley & Sons, Inc.

Herkenham, M.: Laminar organization of thalamic projections to the rat neocortex, Science 207:532, 1980.

Herron, J., editor: Neuropsychology of left-handedness, New York, 1979, Academic Press, Inc.

Jones, E.G., Coulter, J.D., and Wise, S.P.: Commissural columns in the sensory-motor cortex of monkeys, J. Comp. Neurol. 188:113, 1979.

Jones, E.G., and Powell, T.P.S.: An anatomical study of converging sensory pathways within the cerebral cortex of the monkey, Brain 93:793, 1970. A study of the stepwise radiations of auditory, visual, and somatosensory information from the primary receiving areas to parts of the association cortex; done by the straightforward but clever technique of lesioning a primary area, tracing the degenerating fibers, and making lesions where the degeneration terminates.

Jouandet, M.L., and Gazzaniga, M.S.: Cortical field of origin of the anterior commissure of the rhesus monkey, Exp. Neurol. 66:381, 1979.

Jouvet, M.: Neurophysiology of the states of sleep, Physiol. Rev. 47:117, 1967.

Kertesz, A., Lesk, D., and McCabe, P.: Isotope localization of infarcts in aphasia, Arch. Neurol. 34:590, 1977.

LaMotte, R.H., and Mountcastle, V.B.: Disorders in somesthesis following lesions of parietal lobe, J. Neurophysiol. 42:400, 1979.

LeDoux, J.E., Wilson, D.H., and Gazzaniga, M.S.: A divided mind: observations on the conscious properties of the separated hemispheres, Ann. Neurol. 2:417, 1977. An individual with some bilateral language representation may not give the same responses with each hemisphere after section of the corpus callosum.

Libet, B., et al.: Subjective referral of the timing for a conscious sensory experience: a functional role for the somatosensory specific projection system in man, Brain 102:193, 1979. How do we decide when a tactile stimulus occurs? Is it at the instant of physical contact, or when the first electrical activity reaches the postcentral gyrus, or after this activity has rattled around the cortex for awhile? A fascinating and provocative paper that addresses this question experimentally.

Mountcastle, V.B., editor: Medical physiology, ed. 14, St. Louis, 1980, The C.V. Mosby Co. Chapter 10 ("Sleep, wakefulness, and the conscious state," by V.B. Mountcastle) and Chapter 21 ("Higher functions of the nervous system," by G. Werner) are two of several relevant chapters in this excellent textbook.

Mountcastle, V.B., et al.: Posterior parietal association cortex of the monkey: command functions for operations within extrapersonal space, J. Neurophysiol. 38:871, 1975.

Nauta, W.J.H.: The problem of the frontal lobe: a reinterpretation, J. Psychiatr. Res. 8:167, 1971.

Pearlman, A.L., Birch, J., and Meadows, J.C.: Cerebral color blindness: an acquired defect in hue discrimination, Ann. Neurol. 5:253, 1979.

Penfield, W., and Boldrey, E.: Somatic motor and sensory representation in the cerebral cortex of man as studied by electrical stimulation, Brain 60:389, 1937.

Penfield, W., and Rasmussen, T.: The cerebral cortex of man, New York, 1950, Macmillan, Inc. A review of the results of cortical stimulations of a large series of patients and of the results of localized cortical excisions from these patients.

Penfield, W., and Roberts, L.: Speech and brain-mechanisms, Princeton, N.J., 1959, Princeton University Press.

Petre-Quadens, O., and Schlag, J.D., editors: Basic sleep mechanisms, New York, 1974, Academic Press, Inc.

Phelps, M.E., Kuhl, D.E., and Mazziotta, J.C.: Metabolic mapping of the brain's response to visual stimulation: studies in humans, Science 211:1445, 1981. A new, noninvasive technique for studying changes in the rate of glucose utilization in different cortical areas.

Plum, F., and Posner, J.B.: Diagnosis of stupor and coma, ed. 3, Philadelphia, 1980, F.A. Davis Company.

Purpura, D.P.: Dendritic spine "dysgenesis" and mental retardation, Science 186:1126, 1974.

Rubens, A.B., Mahowald, M.W., and Hutton, J.T.: Asymmetry of the lateral (sylvian) fissures in man, Neurology 26:620, 1976.

Russell, I.S., and Ochs, S.: Localization of a memory trace in one cortical hemisphere and transfer to the other hemisphere, Brain 86:37, 1963. We know that inputs spread to both hemispheres under normal circumstances via the corpus callosum. This interesting paper describes what happens if one hemisphere is temporarily inactivated during acquisition of a memory.

Sauerland, E.K., and Harper, R.M.: The human tongue during sleep: electromyographic activity of the genioglossus muscle, Exp. Neurol. 51:160, 1976. If the muscles of your tongue follow the general pattern and become flaccid during REM sleep, then why don't you get into trouble by inhaling it? Read this and find out.

Sperry, R.W.: Lateral specialization in the surgically separated hemispheres. In Schmitt, F.O., and Worden, F.G., editors: The neurosciences: third study program, Cambridge, Mass., 1974, The MIT Press. A general review on results from humans with a sectioned corpus callosum by the principal figure in this type of research.

Szentagothai, J.: The neuron network of the cerebral cortex: a functional interpretation, Proc. R. Soc. Lond. B201:219, 1978.

Teuber, H.-L.: The brain and human behavior. In Held, R., Leibowitz, H.W., and Teuber, H.-L., editors: Handbook of sensory physiology, vol. 8 (Perception), New York, 1978, Springer-Verlag, Inc. An interesting, scholarly, wide-ranging correlation of deficits and brain damage in humans and experimental animals.

Van Essen, D.C.: Visual areas of the mammalian cerebral cortex, Ann. Rev. Neurosci. 2:227, 1979.

Villablanca, J.: Behavioral and polygraphic study of "sleep" and "wakefulness" in chronic decerebrate cats, Electroencephalogr. Clin. Neurophysiol. 21:562, 1966. In the chronic state after a rostral mesencephalic transection, the portions of the CNS both rostral and caudal to the transection are capable of some manifestations of sleep and wakefulness; amazingly enough, they do so with completely independent rhythms.

Wada, J.A., and Davis, A.E.: Fundamental nature of human infant's brain asymmetry, Can. J. Neurol. Sci. 4:203, 1977. We are born not only with built-in anatomical asymmetries but apparently also with built-in physiological asymmetries.

Wada, J., and Rasmussen, T.: Intracarotid injection of sodium amytal for the lateralization of cerebral speech dominance: experimental and clinical observations, J. Neurosurg. 17:266, 1960.

Weinstein, E.A., and Friedland, R.P., editors: Hemi-inattention and hemisphere specialization, Advances in neurology, vol. 18, New York, 1977, Raven Press.

Whitsel, B.L., et al.: Thalamic projections to S-I in macaque monkey, J. Comp. Neurol. 178:385, 1978.

Woolsey, T.A., and van der Loos, H.: The structural organization of layer IV in the somatosensory region (SI) of mouse cerebral cortex: the description of a cortical field composed of discrete cytoarchitectonic units, Brain Res. 17:205, 1970. A special kind of columnar organization described in a delightful paper.

Yamadori, A., et al.: Preservation of singing in Broca's aphasia, J. Neurol. Neurosurg. Psychiatry 40:221, 1977.

CHAPTER 16

OLFACTORY AND LIMBIC SYSTEMS

We seldom perceive things in a completely neutral fashion. Various sights and sounds make us happy, sad, or angry; certain odors can make some individuals positively ecstatic. There is also a two-way connection between these emotional aspects of perception on the one hand and thoughts and memories on the other: appropriate aromas can conjure up images of meals and wines consumed in the past; in addition, the remembrance of something in the past can stir the same emotions that accompanied the original event, and even thinking about something that has not happened can arouse emotions. Assuming that "thinking" depends heavily on the neocortex, it would seem likely that the anatomical substrate for feelings and emotions would at least be closely connected with the neocortex. The same system would also need to be heavily interconnected with the hypothalamus, since sensory inputs that arouse an emotion also initiate autonomic responses such as salivating and gearing up the alimentary tract or pumping adrenalin and diverting blood to skeletal muscles. Finally, the types of stimuli that elicit emotion-laden responses in us—and the responses themselves—are, in a more general sense, crucial to all animals, for these are the drive-related activities central to the preservation of individuals and their species, activities like feeding, defense, and sexual behavior.

The *limbic system* is the name given to the portions of the brain primarily concerned with such responses and behavior. As discussed in some detail later in the chapter, it includes the *cingulate* and *parahippocampal gyri* (Fig. 2-5), the *amygdala*, and the *hippocampal formation*. In view of the preceding discussion, it is not surprising that the components of the limbic system appeared very early in vertebrate phylogeny and that in its connections the limbic system is interposed between the neocortex and the hypothalamus.

The olfactory nerve is the only one that projects directly to the telencephalon; as a result, the telencephalon of primitive vertebrates has been considered to be a processing station for olfactory information and the limbic system to be related to olfactory structures. While there is some reason to think that the brains of all vertebrates are more similar to each other than had previously been suspected (so that all telencephalons play a role in the processing of all types of sensory information), the olfactory and limbic systems are still customarily discussed together. As further recognition of their phylogenetic antiquity, parts of the olfactory and limbic systems are referred to as the *paleocortex* and *archicortex*. Use of the terms varies somewhat from one author to another, but the paleocortex is approximately the same thing as the olfactory cortex, and the archicortex is equivalent to the hippocampal formation. The paleocortex and archicortex, collectively called the *allocortex* or *heterogenetic cortex,* are structurally simpler than the neocortex and have fewer than six layers (in most areas, only three layers).

OLFACTORY SYSTEM
Olfactory epithelium

The olfactory system begins peripherally with the *olfactory epithelium*, a pigmented, yellowish patch of cells that occupies about 2.5 sq cm of the roof and adjacent walls of the nasal cavity on each side. Each patch of olfactory epithelium consists of about 25 million receptor cells interspersed with supporting cells and small glands (called *Bowman's glands*). Sensory endings of the trigeminal nerve are also found in the olfactory epithelium. The trigeminal endings are responsible for the noxious sensation (not really one of smell) elicited by irritants like concentrated ammonia. The *olfactory receptors* are bipolar neurons, each with a single slender

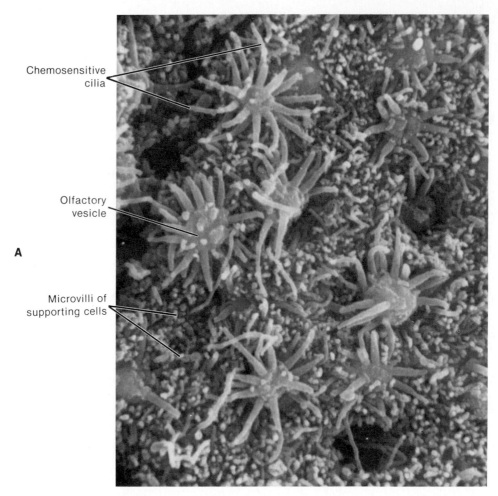

Chemosensitive cilia

Olfactory vesicle

A

Microvilli of supporting cells

Fig. 16-1. Olfactory receptors. **A,** Scanning electron micrograph of the exposed surface of the olfactory epithelium; interspersed in a carpet of microvilli are olfactory vesicles, giving rise to the chemosensitive cilia of the olfactory receptors. **B,** Schematic drawing of a single olfactory receptor. (**A,** from Tissues and organs: a text-atlas of scanning electron microscopy by Richard G. Kessel and Randy H. Kardon. W.H. Freeman and Company. Copyright © 1979.)

dendrite emerging from one end of its cell body and an axon emerging from the other end (Fig. 16-1). The dendrite extends to a bulbous termination, the *olfactory vesicle*, from which a series of cilia spread out over the surface of the epithelium in a layer of mucus secreted by the supporting cells and Bowman's glands. Substances to be smelled dissolve in the mucous layer and stimulate the chemosensitive cilia of the olfactory receptors.

The unmyelinated axons of the olfactory receptors are among the finest (only 0.2 μm in diameter) and most slowly conducting axons in the entire central nervous system. They collect into a series of about 20 small bundles, the *olfactory fila* (Latin, filum = thread), which pass through the holes in the cribriform plate of the ethmoid bone and end in the *olfactory bulb*. Collectively the olfactory fila make up the first cranial nerve.

Olfactory bulb

Animals that depend heavily on their sense of smell (called *macrosmatic* animals; Greek, osme = odor) have a well-developed central olfactory apparatus, including a neatly laminated olfactory bulb. In *microsmatic* humans, this lamination is not so apparent, and the olfactory bulb is relatively small and poorly developed. Its most prominent cell type is the *mitral cell*, which has a triangular cell body and was named for its fancied resemblance to a bishop's miter. A mitral cell is configured like a neocortical pyramidal cell in reverse (Fig. 16-2): an axon emerges from its apex and moves toward

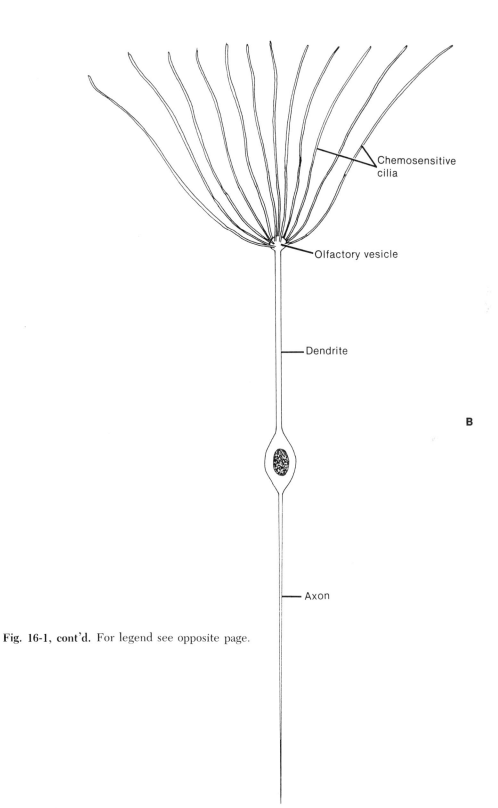

Chemosensitive cilia

Olfactory vesicle

Dendrite

B

Axon

Fig. 16-1, cont'd. For legend see opposite page.

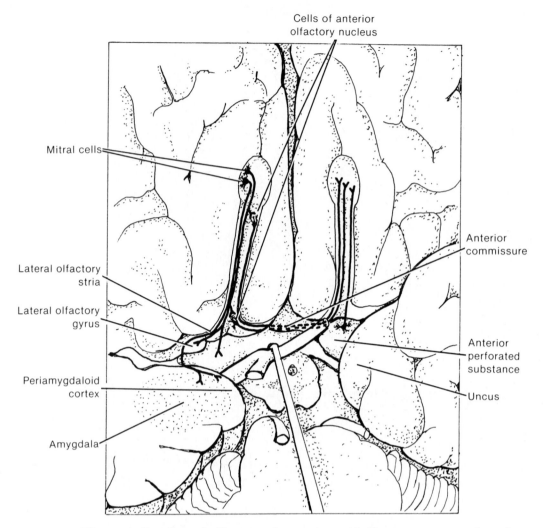

Fig. 16-2. Olfactory bulb and initial olfactory pathways. Axons of olfactory receptors end on the dendrites of mitral and tufted cells, which in turn send their axons out through the olfactory tract. Collaterals of fibers in the olfactory tract end on cells of the anterior olfactory nucleus. Efferents to the olfactory bulb, shown on the right side of the diagram, arise in the anterior olfactory nucleus (of both sides) and in the vicinity of the anterior perforated substance. (Compare with Fig. 16-3.)

the interior of the bulb to enter the *olfactory tract*, while a dendrite emerges from its base, ascends to the surface of the bulb, and receives contacts from the incoming axons of olfactory receptors. These dendrites spread out in large spherical arborizations 100 to 200 μm in diameter called *glomeruli*. Olfactory axons terminate in these glomeruli with a great deal of convergence; it is estimated that there are 1,000 olfactory receptors for each mitral cell in the rabbit. The olfactory bulb also contains interneurons (most of them called *granule cells* here as in other regions of the CNS) and a collection of *tufted cells*, which are smaller than mitral cells but also send their dendrites into the glomeruli and their axons into the olfactory tract. The olfactory bulb, like

other sensory relays in the CNS, also receives a contingent of efferent fibers that are assumed to regulate or tune its sensitivity in some way. Some of these efferents arise in the vicinity of the *anterior perforated substance*. Others arise from the *anterior olfactory nucleus*, a collective name for clusters of cells scattered all along the olfactory tract.

Axons of mitral and tufted cells proceed caudally in the olfactory tract, giving off collaterals to cells of the anterior olfactory nucleus along the way. Fibers from the anterior olfactory nucleus then project to both olfactory bulbs (Fig. 16-2). At the junction between the orbital frontal cortex and the anterior perforated substance, the olfactory tract diverges to form the *olfactory trigone*

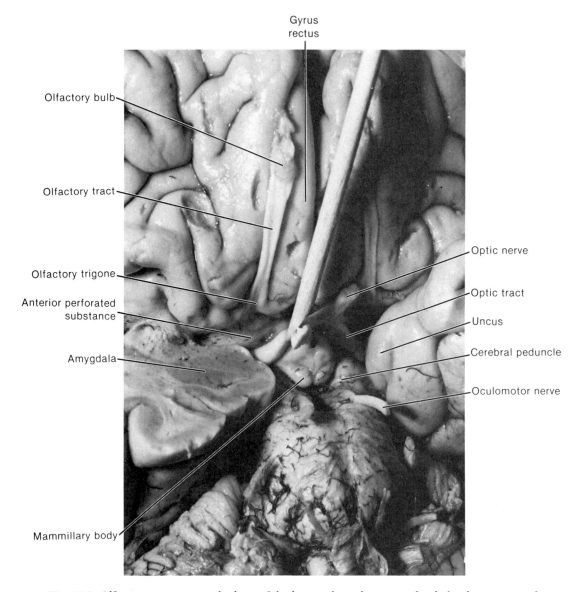

Gyrus
rectus

Olfactory bulb

Olfactory tract

Olfactory trigone

Anterior perforated
substance

Amygdala

Mammillary body

Optic nerve

Optic tract

Uncus

Cerebral peduncle

Oculomotor nerve

Fig. 16-3. Olfactory structures at the base of the brain. The right temporal pole has been removed and the optic chiasm retracted.

(Fig. 16-3). The two sides of this triangle are formed by the *medial* and *lateral olfactory striae,* and its base merges with the anterior perforated substance. Fibers from the anterior olfactory nucleus enter the medial olfactory stria, cross the midline through the anterior part of the anterior commissure, and project to the contralateral olfactory bulb. Some fibers from the olfactory bulb continue straight back through the olfactory trigone and end in the adjacent portion of the anterior perforated substance, but most of them enter the lateral olfactory stria. The lateral stria is therefore the principal central projection pathway for the olfactory system.

Central connections

The lateral olfactory stria travels along the lateral edge of the anterior perforated substance covered by a thin layer of gray matter called the *lateral olfactory gyrus.* When it reaches the posterior border of the anterior perforated substance, it curves up onto the surface of the temporal lobe in the vicinity of the uncus and disappears. Along this course, it terminates in two places (Fig. 16-4): in the *primary olfactory cortex* and in a portion of the amygdala. There is no thalamic relay for the olfactory system. The primary olfactory cortex consists of the lateral olfactory gyrus and a small portion of the

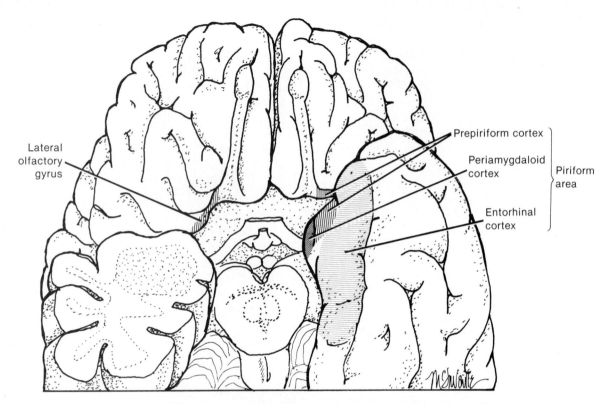

Fig. 16-4. Diagram of the base of the brain showing the location of the primary olfactory cortex (vertical lines and stippling) and the olfactory association cortex (horizontal lines). Fibers of the olfactory tract also terminate directly in a portion of the amygdala.

uncus and is itself subdivided into two portions. The lateral olfactory gyrus, together with part of the olfactory region of the uncus, is called the *prepiriform cortex.* The remainder of the olfactory region of the uncus is called the *periamygdaloid cortex,* since it is continuous with the underlying amygdala.

These primary receiving sites for olfactory information project in turn to the rest of the amygdala and to the *olfactory association cortex,* which occupies the anterior part of the parahippocampal gyrus and corresponds to Brodmann's area 28 (Fig. 15-12). This area, commonly referred to as the *entorhinal cortex,* lies adjacent to the primary olfactory cortex and may in fact receive projections directly from the olfactory tract, in addition to projections from the primary olfactory cortex. As will be seen later in this chapter, the entorhinal cortex does considerably more than serve as the olfactory association cortex. The prepiriform, periamygdaloid, and entorhinal cortices taken together are sometimes referred to as the *piriform area* or *piriform lobe,* because this portion of the telencephalon in some lower vertebrates is relatively large and pear-shaped.

The olfactory system is unusual in a number of respects. It has already been noted that it is the only

sensory system that projects directly to the telencephalon without a thalamic relay. You also may have noticed that central olfactory projections, at least up to the level of the association cortex, are uncrossed. This implies a strange state of affairs in which each cerebral hemisphere is concerned with the contralateral visual field, the contralateral half of the body, and substances entering the *ipsilateral* nostril. That this is indeed the case has been shown in experiments with patients who had undergone section of the corpus callosum as described in Chapter 15. Although such patients can only name (that is, speak about) things in the right visual field or the right hand, they can only name odors presented to the left nostril. Furthermore, if an identifiable odor is presented to one nostril, they can pick out the corresponding object by feeling around with the contralateral, but not the ipsilateral, hand.

Some functional aspects of the olfactory system

Although our sense of smell is exquisitely sensitive and allows some remarkable discriminations, it is less well developed in humans (and less important in everyday life) than in many other species. As a consequence of some head injuries, the olfactory fila may be torn loose from the olfactory bulb. Someone deprived of the sense of smell (that is, rendered *anosmatic*) by this or some other means is likely to complain less of loss of olfaction than of the fact that food tastes bland. (Much of what we attribute to our sense of taste actually depends on the aromas of what we eat and drink.) However, testing olfaction can sometimes provide useful diagnostic clues. For example, tumors growing at the base of the skull beneath the orbital surface of the frontal lobe can become quite large before they cause any symptoms other than a unilateral anosmia.

The piriform area has been directly identified as the functional olfactory cortex in humans, since electrical stimulation there causes olfactory sensations. Clues pointing in the same direction were provided in the nineteenth century by the British neurologist Hughlings Jackson, who noted that epileptic seizures that originate in the vicinity of the uncus may begin with an illusion of smell or taste, most often an unpleasant one. The seizure may go on to include motor phenomena such as chewing movements or smacking of the lips and alterations of consciousness such as a "dreamy state" or a feeling of déjà vu. Seizures of this type are still known as *uncinate fits*.

LIMBIC SYSTEM

In 1878, Broca pointed out that a general feature of mammalian brains is a great horseshoe-shaped rim of cortex surrounding the junction between the diencephalon and each cerebral hemisphere (Fig. 2-5). The ends of the arc are joined by olfactory areas at the base of the brain so that a complete loop is formed with the olfactory tract and bulb extending anteriorly like the handle of a tennis racket. He referred to this ring of cortex at the margin of the hemisphere as the *limbic lobe* (Latin, limbus = border) and suggested that the entire lobe might be concerned with the sense of smell. However, the limbic lobe includes the cingulate and parahippocampal gyri and the hippocampal formation, and it soon became apparent that olfaction is not the primary responsibility of these areas. For example, although dolphins have no olfactory bulbs and are thought to be completely anosmatic, they nevertheless have well-developed hippocampi. A few rare cases have been reported of humans with congenital absence of the olfactory bulb and tracts but with apparently normal limbic lobes. Finally, more recent anatomical and physiological experiments have shown that, aside from the already mentioned olfactory areas at the base of the brain, the limbic lobe does not receive a particularly large amount of olfactory input.

The limbic lobe does, however, fit many of the previously described criteria for an anatomical substrate for drive-related and emotional behavior. As will be seen in the remainder of this chapter, the limbic cortex is connected in one direction with widespread neocortical areas and in another direction with the hypothalamus. Physiological evidence has supported this view, and the conglomerate of the limbic lobe, its connections, and a few additional structures has come to be referred to as the *limbic system*. There is, unfortunately, no universal agreement on the total list of structures that should be included in the term "limbic system," but the concept should be clear by the end of this chapter. All authors would include the cingulate and parahippocampal gyri,* the hippocampal formation, the amygdala, and the *septal area* (located at the base of the septum pellucidum) (Fig. 16-5); most would include the hypothalamus, parts of the midbrain reticular formation, and the olfactory areas. Beyond that, the boundaries get fuzzy; some authors include various of the thalamic and neocortical regions interconnected with undisputed limbic components, while others do not.

The interconnections of limbic components are numerous and complex, but the overall concept of the system is not. The output end (in terms of programming or triggering behavioral outputs) is a continuous core of neural tissue extending from the septal area through the hypothalamus and into the midbrain reticular formation. The *medial forebrain bundle* (Figs. 10-16 and 10-17) is its principal longitudinal fiber pathway.† Two major limbic subsystems feed into this common output. The first (Fig. 16-6) is centered around the hippocampal formation, utilizes the cingulate and parahippocampal gyri as its liaison with the neocortex generally, and has a

---

*Some authors consider the cingulate and parahippocampal gyri to be intermediate in structure between the archi- and paleocortex on the one hand and the neocortex on the other; they refer to these two gyri as the *mesocortex* or *juxtallocortex*.

†Activation of these output structures is also apparently responsible for triggering some of the feelings that are one object of drive-related behavior. Animals with electrodes implanted in certain CNS locations, if given control of the button that turns on stimulation through these electrodes, will push the button with great zest. Electrode locations that elicit self-stimulation are widespread in the limbic system, but the most effective sites are in the septal area and along the medial forebrain bundle; animals with electrodes there will stimulate themselves at great rates for long periods and may be willing to forego food or sleep or to endure painful stimuli to press the button. Sites with the opposite effect (that is, sites at which animals will try hard to avoid being stimulated) are fewer and are principally located in the vicinity of the periaqueductal gray matter of the midbrain. These results have been generally confirmed for humans. Direct stimulation of the septal area, as an experimental treatment for certain psychiatric disorders, often yields a feeling of well-being, which is diffuse and hard to define but definitely pleasant. Stimulation near the periaqueductal gray matter sometimes causes unbearable feelings of horror and pain—an indication of the complexity of this region, since stimulation at very nearby sites can cause analgesia (see Chapter 8).

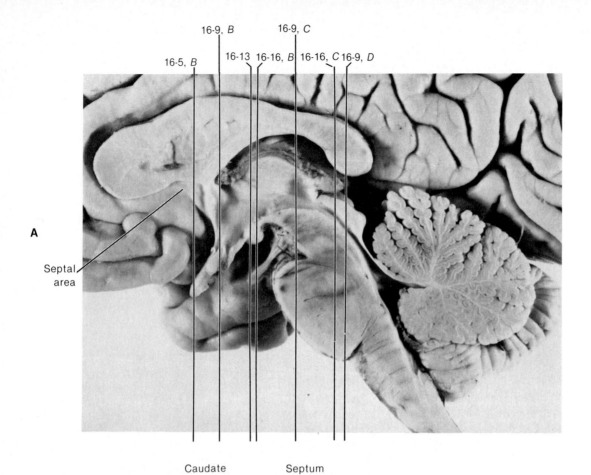

A

16-5, *B* 16-9, *B* 16-13 16-16, *B* 16-16, *C* 16-9, *D* 16-9, *C*

Septal
area

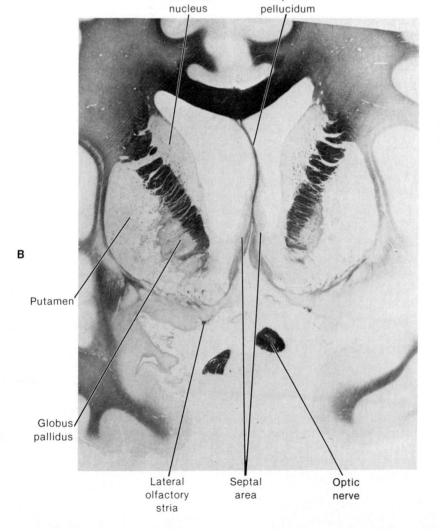

B

Caudate
nucleus

Septum
pellucidum

Putamen

Globus
pallidus

Lateral
olfactory
stria

Septal
area

Optic
nerve

Fig. 16-5. The septal area seen on the medial surface of a hemisected brain (**A**) and in a coronal section (**B**). Planes of various sections used in this chapter are indicated by the corresponding figure number in **A**.

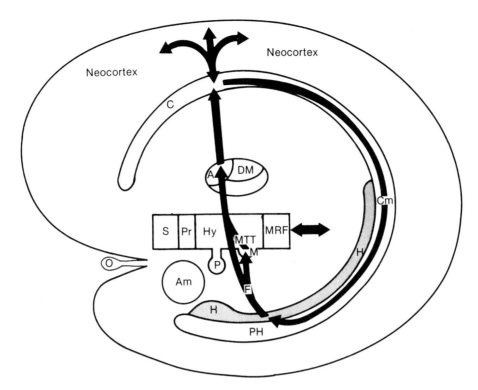

Fig. 16-6. Schematic outline of hippocampal participation in the limbic system. The hippocampal formation is interposed between neocortex generally (through connections with the cingulate and parahippocampal gyri) and the septal–hypothalamic output core of the limbic system. Since the anterior thalamic nucleus is closely related to the cingulate gyrus, it plays a prominent role in hippocampal circuits, as does the mammillary body. Abbreviations used in this and later figures: A, Anterior nucleus of thalamus; Am, amygdala; C, cingulate gyrus; Cm, cingulum; DM, dorsomedial and midline nuclei of thalamus; F, fornix; H, hippocampal formation; Hy, hypothalamus (exclusive of mammillary bodies); M, mammillary body; MRF, midbrain reticular formation; MTT, mammillothalamic tract; O, olfactory bulb; P, pituitary gland; PH, parahippocampal gyrus; Pr, preoptic area; S, septal area.

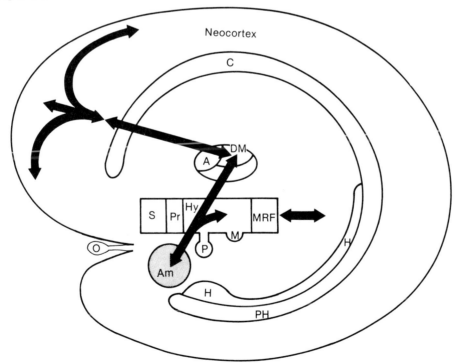

Fig. 16-7. Schematic outline of amygdalar participation in the limbic system. The amygdala is interposed between neocortex generally (through connections with orbital and other prefrontal cortex) and the septal–hypothalamic output core of the limbic system. Since the dorsomedial thalamic nucleus is closely related to the prefrontal cortex, this nucleus plays a prominent role in circuits formed by the amygdala. Abbreviations: see Fig. 16-6.

close relationship with the anterior thalamic nucleus and the mammillary body. The second (Fig. 16-7) is centered around the amygdala, utilizes prefrontal (especially orbital) and anterior temporal cortex as its liaison with the neocortex generally, and has a close relationship with the dorsomedial nucleus of the thalamus.

Hippocampal formation

The paleocortex and archicortex occupy most of the surface of each cerebral hemisphere in lower vertebrates. As the area devoted to the neocortex expands through phylogeny, the archicortex moves dorsally and then rolls around onto the medial surface of the hemisphere, while the paleocortex moves ventrally onto the base of the brain. With the continued expansion of the hemisphere in primates, the hippocampal formation becomes one more structure that is carried around in a great arc and ends up in the temporal lobe as the floor of the inferior horn of the lateral ventricle (Fig. 16-8). Traces of its heritage are revealed by a thin strand of rudimentary gray matter (the *hippocampal rudiment* or *indusium griseum*), continuous with the hippocampal formation, which is left behind on the dorsal surface of the corpus callosum and by the long, curved course of the fornix, the principal hippocampal output pathway (Fig. 16-9).

The hippocampal formation is a curved and recurved sheet of cortex folded into the medial surface of the temporal lobe. Transverse sections (Fig. 16-8) reveal that it has three distinct zones: the *dentate gyrus,* the *hippocampus* proper,* and the *subiculum.* In such sections, the dentate gyrus and the hippocampus have the form of two interlocking C's. The subiculum is a transitional zone continuous with the hippocampus at one of its edges and with the cortex of the parahippocampal gyrus at the other edge. The entire hippocampal formation has a length of about 5 cm in the inferior horn from its anterior end at the amygdala to its tapering posterior end near the splenium of the corpus callosum. Along this course numerous small blood vessels enter the hippocampal formation from the adjacent subarachnoid space by penetrating the dentate gyrus, thus giving this gyrus the beaded or toothed appearance for which it was named.

Histology. The hippocampus and the dentate gyrus are three-layered, with a superficial *molecular layer* and

---

*Also called *Ammon's horn* (or *cornu ammonis,* after an Egyptian deity with ram's horns) because of the way the hippocampi curve downward and outward from the hippocampal rudiment into the temporal lobes. Hippocampal nomenclature has a long, colorful, and not entirely logical history, as discussed by F.T. Lewis in "The significance of the term *hippocampus*" (J. Comp. Neurol. **35**:213, 1923-1924). Many authors now use the term "hippocampus" to refer to the entire hippocampal formation.

a deep *polymorphic layer,* both similar to the layers of the same name in the neocortex. The intermediate stratum is a *granule cell layer* in the dentate gyrus and a *pyramidal cell layer* in the hippocampus. The molecular layer of the hippocampus faces the dentate gyrus, and the hippocampal equivalent of subcortical white matter is a layer of fibers called the *alveus* that lies just beneath the ependymal lining of the ventricle (Fig. 16-8). The molecular layer of the dentate gyrus faces the subarachnoid space, and its output fibers, which do not leave the hippocampal formation, project directly into the hippocampus. The subiculum, as mentioned previously, is the zone of transition from the hippocampus to the parahippocampal gyrus and changes gradually from a three-layered to a six-layered cortex.

The alveus contains both afferents to and efferents from the hippocampal formation. These fibers collect into a bundle called the *fimbria* (Latin = fringe) *of the hippocampus* at the edge of the choroid fissure (Fig. 16-8). When the hippocampal formation ends near the splenium of the corpus callosum, the fimbria becomes a detached bundle called the *crus of the fornix.* The two crura converge and join in the midline to form the *body of the fornix,* which travels forward at the inferior edge of the septum pellucidum (Fig. 16-9). At the interventricular foramen, the fornix turns inferiorly and posteriorly, diverging into the *columns of the fornix,* which then pass through the middle of the hypothalamus toward the mammillary bodies (Figs. 10-10 and 10-15).

The connections of the hippocampal formation have been mapped in ruthless detail and in three dimensions. Proceeding around its C shape (as seen in transverse sections), the hippocampus has been divided into several zones, all of whose connections differ somewhat from each other and from those of the subiculum and dentate gyrus. Along the course of the hippocampal formation through the temporal lobe, its connections change. Finally, afferents from different sources end at different levels on the apical dendrites of hippocampal pyramidal cells. This high degree of order has made the hippocampal formation very attractive for anatomical and physiological research, particularly in studies of neural plasticity and regeneration. However, to keep matters manageable the following account will treat the hippocampal formation, by and large, as a uniform structure.

Hippocampal afferents. By far the most prominent source of afferents to the hippocampal formation is the adjacent entorhinal cortex (Figs. 16-4 and 16-10). If the entorhinal cortex only received olfactory inputs this would not be very impressive, but it also receives projections from the cingulate gyrus (via the cingulum), from the orbital cortex (via the uncinate fasciculus), and from other areas of the temporal lobe. Through these cortical connections the hippocampal formation

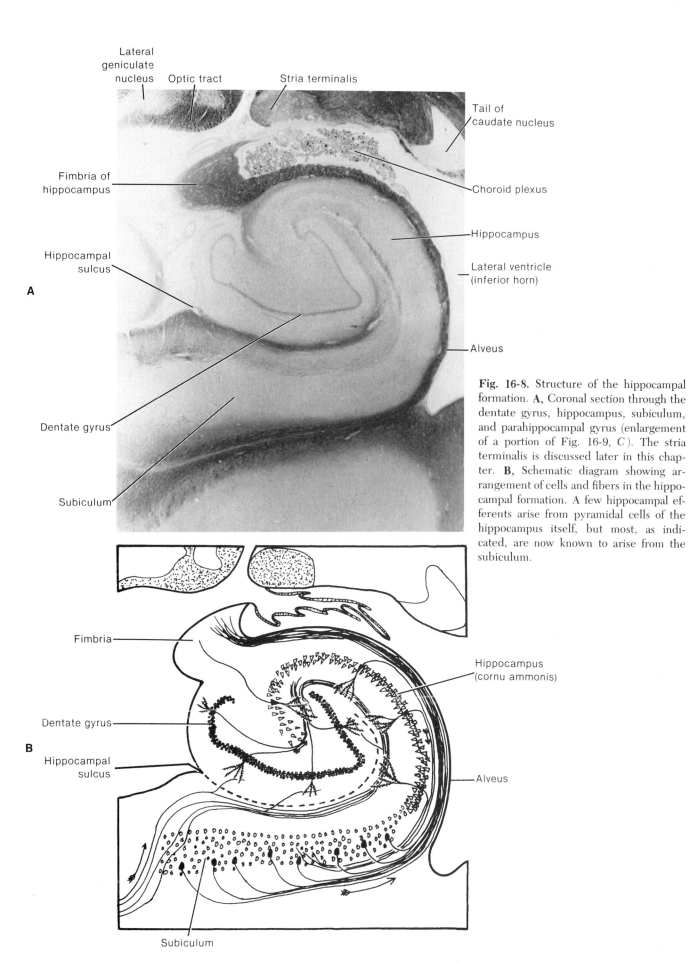

Lateral geniculate nucleus

Optic tract

Stria terminalis

Tail of caudate nucleus

Fimbria of hippocampus

Choroid plexus

Hippocampus

Hippocampal sulcus

Lateral ventricle (inferior horn)

A

Alveus

Dentate gyrus

Subiculum

Fig. 16-8. Structure of the hippocampal formation. **A,** Coronal section through the dentate gyrus, hippocampus, subiculum, and parahippocampal gyrus (enlargement of a portion of Fig. 16-9, *C*). The stria terminalis is discussed later in this chapter. **B,** Schematic diagram showing arrangement of cells and fibers in the hippocampal formation. A few hippocampal efferents arise from pyramidal cells of the hippocampus itself, but most, as indicated, are now known to arise from the subiculum.

Fimbria

Hippocampus (cornu ammonis)

Dentate gyrus

B

Hippocampal sulcus

Alveus

Subiculum

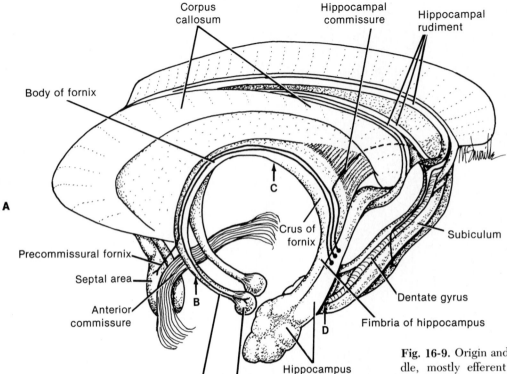

A

Corpus callosum

Hippocampal commissure

Hippocampal rudiment

Body of fornix

C

Crus of fornix

Subiculum

Precommissural fornix

Septal area

B

Anterior commissure

D

Dentate gyrus

Fimbria of hippocampus

Column of fornix

Mammillary body

Hippocampus

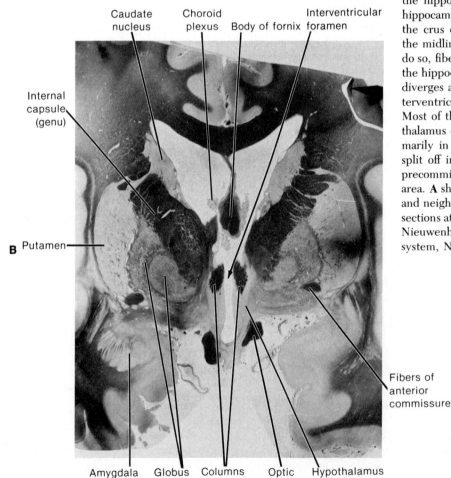

Caudate nucleus

Choroid plexus

Body of fornix

Interventricular foramen

Internal capsule (genu)

B Putamen

Fibers of anterior commissure

Amygdala

Globus pallidus

Columns of fornix

Optic tract

Hypothalamus

Fig. 16-9. Origin and course of the fornix. This bundle, mostly efferent fibers from the hippocampal formation, begins as fibers that collect on the ventricular surface of the hippocampus as the alveus. The fibers then move medially to form the fimbria of the hippocampus and then part company with the hippocampal formation near the splenium to become the crus of the fornix. The two crura converge on the midline, forming the body of the fornix; as they do so, fibers are exchanged between the two crura in the hippocampal commissure. The body of the fornix diverges again near the anterior commissure and interventricular foramen into the columns of the fornix. Most of these fibers continue on through the hypothalamus as the postcommissural fornix, ending primarily in the mammillary bodies. Some, however, split off in front of the anterior commissure as the precommissural fornix, ending primarily in the septal area. **A** shows this course in a dissection of the fornix and neighboring structures. **B, C,** and **D** are coronal sections at the levels indicated in **A**. (**A** modified from Nieuwenhuys, R., et al.: The human central nervous system, New York, 1978, Springer-Verlag, Inc.)

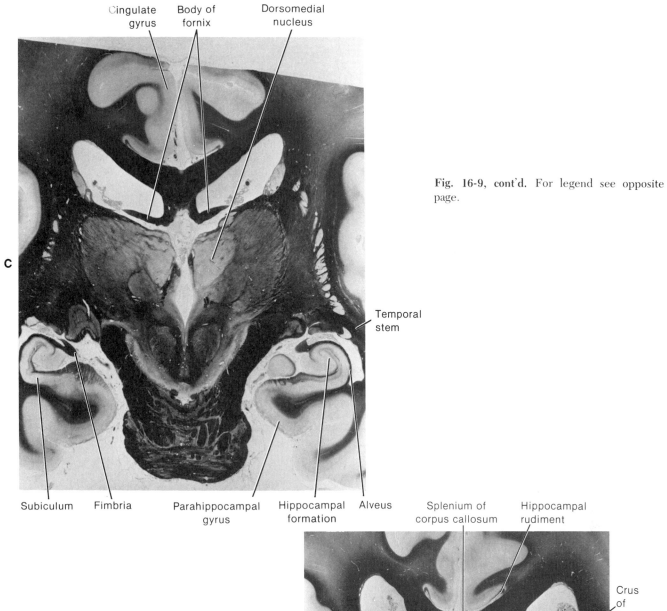

C

Cingulate gyrus   Body of fornix   Dorsomedial nucleus

Temporal stem

Subiculum   Fimbria   Parahippocampal gyrus   Hippocampal formation   Alveus

Fig. 16-9, cont'd. For legend see opposite page.

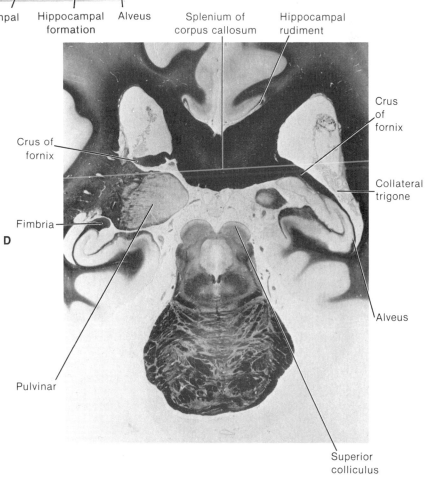

D

Splenium of corpus callosum   Hippocampal rudiment

Crus of fornix

Crus of fornix

Collateral trigone

Fimbria

Alveus

Pulvinar

Superior colliculus

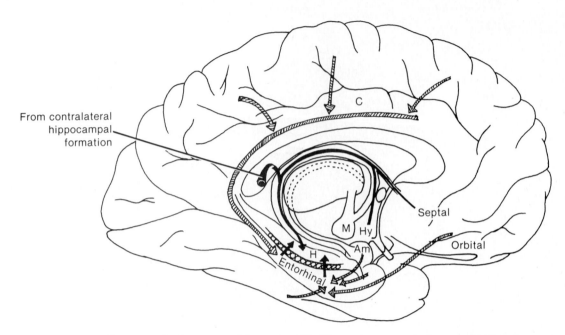

Fig. 16-10. Afferents to the hippocampal formation *(H)*. The major source is the entorhinal cortex, which in turn collects inputs from the cingulate, temporal, and orbital cortices and from the amygdala and olfactory cortex. Other hippocampal inputs arrive from the septal area and hypothalamus *(Hy)* and from the contralateral hippocampal formation, all via the fornix. Indirect afferents are indicated by hatched pathways. Other abbreviations: see Fig. 16-6.

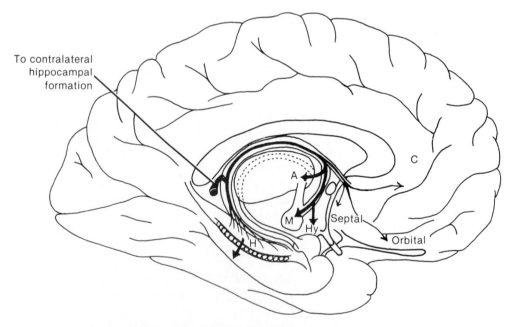

Fig. 16-11. Efferents from the hippocampal formation *(H)*. The major efferent pathway is the fornix, through which fibers reach an assortment of anteriorly situated forebrain structures. Some fibers project directly from the subiculum to the entorhinal cortex. Abbreviations: see Fig. 16-6.

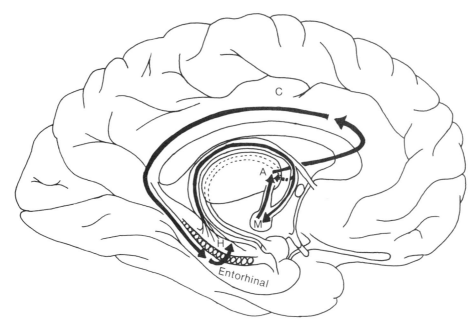

Fig. 16-12. The Papez circuit. The shortcut from the hippocampal formation directly to the anterior thalamic nucleus (not part of the original circuit) is indicated by an interrupted line. Abbreviations: see Fig. 16-6.

has access to virtually all types of sensory information. In addition, some septal and hypothalamic fibers reach the hippocampal formation through the fornix. Finally, some fibers arrive from the contralateral hippocampal formation by passing from one crus of the fornix to the other beneath the splenium of the corpus callosum in the *hippocampal commissure* (Fig. 16-9).

Hippocampal efferents. The hippocampal formation sends some fibers directly back to the entorhinal and cingulate cortex, but its principal output pathway is the fornix (Fig. 16-11).* Fornix fibers arch forward under the corpus callosum along the path depicted in Fig. 16-9 (except for those that cross in the hippocampal commissure). At the level of the interventricular foramen, some fibers split off in front of the anterior commissure as the *precommissural fornix.* Most of these end nearby in the septal and preoptic areas, but some continue on to reach orbital and anterior cingulate cortex. The remaining fibers of the fornix (the *postcommissural fornix*) do one of two things: some turn sharply posteriorly and end in the anterior thalamic nucleus; the rest travel through the hypothalamus in the column of the fornix and end mainly in the mammillary body (although some

end in other hypothalamic areas or in the midbrain reticular formation). Since the mammillothalamic tract ends in the anterior nucleus, the hippocampal formation can influence this part of the thalamus both directly and indirectly.

The anterior thalamic nucleus projects to the cingulate gyrus, thus completing a great loop through the diencephalon and telencephalon (Fig. 16-12). Beginning in the hippocampal formation, the pathway proceeds through the fornix to the mammillary body, from there in sequence to the anterior thalamic nucleus, the cingulate gyrus, and part of the parahippocampal gyrus (the entorhinal cortex), and finally back to the hippocampal formation. James Papez pointed out in 1937 that this loop provided for interactions among the neocortex, limbic structures, and the hypothalamus and proposed that it might be the anatomical substrate of emotional experience. While undoubtedly a great oversimplification (for one thing, hippocampal connections are considerably more complex than this loop would indicate), this idea provided the impetus for a great deal of research into the structure and function of the limbic system; the loop is still known as the *Papez circuit.*

Hippocampal function. A variety of changes in autonomic and endocrine function have been described as resulting from hippocampal stimulation or damage in experimental animals, consistent with the connections between the hippocampal formation and the septal nuclei and hypothalamus; a number of behavioral changes

---

*It was a longstanding anatomical tenet that the efferent fibers in the fornix are the axons of the prominent pyramidal cells of the hippocampus. However, recent work has shown that most of these axons actually end locally in the subiculum. The hippocampus proper provides part of the output to the septal area, but the bulk of the output from the hippocampal formation arises in the subiculum.

have been described as well. Despite this, however, it has not yet been possible to derive one general function or set of functions for the hippocampal formation. The only single role ascribed to it in humans has to do with learning and memory. Neurosurgeons discovered (by accident) in the early 1950s that after bilateral removal of the medial parts of the temporal lobe (or after unilateral removal from patients with preexisting damage on the other side), humans have a striking memory deficit. After such surgery, patients are unable to form new memories. There is typically some retrograde amnesia for events that occurred before the surgery, but beyond some point in the past, early memories are intact. However, a new item like a list of numbers or a dictated phrase disappears at the first distraction, although it can be retained for a little while if the patient has nothing else to do but concentrate on that item. Intelligence is more or less undisturbed, but nevertheless, this is an enormously debilitating problem. Imagine being perpetually unable to remember new acquaintances; unable to keep track of events in the lives of relatives and old friends; unable to complete simple tasks because of inability to remember why they were begun; unable to read a story, because there is no memory of sentences preceding the current one.

Since the hippocampal formation is a major part of the medial temporal lobe, and since the memory deficit occurs in cases where little appears to be damaged other than the two hippocampal formations, the function of laying down or consolidating new memories is now attributed to this portion of the limbic system.

Damage to the mammillary bodies (which occurs in the course of widespread damage to the periaqueductal and periventricular gray as a result of chronic alcoholism) is correlated with a similar memory deficit. The condition is called *Korsakoff's psychosis*. Patients so afflicted may have relatively intact intelligence but an inability to form new memories. They typically make up answers as they go along, concealing to some extent the memory loss (hence a wonderful alternate name for Korsakoff's psychosis: the *amnestic confabulatory syndrome*). This led to the appealing notion that the entire Papez circuit is involved in learning and memory. Unfortunately, things are rarely as simple as they seem; bilateral destruction of the cingulum causes no particular memory loss,* and destruction of the fornix rarely, if ever, causes one. In addition, there have been cases in which destruction of the mammillary bodies was not accompanied by memory loss. Some investigators

claim that the only common factor in all cases of Korsakoff's psychosis is bilateral damage to the medial thalamus (that is, the dorsomedial nuclei). Finally, there is a disturbing fact about the generally accepted central role of the hippocampal formation in human memory: careful, selective, bilateral ablation of the hippocampal formations of experimental animals does not result in the obvious memory deficits seen in humans. Certain types of learning disabilities can be demonstrated in these animals, but most tasks are learned as well or nearly as well as they were before the surgery. Some investigators think that this apparent dilemma can be explained on the basis of rapid change in hippocampal function during mammalian evolution; others think that it arises from the fact that we communicate differently with animals than with humans so that we are actually measuring two different things when we study the learning abilities of animals and the memory of humans. Still other investigators think that some other part of the temporal lobe close to the hippocampal formation is actually of major importance for learning and that this other structure is also damaged in lesions of the medial temporal lobe. For example, the *temporal stem* (Fig. 16-9) is a sheet of white matter that carries much of the neural traffic between anterior parts of the temporal lobe and the rest of the brain. It would probably be damaged by any process that damaged the entire hippocampal formation in humans but could be spared by the selective lesions that can be made in experimental animals.

Amygdala

The amygdala is a collection of nuclei lying beneath the uncus of the temporal lobe at the anterior end of the hippocampal formation and the inferior horn of the lateral ventricle (Fig. 16-13). It merges with the periamygdaloid cortex, which forms part of the surface of the uncus. The amygdala also abuts the tail of the caudate nucleus as the latter ends in the temporal lobe (Fig. 13-4) and was considered at one time to be one of the basal ganglia, which by definition comprised all subcortical gray masses of the telencephalon. However, as will be seen, the connections of the amygdala are typical for part of the limbic system and quite unlike those of the corpus striatum.

Afferents to the amygdala. The amygdala receives a great deal of sensory input in a highly processed form. Single amygdalar cells may respond to various combinations of many different sensory modalities, including somatosensory, visual, auditory, and all types of visceral inputs. The afferents carrying this information arise in several locations (Fig. 16-14) and reach the amygdala by traveling in the reverse direction along the paths followed by amygdalar efferents (described in the next section).

---

*Interestingly, bilateral section of the cingulum causes emotional changes similar to those seen after prefrontal leukotomy—a type of change that might be expected after damage to the limbic system. This operation has been used on an experimental basis as a treatment for intractable pain and for certain psychiatric disorders.

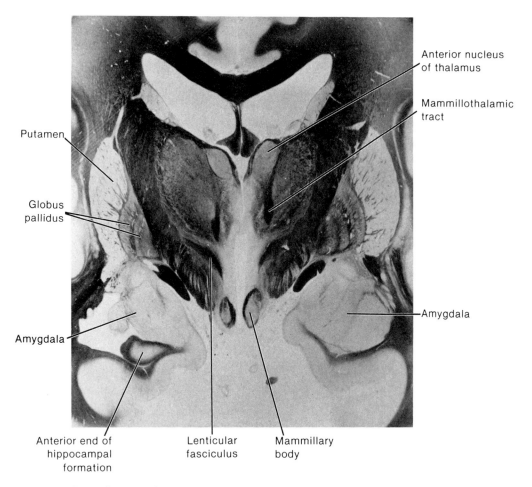

Putamen

Globus
pallidus

Amygdala

Anterior end of
hippocampal
formation

Lenticular
fasciculus

Mammillary
body

Anterior nucleus
of thalamus

Mammillothalamic
tract

Amygdala

Fig. 16-13. Coronal section through the amygdala. Note the fairly direct route beneath the lentiform nucleus that is available for fibers interconnecting the amygdala and various diencephalic and telencephalic structures (the ventral amygdalofugal pathway).

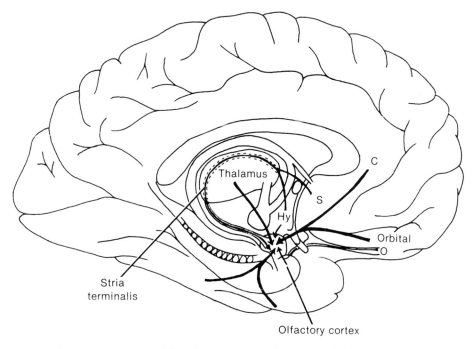

Thalamus

Hy

C

S

Orbital

O

Stria
terminalis

Olfactory cortex

Fig. 16-14. Afferents to the amygdala. These arrive via four routes: (1) from the hypothalamus and septal area through the stria terminalis, (2) from the thalamus and hypothalamus and from orbital and anterior cingulate cortex through the ventral pathway, (3) from the olfactory bulb through the lateral olfactory stria, as well as from olfactory cortex, and (4) directly from temporal neocortical areas. Abbreviations: see Fig. 16-6.

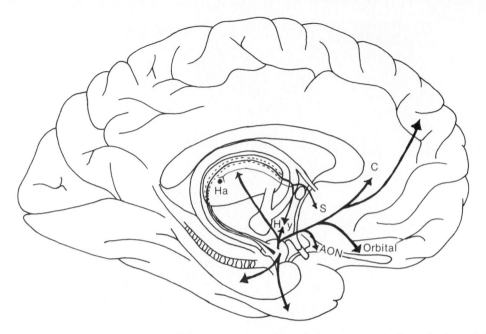

Fig. 16-15. Efferents from the amygdala. Some project through the stria terminalis to the hypothalamus, the septal area, and the habenula *(Ha);* others project through the ventral amygdalofugal pathway to the hypothalamus, the dorsomedial thalamic nucleus, widespread areas of the prefrontal and insular cortices, and various olfactory structures; still others project directly to the entorhinal cortex and other areas of the temporal lobe. *AON,* anterior olfactory nucleus. Other abbreviations: see Fig. 16-6.

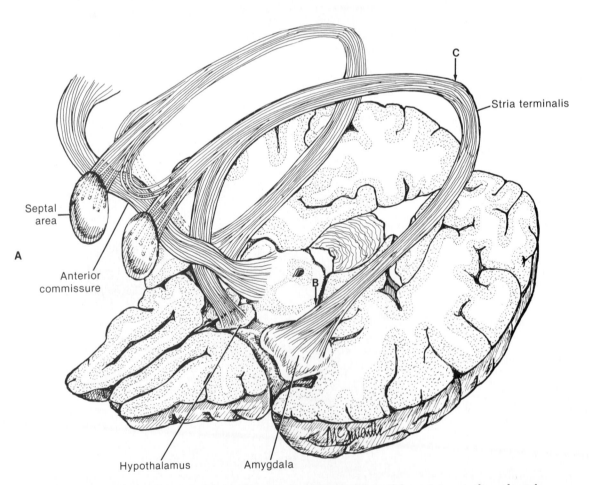

Fig. 16-16. Origin and course of the stria terminalis. **A,** A dissection of the stria terminalis and neighboring structures indicating the course of some of its fibers. **B** and **C,** Coronal sections at the levels indicated in **A.** (**A** suggested by a drawing in Isaacson, R.L.: The limbic system, New York, 1974, Plenum Press.)

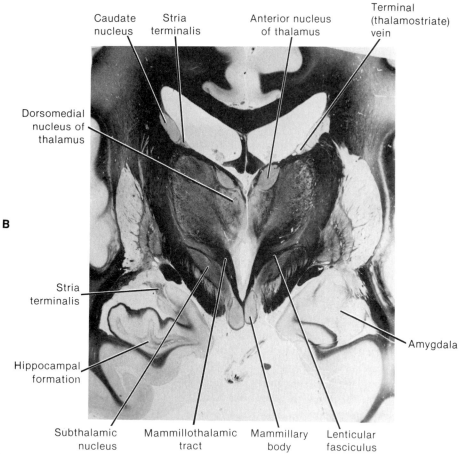

Caudate nucleus   Stria terminalis   Anterior nucleus of thalamus   Terminal (thalamostriate) vein

Dorsomedial nucleus of thalamus

B

Stria terminalis

Hippocampal formation

Amygdala

Subthalamic nucleus   Mammillothalamic tract   Mammillary body   Lenticular fasciculus

Fig. 16-16, cont'd. For legend see opposite page.

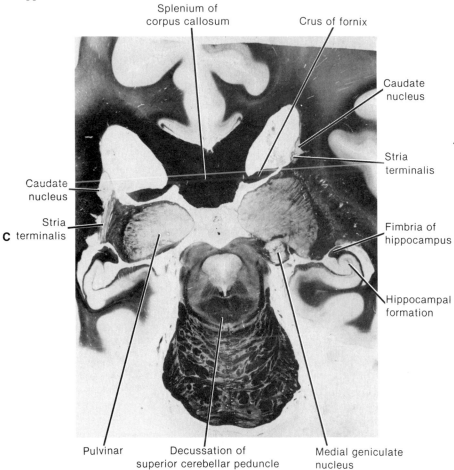

Splenium of corpus callosum   Crus of fornix

Caudate nucleus

Stria terminalis

Caudate nucleus

Stria terminalis

C

Fimbria of hippocampus

Hippocampal formation

Pulvinar   Decussation of superior cerebellar peduncle   Medial geniculate nucleus

Olfactory inputs are especially prominent. Some olfactory tract fibers end in part of the amygdala (the *cortico-medial* nuclear group), and this part in turn projects to the rest of the amygdala; olfactory inputs also arise in the piriform cortex. Additional visceral information reaches the amygdala indirectly from the hypothalamus and septal area and also by more direct routes; for example, the pontine taste area has recently been shown to project to the amygdala, and it seems likely that the same may be true of other visceral nuclei in the brainstem. The orbital, anterior temporal, and anterior cingulate cortices also project to the amygdala and are probably responsible for most of the auditory, visual, and somatosensory information that reaches this structure. Finally, the amygdala may receive some fibers from the dorsomedial nucleus of the thalamus, although recent work has cast some doubt on this connection.

Efferents from the amygdala. Fibers leave the amygdala through two major pathways to reach many of the same areas that send afferents to it (Fig. 16-15). The first pathway is the *stria terminalis*, which arches around from the temporal lobe toward the interventricular foramen in company with the caudate nucleus and the thalamostriate (or terminal) vein. In the body of the lateral ventricle, the stria terminalis lies in the groove between the caudate nucleus and the thalamus (Fig. 16-16). Fibers of the stria terminalis distribute mainly to the septal area and the hypothalamus; a few turn caudally into the stria medullaris thalami and reach the habenula, while some remarkably long ones cross the midline in the anterior commissure and arch around to the contralateral amygdala.

The second efferent route goes by the awkward name of the *ventral amygdalofugal pathway* (particularly awkward since it also contains many afferents to the amygdala). These fibers pass underneath the lenticular nucleus (Fig. 16-13) and spread out to blanket the base of the brain, ending in the septal area and the hypothalamus, in olfactory regions like the anterior olfactory nucleus, the anterior perforated substance, and the prepiriform cortex, and in the orbital and anterior cingulate cortices. Many of these fibers turn dorsally in the diencephalon and reach the dorsomedial nucleus of the thalamus. Finally, some amygdalar efferents enter neither the stria terminalis nor the ventral pathway but rather pass directly to entorhinal cortex and other cortical areas of the anterior temporal lobe.

Amygdalar function. As complex as the connections of the amygdala appear, they are dominated by extensive interconnections with the septal area and hypothalamus on the one hand and with prefrontal cortex, both directly and indirectly (via the dorsomedial nucleus), on the other. This puts it in a position to influence both drive-related behavior patterns and the subjective feelings that accompany these activities. In the first of these two roles, the amygdala can be considered a sort of higher-order modulating influence on the hypothalamus. Almost any visceral or somatic activity that can be elicited by stimulating the hypothalamus (including such things as feeding or cardiovascular and respiratory changes) can also be elicited by stimulating some point in the amygdala. The responses to amygdalar stimulation tend to be more "natural" than those to hypothalamic stimulation, building up gradually and then decaying slowly at the end of the stimulus. Conversely, syndromes such as the aphagia or hyperphagia that follow selective lesions of parts of the hypothalamus can also be caused by amygdalar lesions, although in this case the syndromes are less severe.

The role of the amygdala in subjective feelings (presumably involving interactions with both the prefrontal cortex and the hypothalamus) has also been indicated in electrical studies. When an animal's amygdala is stimulated, it most often stops whatever it was doing and becomes very attentive. This may be followed by responses of defense, raging aggression, or fleeing. Amygdalar stimulation in humans can cause a variety of emotions, but the most common is fear accompanied by all its normal autonomic manifestations (dilation of the pupils, release of adrenalin, increased heart rate, etc.). Conversely, bilateral destruction of the amygdala causes a great decrease in aggression, and as a result the animals are tame and placid.

Some functional aspects of the limbic system

One classic technique for studying the function of a structure is to remove it or destroy it and then see what happens. Removing the temporal lobe back to the level of the primary auditory cortex should certainly incapacitate the limbic system to a great extent, since the amygdala and most of the hippocampal formation and parahippocampal gyrus would be lost. When this is done to animals bilaterally, a constellation of deficits results called the *Klüver-Bucy syndrome* for the investigators who first described it.

1. The animals are fearless and placid, showing an absence of emotional reactions. They do not respond to threats, to social gestures by other animals, or to objects they would normally flee from or attack.
2. Male animals become hypersexual and are impressively indiscriminate in their choice of sex partners. They are likely to mount other animals of the same sex, animals of whatever species may be available, or inanimate objects.
3. They show an inordinate degree of attention to all sensory stimuli, as though ceaselessly curious. They respond to every object within sight or reach

by sniffing it and examining it orally. If the object can in any sense be considered edible, they eat it. Partly because of this, they eat much more than normal animals.

4. Although they incessantly examine all objects in sight, they recognize nothing and may pick up the same thing over and over. This was called "psychic blindness" by Klüver and Bucy and would now be called visual agnosia.

The Klüver-Bucy syndrome has been fractionated to some extent, and different parts of it can be attributed to the loss of different structures. Thus the placidity results from destruction of the amygdala, the hypersexuality from loss of the piriform cortex, and the visual agnosia from damage to visual processing areas on the inferior surface of the temporal lobe. The composite syndrome is tremendously detrimental.* Leaving aside the visual agnosia, it is as though the animal still had intact all the behavior patterns central to satisfying basic drives but could no longer tell when and in what context to use them.

---

*"A monkey which approaches every enemy to examine it orally will conceivably not survive longer than a few hours if turned loose in a region with a plentiful supply of enemies. We doubt that a monkey would be seriously hampered under natural conditions, in the wild, by a loss of its prefrontal region, its parietal lobes or its occipital lobes, as long as small portions of the striate cortex remained intact." (Klüver, H., and Bucy, P.C.: Preliminary analysis of functions of the temporal lobes in monkeys, Arch. Neurol. Psychiatr. **42**:979, 1939.)

ADDITIONAL READING

Andy, O.J., and Stephan, H.: The septum in the human brain, J. Comp. Neurol. 133:383, 1968. *There is a tendency to think of the septal area as small and rudimentary in humans, but this paper argues that in fact it reaches its highest development in us.*

DeFrance, J.F., editor: The septal nuclei, advances in behavioral biology, vol. 20, New York, 1976, Plenum Press.

Gordon, H.W., and Sperry, R.W.: Lateralization of olfactory perception in the surgically separated hemispheres of man, Neurophyschologia 7:111, 1969.

Graziadei, P.P.C., et al.: Neurogenesis of sensory neurons in the primate olfactory system after section of the fila olfactoria, Brain Res. 186:289, 1980. *Olfactory receptor neurons can be replaced after injury, which makes them highly unusual neurons.*

Herzog, A.G., and van Hoesen, G.W.: Temporal neocortical afferent connections to the amygdala in the rhesus monkey, Brain Res. 115:57, 1976.

Horel, J.A.: The neuroanatomy of amnesia: a critique of the hippocampal memory hypothesis, Brain 101:403, 1978. *A very convincing argument and interesting review from one group that thinks the hippocampus is not the crucial structure for learning and memory.*

Isaacson, R.L.: The limbic system, New York, 1974, Plenum Press.

Isaacson, R.L., and Pribram, K.H., editors: The hippocampus, New York, 1975, Plenum Press.

Kaada, B.R.: Stimulation and regional ablation of the amygdaloid complex with reference to functional representations. In Eleftheriou, B.E., editor: The neurobiology of the amygdala, New York, 1972, Plenum Press.

Klüver, H., and Bucy, P.C.: Preliminary analysis of functions of the temporal lobes in monkeys, Arch. Neurol. Psychiatr. 42:979, 1939. *Still interesting reading.*

Krettek, J.E., and Price, J.L.: Projections from the amygdaloid complex to the cerebral cortex and thalamus in the rat and cat, J. Comp. Neurol. 172:687, 1977.

Krettek, J.E., and Price, J.L.: Projections from the amygdaloid complex and adjacent olfactory structures to the entorhinal cortex and to the subiculum in the rat and cat, J. Comp. Neurol. 172:723, 1977.

Lewis, F.T.: The significance of the term *hippocampus*, J. Comp. Neurol. 35:213, 1923-24. *A caustic but interesting paper concerning "the flight of fancy which led Arantius, in 1587, to introduce the term 'hippocampus.' . . . recorded in what is perhaps the worst anatomical description extant. It has left its readers in doubt whether the elevations of cerebral substance were being compared with fish or beast, and no one could be sure which end was the head."*

Machne, X., and Segundo, J.P.: Unitary responses to afferent volleys in amygdaloid complex, J. Neurophysiol. 19:232, 1956. *Single cells that respond equally well to a brief shock to the sciatic nerve and to a whiff of something.*

Malamud, N.: Psychiatric disorder with intracranial tumors of limbic system, Arch. Neurol. 17:113, 1967.

Norgren, R.: Taste pathways to hypothalamus and amygdala, J. Comp. Neurol. 166:17, 1976.

Pandya, D.N., van Hoesen, G.W., and Domesick, V.B.: A cinguloamygdaloid projection in the rhesus monkey, Brain Res. 61:369, 1973.

Papez, J.W.: A proposed mechanism of emotion, Arch. Neurol. Psychiat. 38:725, 1937. *The evidence wasn't very strong by today's standards, but the idea has been extremely influential anyway.*

Penfield, W., and Mathieson, G.: Memory: autopsy findings and comments on the role of hippocampus in experiential recall, Arch. Neurol. 31:145, 1974. *The conventional hippocampus-memory hypothesis in a well-written account by one of the neurosurgeons who made the unfortunate discovery.*

Rosene, D.L., and van Hoesen, G.W.: Hippocampal efferents reach widespread areas of cerebral cortex and amygdala in the rhesus monkey, Science 198:315, 1977.

Shepherd, G.M.: The synaptic organization of the brain, ed. 2, New York, 1979, Oxford University Press. *Chapter 8, olfactory bulb; Chapter 13, olfactory cortex; Chapter 14, hippocampus.*

Swanson, L.W., and Cowan, W.M.: Hippocampo-hypothalamic connections: origin in subicular cortex, not Ammon's horn, Science 189:303, 1975.

Turner, B.H., Gupta, K.C., and Mishkin, M.: The locus and cytoarchitecture of the projection areas of the olfactory bulb in *Macaca mulatta*, J. Comp. Neurol. 177:381, 1978.

Van Hoesen, G.W., and Pandya, D.P.: Some connections of the entorhinal (area 28) and perirhinal (area 35) cortices of the rhesus monkey, III: efferent connections, Brain Res. 95:39, 1975.

Van Hoesen, G.W., Rosene, D.L., and Mesulam, M.-M.: Subicular input from temporal cortex in the rhesus monkey, Science 205:608, 1979.

Victor, M., Adams, R.D., and Collins, G.H.: The Wernicke-Korsakoff syndrome: a clinical and pathological study of 245 patients, 82 with post-morten examination, Philadelphia, 1971, F.A. Davis Company.

Weiskrantz, L.: A comparision of hippocampal pathology in man and other animals. In Functions of the septo-hippocampal system, Ciba Foundation Symposium 58, new series, New York, 1977, Elsevier North-Holland, Inc.

INDEX